KU-548-211

Psychiatry
Lecture Notes

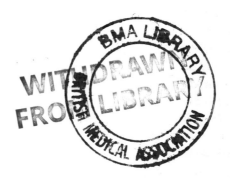

WITHDRAWN
FROM LIBRARY

BRITISH MEDICAL ASSOCIATION
0768351

Psychiatry
Lecture Notes

Gautam Gulati

MBBS, MRCPsych, PGDipLATHE(Oxon), FHEA
Honorary Senior Clinical Lecturer in Forensic Psychiatry,
University of Oxford & Consultant Forensic Psychiatrist,
Oxford Health NHS Foundation Trust, UK

Mary-Ellen Lynall

MA (Cantab.)
Graduate-entry medical student, Magdalen College, University of Oxford, UK
Retained Lecturer in Neuroscience, Somerville College, University of
Oxford, UK

Kate Saunders

BM, BCh, MA, MRCPsych, PGDipLATHE, FHEA
University of Oxford Department of Psychiatry, Warneford Hospital, UK

Eleventh Edition

WILEY Blackwell

This edition first published 2014 © 2014 by John Wiley & Sons, Ltd

Previous editions 1964, 1968, 1972, 1974, 1979, 1984, 1989, 1998, 2005, 2010

Registered office: John Wiley & Sons, Ltd, The Atrium, Southern Gate, Chichester, West Sussex, PO19 8SQ, UK

Editorial offices: 9600 Garsington Road, Oxford, OX4 2DQ, UK
The Atrium, Southern Gate, Chichester, West Sussex, PO19 8SQ, UK
350 Main Street, Malden, MA 02148-5020, USA

For details of our global editorial offices, for customer services and for information about how to apply for permission to reuse the copyright material in this book please see our website at www.wiley.com/wiley-blackwell

The right of the author to be identified as the author of this work has been asserted in accordance with the UK Copyright, Designs and Patents Act 1988.

All rights reserved. No part of this publication may be reproduced, stored in a retrieval system, or transmitted, in any form or by any means, electronic, mechanical, photocopying, recording or otherwise, except as permitted by the UK Copyright, Designs and Patents Act 1988, without the prior permission of the publisher.

Designations used by companies to distinguish their products are often claimed as trademarks. All brand names and product names used in this book are trade names, service marks, trademarks or registered trademarks of their respective owners. The publisher is not associated with any product or vendor mentioned in this book. It is sold on the understanding that the publisher is not engaged in rendering professional services. If professional advice or other expert assistance is required, the services of a competent professional should be sought.

The contents of this work are intended to further general scientific research, understanding, and discussion only and are not intended and should not be relied upon as recommending or promoting a specific method, diagnosis, or treatment by health science practitioners for any particular patient. The publisher and the author make no representations or warranties with respect to the accuracy or completeness of the contents of this work and specifically disclaim all warranties, including without limitation any implied warranties of fitness for a particular purpose. In view of ongoing research, equipment modifications, changes in governmental regulations, and the constant flow of information relating to the use of medicines, equipment, and devices, the reader is urged to review and evaluate the information provided in the package insert or instructions for each medicine, equipment, or device for, among other things, any changes in the instructions or indication of usage and for added warnings and precautions. Readers should consult with a specialist where appropriate. The fact that an organization or Website is referred to in this work as a citation and/or a potential source of further information does not mean that the author or the publisher endorses the information the organization or Website may provide or recommendations it may make. Further, readers should be aware that Internet Websites listed in this work may have changed or disappeared between when this work was written and when it is read. No warranty may be created or extended by any promotional statements for this work. Neither the publisher nor the author shall be liable for any damages arising herefrom.

Library of Congress Cataloging-in-Publication Data
Gulati, Gautam, 1979- author.
Lecture notes. Psychiatry / Gautam Gulati, Mary-Ellen Lynall, Kate Saunders. — Eleventh edition.
p. ; cm.
Psychiatry
Preceded by: Lecture notes. Psychiatry. 10th ed. / Paul Harrison, John Geddes, Michael Sharpe. 2010.
Includes bibliographical references and index.
ISBN 978-1-118-37820-5 (pbk.)
I. Lynall, Mary-Ellen, 1986- author.   II. Saunders, Kate, 1978- author.   III. Harrison, P. J. (Paul J.), 1960- Lecture notes. Psychiatry. Preceded by (work):   IV. Title. V. Title: Psychiatry.
[DNLM: 1. Mental Disorders–Handbooks.   2. Psychiatry–Handbooks.   WM 34]
RC457.2
616.89–dc23

2013023531

A catalogue record for this book is available from the British Library.

Wiley also publishes its books in a variety of electronic formats. Some content that appears in print may not be available in electronic books.

Cover image: iStockphoto.com/geopaul
Cover design by Grounded Design Ltd

Set in 8.5/11pt Utopia Std by Aptara® Inc., New Delhi, India
Printed and bound in Malaysia by Vivar Printing Sdn Bhd

1   2014

Contents

BMA LIBRARY
BRITISH MEDICAL ASSOCIATION

Foreword

When Paul Harrison, Mike Sharpe and I were offered the chance to take over the eighth edition of *Lecture Notes in Psychiatry* in 1997, we spent a great deal of time together thinking through the structure of a book that would portray psychiatry as the evidence-based, patient-oriented branch of medicine that we knew it could be. Our thinking was inspired by the advances in evidence-based medicine led in Oxford by David Sackett, Muir Gray and Iain Chalmers and the Cochrane Collaboration. We wanted to apply the principles of clinical epidemiology – not just in our recommendations around use of treatments but also to challenge traditional approaches to history and examination taking in psychiatry. For decades, students had been taught that the only way to do a proper psychiatric assessment was to do a 'full' history and examination – an approach that is both inefficient and incompatible with real-world clinical practice.

The Oxford University Department of Psychiatry is proud of its heritage of producing and updating its suite of textbooks, a process initiated by Michael Gelder when he was the first Head of Department. We are therefore delighted that Gautam Gulati, Mary-Ellen Lynall and Kate Saunders have taken on the task of updating and revising *Lecture Notes in Psychiatry*. To an extent, all textbooks are out of date as soon as they are published but even with the developments in information technology, a concise, portable, paper textbook containing an up-to date synthesis of current knowledge occupies its own niche and still has a major role in training. Frequent revisions and updating are, however, critical to keep them accurate and useful. This is hard work of course and after three editions, Paul, Mike and I felt that we could not face revising the book again! It is marvellous to see that Gautam, Mary-Ellen and Kate have done so with such aplomb, keeping what remains useful from earlier editions but updating it with great skill.

John Geddes

Preface

The skills, attitudes and knowledge inherent in learning psychiatry are relevant to all doctors – and to all other health professionals. We have written this book with medical students and psychiatric trainees in mind, but anticipate it being a useful resource for any health professional interested in the subject.

We describe a practical approach towards psychiatry. Chapter 1 outlines the principles behind the practice of modern psychiatry and introduces the psychiatric assessment. Our guide to assessment comprises a *basic psychiatric assessment* (Chapter 2), followed by *diagnosis-specific assessments* (Chapter 3) and a guide to *risk assessment* (Chapter 4). Chapter 5 describes how to draw everything together and communicate the information to others. The recommendations in these chapters are summarized in a set of 'quick guides', included at the front of the book for easy reference.

The middle chapters cover the principles of aetiology (Chapter 6), treatment (Chapter 7) and psychiatric services (Chapter 8). The main psychiatric disorders of adults are covered in Chapters 9–15, followed by childhood disorders (Chapter 16) and learning disability (Chapter 17). Chapter 18 discusses psychiatry in non-psychiatric medical settings – the place where most psychiatry actually happens. Chapter 19 (Mental health and the law) is a new addition to the book and one you are likely to find useful in whichever setting you work.

Given our illustrious predecessors, we were humbled to be asked to write the 11th edition of *Lecture Notes*. Indeed we aimed to build upon the last edition of the book written so eloquently by Paul Harrison, John Geddes and Michael Sharpe.

To facilitate learning, we have added learning objectives at the start of each chapter and highlighted key points towards the end. Multiple-choice questions have been added, along with detailed explanations of the answers, to allow the reader to consolidate key points. Links to key papers and guidelines have been added for readers keen to know more about a particular disorder.

We hope we have done justice to the work started by Paul, John and Michael in keeping this *Lecture Series* book both informative and enjoyable.

We thank Jonathan Price, who was instrumental in drawing our team together and in setting the direction in the early days of our writing. We are grateful to colleagues who have generously shared their expertise with us.

The book is dedicated to Annette Lynall, John Conway, Catherine Sage, and the memory of Graham (Matthew) Jay and Colonel S. Gulati.

Gautam Gulati
Mary-Ellen Lynall
Kate Saunders

Acknowledgements

We would like to thank the following people for their contribution to this book.

Professor Paul Harrison (University of Oxford), **Professor John Geddes** (University of Oxford) and **Professor Michael Sharpe** (University of Edinburgh) who edited the 10th edition of this book.

Dr Jonathan Price (University of Oxford) for bringing the author team together, and for helping set the direction in the early days of our work on this edition of the book.

Dr Ruth Reed (Oxford Health NHS Foundation Trust) for her contribution to the chapter on Childhood disorders.

Dr Valerie Elizabeth Murphy (Southern Health NHS Foundation Trust and University of Oxford) for her contribution to the chapter on Learning disabilities.

Dr Robert Cornish (Oxford Health NHS Foundation Trust) for his contribution to the chapter on Psychiatric specialties.

Dr Borys Borvin (Oxford Health NHS Foundation Trust) for his contribution to the chapter on Substance misuse.

Dr Suzanne Coghlan (Oxford Health NHS Foundation Trust) for her contribution to the chapter on Neuroses.

Dr Elizabeth Naomi Smith (Oxford Health NHS Foundation Trust) for her contribution to the chapter on Psychiatry in other settings.

Dr Charlotte Allan (Oxford Health NHS Foundation Trust) for her contribution to the chapter on Dementia, delirium and neuropsychiatry.

Karen Moore (Senior Development Editor at Wiley) for her help and advice with editorial aspects.

Quick guides

History-taking checklist

Before you begin:
- Information (referral letters, notes), location, safety
- Introduction, consent, establish expectations

Basic details:
- Method of referral, status under the Mental Health Act (where appropriate)
- Age, marital status, occupation, current living arrangements

Presenting complaint(s):
- Main symptom: 'NOTEPAD': Nature, Onset, Triggers, Exacerbating/relieving, Progression, Associated symptoms, Disability
- Other symptoms or problems, important negatives
- Impact of symptoms (biological, psychological, social)
- How others perceived symptoms/state
- Treatment received to date

Past psychiatric history:
- Formal care: community psychiatric care? In-patient treatment? Detention?
- Treatments and response
- Self-harm or harm to others

Treatment/drug history:
- Prescribed biological and psychological treatments
- Non-prescribed treatments
- Adherence, side effects
- Any recent changes?
- Allergies

Family history:
- Parents, siblings and children: age, occupation, health and quality of relationship with patient
- For children: name, DOB, school, any other professional involvement
- Family history of mental illness, suicide, self-harm or substance misuse
- Any recent family events

Personal history and premorbid personality:
- Pregnancy, birth and developmental milestones normal?
- Childhood: emotional problems, serious illnesses, parental separation
- Education: enjoyed school, bullying, finished school, special education classes?
- Occupational history: job changes, military service
- Intimate relationships (psychosexual history): partners, quality of relationships, sexual problems, abuse
- Traumatic events including exposure to self-harm/suicide
- Premorbid personality: character, interests, beliefs, habits

(continued)

Psychiatry Lecture Notes, Eleventh Edition. Gautam Gulati, Mary-Ellen Lynall and Kate Saunders. © 2014 John Wiley & Sons, Ltd. Published 2014 by John Wiley & Sons, Ltd.

Social history (current circumstances):
- Self-care
- Family and social support
- Caring responsibilities
- Living arrangements
- Finances: problems? benefits?
- Description of a typical day

Substance use: smoking, alcohol, illicit drugs:
- Which substances, quantity, how and when?
- Evidence of dependence? Periods of abstinence?
- Impact on life, esp. related offences

Forensic history:
- Contact with police, charges, convictions, imprisonment
- How do these relate to episodes of illness?

Past medical history:
- Current and past illnesses, surgery, admissions
- (Menstrual and obstetric history)

Risk assessment:
- Risks to self (self-harm, self-neglect…)
- Risks to others (staff, family, work…)
- Driving
- Child protection considerations

Corroborative history if appropriate

Proceed to **Mental State Examination**

Mental State Examination checklist

Appearance and behaviour
- Appearance
- Body language/abnormal movements
- Eye contact/rapport

Speech
- Quantity and spontaneity
- Volume and rate
- Tone, prosody
- Articulation and intelligibility

Mood
- Subjective
- Objective: mood, constancy, congruity

Thoughts
- Form/flow: any classic patterns? (formal thought disorder, flight of ideas)
- Content:
  abnormal beliefs: delusions and over-valued ideas
  preoccupations and obsessions
  phobias
  morbid thoughts: harm to self or others

Perceptions
- Illusions and hallucinations (esp. visual, auditory)
- Derealization and depersonalization

Cognition
- Orientation (time, place, person)
- Conscious level
- Specific domains: attention, memory, language, visuo-spatial

Insight
- That they are unwell
- That they recognize their symptoms to be those of illness
- That the illness needs treatment
- Willingness to comply with treatment plan
- Capacity to consent to treatment plan

Structure of a psychiatric case presentation

For an example of a case presented in both oral and written form, see pages 51–52.

Demographic details:
- Name, age, sex, occupation
- Dates of referral, assessment, admission, detention, discharge
- Current Mental Health Act status

Presenting complaint(s):
- Nature, onset, progression, treatments to date
- Mental state at presentation

Background history:
- Past psychiatric history and past medical history: diagnoses, admission and treatments
- Family history
- Personal and social history including job record, relationships, children, premorbid personality
- Use of alcohol and drugs
- Forensic history

Mental State Examination:
- Appearance and behaviour
- Speech
- Mood
- Thoughts
- Perceptions
- Cognition
- Insight

Risk assessment:
- Risks to self
- Risks to others

Physical examination

Investigations

Differential diagnosis: List the possible diagnoses, giving the most likely diagnosis first and citing evidence for and against the top differentials

(continued)

Aetiology, divided into either or both of:
- Predisposing, precipitating, perpetuating and protective factors
- Biological, psychological and social factors

Management and progress:
- General aspects of management including setting of care
- Acute management: biological, psychological and social aspects
- Maintenance (long-term) management
- Current symptoms and problems

Prognosis:
- Short-term
- Long-term

Getting started

Psychiatry can seem disconcertingly different from other specialties, especially if your first experience is on a psychiatric in-patient unit. How do I approach a patient? What am I trying to achieve? Is he or she dangerous? How does psychiatry relate to the rest of medicine? This chapter is meant to help orientate anyone facing this situation. Like the rest of the book, it is based on three principles:

- Psychiatry is part of medicine.
- Psychiatric knowledge, skills and attitudes are relevant to all doctors.
- Psychiatry should be as effective, pragmatic and evidence-based as every other medical specialty.

What is psychiatry?

'Psychiatry is ... weird doctors in Victorian asylums using bizarre therapies on people who are either untreatably mad or who are not really ill at all.' Although remnants of such ill-informed stereotypes persist, the reality of modern psychiatry is very different and rather more mundane! Psychiatry is, in fact, fundamentally similar to the rest of medicine: the treatments used are primarily evidence-based, with success rates comparable with those in other specialties. Psychiatric patients are not a breed apart – psychiatric diagnoses are common in medical patients, and most patients with psychiatric disorders are treated in primary care. And psychiatrists are no stranger than other doctors, probably.

Psychiatric disorders may be defined as illnesses that are conventionally treated with treatments used by psychiatrists, just as surgical conditions are those thought best treated by surgery. The specialty designation does not indicate a profound difference in the illness or type of patient. In fact it can change as new treatments are developed; peptic ulcer moved from being a predominantly surgical to a medical condition once effective drug treatments were developed.

Similarly, conditions such as dementia may move between psychiatry and neurology.

The conditions in which psychiatrists have developed expertise have tended to be those that either manifest with disordered psychological functioning (emotion, perception, thinking and memory) or those that have no clearly established biological basis. However, scientific developments are showing us that these so-called psychological disorders are associated with abnormalities of the brain, just as so-called medical disorders are profoundly affected by psychological factors. Consequently, the delineation between psychiatry and the rest of medicine can increasingly be seen as only a matter of convenience and convention.

Traditional assumptions, however, continue to influence both service organization (with psychiatric services usually being planned and often situated separate from other medical services) and terminology (see below).

Where is psychiatry going?

Psychiatry is evolving rapidly, and three themes permeate this book:

- *Psychiatry, like the rest of medicine, is becoming less hospital based.* Most psychiatric problems are seen and treated in primary care, with many others handled in the general hospital. Only a minority are managed by specialist psychiatric services. So psychiatry should be learned and practised in these other settings too.
- *Psychiatry is becoming more evidence-based.* Diagnostic, prognostic and therapeutic decisions should, of course, be based on the best available evidence. It may come as a surprise to discover that current psychiatric interventions are as evidence-based (and sometimes more so) as in other specialties.

Psychiatry Lecture Notes, Eleventh Edition. Gautam Gulati, Mary-Ellen Lynall and Kate Saunders. © 2014 John Wiley & Sons, Ltd. Published 2014 by John Wiley & Sons, Ltd.

- *Psychiatry is becoming more neuroscience based.* Developments in brain imaging and molecular genetics are beginning to make real progress in the neurobiological understanding of psychiatric disorders. These developments are expanding the knowledge base and range of skills that the next generation of doctors will need. These developments do not, however, make the other elements of psychiatry – psychology and sociology, for example – any less important, as we will see later.

Why study psychiatry?

Studying psychiatry is worthwhile for all trainee doctors, and other health practitioners, because the knowledge, skills and attitudes acquired are applicable to every branch of medicine. Specifically, studying psychiatry will give you:

- A basic knowledge of the common and the 'classic' psychiatric disorders.
- A working knowledge of psychiatric problems encountered in all medical settings.
- The ability to effectively assess someone with a 'psychiatric problem'.
- Skills in the assessment of psychological aspects of medical conditions.
- A holistic or 'biopsychosocial' perspective from which to understand all illness.

Useful knowledge

Formerly, patients with severe psychiatric disorders were often institutionalized and their management was exclusively the domain of psychiatrists. The advent of community care means that other doctors, especially GPs, encounter and participate in the management of such patients, so all doctors need basic information about these 'specialist' psychiatric disorders. Equally, all doctors need to recognize and treat the more common psychiatric illnesses, such as anxiety and depressive disorders. These are extremely prevalent in all medical settings, yet they are all too often overlooked and ineffectively treated.

Useful skills

Most psychiatric disorders are diagnosed from the history, and many treatments are based on listening and talking. So, psychiatrists have had to acquire particular expertise in interviewing patients, in assessing their state of mind and in establishing a therapeutic doctor–patient relationship – with patients who may pose challenges in this respect because of the nature of their problems. These skills remain important in all medical practice. For example, all doctors should be able to:

- Make the patient feel comfortable enough to express their symptoms and feelings clearly.
- Use basic psychotherapeutic skills – for example, knowing how to help a distressed patient and how best to communicate bad news.
- Discuss and prescribe antidepressants and other common psychotropic drugs with confidence.

Without these 'soft' skills, the 'hard' skills of technological, evidence-based medicine cannot be fully effective. An impatient, non-empathic doctor is less likely to elicit the symptoms needed to make the correct diagnosis, and their patient is less likely to adhere to the treatment plan they prescribe.

Useful attitudes

Psychiatric diagnoses are still associated with stigma and misunderstanding. These stem largely from the misconception that illnesses that do not have established 'physical' (or 'organic') pathology are 'mental', and that such 'mental' illness is not real, represents inadequacies of character, or is the person's own fault. Studying psychiatry will help you to challenge these attitudes. You will see many patients with severe symptoms in whom no 'organic' pathology has been established, but who have real symptoms and disability. You will be repeatedly reminded of the stigma that patients with psychiatric problems experience from the public, and sometimes from their relatives and even, sadly, from health professionals. Finally, you will be confronted with the reality of human frailty. Recognizing these issues and dealing with them appropriately – by developing positive, educated and effective attitudes – is another important consequence of studying psychiatry. You might conclude, as we have done that:

- Suffering is real even when there is no 'test' to prove it.
- Psychological and social factors are relevant to all illnesses and can be scientifically studied.
- Much harm is done by negative attitudes towards patients with psychiatric diagnoses.

Your own experience and personality will influence your relationship with patients – your positive attributes as well as your vulnerabilities and prejudices.

How to start psychiatry

The psychiatric interview

The first, key skill to learn is how to listen and talk to patients, in that order. The *psychiatric interview* has two functions:

- It forms the main part of the psychiatric assessment by which diagnoses are made.
- It can be used therapeutically – in the psychotherapies, the communication between patient and therapist is the currency of treatment (Chapter 7).

Psychiatric assessment

Because of its central importance, the principles of psychiatric assessment are outlined here. The practicalities are described in the next two chapters. Psychiatric assessment has three goals:

1 To elicit the information needed to make a diagnosis, since a diagnosis provides the best available framework for making clinical decisions. This may seem obvious, but it hasn't always been so in psychiatry.
2 To understand the causes and context of the disorder.
3 To form a therapeutic relationship with the patient.

Though these goals are the same in all of medicine, the balance of psychiatric assessment differs in several ways. Firstly, the interview provides a greater proportion of diagnostic information. Physical examination and laboratory investigations usually play a lesser, though occasionally crucial, role. Secondly, the interview includes a detailed examination of the patient's current thoughts, feelings, experiences and behaviour (the *mental state examination*), in addition to the standard questioning about the presenting complaint and past history (the *psychiatric history*). Thirdly, a greater wealth of background information about the person is collected than in other specialties (the *context*).

Psychiatric assessments have a reputation for being excessively long. We take a pragmatic approach to the process of assessment. A *basic psychiatric assessment* is used to collect the essential diagnostic and contextual information (Chapter 2). Then, more detailed *diagnosis-specific assessments* are used if anything has led you to hypothesize that the patient has a particular disorder (Chapter 3). This two-stage *basic and diagnosis-specific* approach considerably shortens most assessments – to 45 minutes or less. It also happens to be what psychiatrists actually do – as opposed to what they tell their students to do.

Diagnostic categories

Solving a problem is always easier when you know the range of possible answers. Similarly, before embarking on your first assessment, it helps to know the major psychiatric diagnoses and their cardinal features. Table 1.1 is a simplified guide. As you gain experience, aim for more specific diagnoses that correspond to those listed in the *International*

Table 1.1 A basic guide to psychiatric classification

Category	Examples of disorders	Basic characteristics	Common presentations
Organic disorder	Dementia, delirium	Defined by 'organic' cause	Forgetfulness, confusion
Psychosis	Schizophrenia	Delusions, hallucinations	Bizarre ideas, odd behaviour
Mood disorders	Depression	Low mood	Tearful, fed up, somatic complaints
Neurosis	Anxiety disorders	Emotional disturbance	Worried, tired, stressed
Somatoform disorders	Somatization disorder	Unexplained physical symptoms	Chronic pain, fear of disease
Substance misuse	Opiate dependence	Effects of the drug	Addiction, withdrawal, depression
Personality disorder	Dissocial, histrionic	Dysfunctional personality traits	Exacerbation of traits when stressed
Learning disability	Down's syndrome, autism	Congenitally low IQ	Developmental delay, physical appearance

Classification of Diseases, 10th revision (ICD-10), which are used in this book (see Appendix 1). There is an alternative to ICD-10, published by the American Psychiatric Association, called the *Diagnostic and Statistical Manual of Mental Disorders*. It is widely used in research, and the controversial 5th edition (DSM-5) was published in 2013. The two systems are broadly similar. Whatever the classification, remember the underused category of 'no psychiatric disorder'. A term such as 'nervous breakdown' has no useful psychiatric meaning – it may describe almost any of the categories in Table 1.1.

Psychiatric classification

The classification of psychiatric disorders has several problems that you should be aware of before you start:

- *Most diagnoses are syndromes, defined by combinations of symptoms, but some are based on aetiology or pathology.* For example, depression can be caused by a brain tumour (diagnosis: organic mood disorder), or after bereavement (diagnosis: abnormal grief reaction) or without clear cause (diagnosis: depressive disorder). This combination of different sorts of category leads to some conceptual and practical difficulties, which will become apparent later.
- *Comorbidity: many patients suffer from more than one psychiatric disorder* (or a psychiatric disorder and a medical disorder). The comorbid disorders may or may not be causally related, and may or may not both require treatment. As a rule, comorbidity complicates management and worsens prognosis.
- *Hierarchy: not all diagnoses carry equal weight.* Traditionally, organic disorder trumps everything (i.e. if it is present, coexisting disorders are not diagnosed), and psychosis trumps neurosis. This principle is no longer applied consistently, partly because it is hard to reconcile with the frequency and clinical importance of comorbidity.
- *Categories versus dimensions.* The current system assumes there are distinctions between one disorder and another, and between disorder and health. However, such cut-offs are notoriously difficult to demonstrate, either aetiologically or clinically, whereas there is good evidence that there are continuums – for example, between bipolar disorder and schizophrenia, and for the occurrence of psychotic symptoms in 'normal' people. However,

clinical practice requires 'yes/no' decisions to be made (e.g. as to what treatment to recommend) and so a categorical approach persists.
- *Psychiatric classification is not an exact science.* All classifications have drawbacks, and psychiatry has more than its share, as illustrated by the above points. Nevertheless, despite the imperfections, rational clinical practice requires a degree of order to be created, and most of the current diagnostic categories at least have good reliability, and utility in predicting treatment response and prognosis.

After the assessment: summarizing and communicating the information

Completion of the psychiatric assessment is followed by several steps:

- *Make a (differential) diagnosis*, according to ICD-10 categories (Appendix 1), using your knowledge of the key features of each psychiatric disorder.
- *Attempt to understand how and why the disorder has arisen* (Chapter 6).
- *Develop a management plan*, based on an awareness of the best available treatment (Chapter 7), how psychiatric services are organized (Chapter 8) and the patient's characteristics, including their risk of harm to self or others (Chapter 4).
- *Communicate your understanding of the case* (Chapter 5).

 KEYPOINTS

- Psychiatry is a medical specialty. It mostly deals with conditions in which the symptoms and signs predominantly relate to emotions, perception, thinking or memory. It also encompasses learning disability and the psychological aspects of the rest of medicine.
- Knowledge, skills and attitudes learned in psychiatry are relevant and valuable in all medical specialties.
- Be alert to the possibility of psychiatric disorder in all patients, and be able to recognize and elicit the key features.
- The major diagnostic categories are: neurosis, mood disorder, psychosis, organic disorder, substance misuse and personality disorder.

The basic psychiatric assessment

Learning objectives

✓ To understand the structure of a typical psychiatric assessment, including the history and mental state examination

✓ To develop a practical approach to the initial assessment of patients who present to psychiatric services, and to patients in other settings in whom you suspect a psychiatric problem

✓ To learn basic psychiatric terminology

Approaching a psychiatric assessment

The principles and goals of psychiatric assessment were outlined in Chapter 1. A 'traditional' first assessment interview includes an extensive search for symptoms and detailed, wide-ranging questions about the patient's life history. Though comprehensive, this approach can take over an hour, which in many situations is unrealistic. We suggest a more flexible approach to assessment in which screening questions and other basic information (*the basic psychiatric assessment*; this chapter) are used to identify possible diagnoses, which are then confirmed or excluded by more focused assessment (*diagnosis-specific assessments*; Chapter 3). For a checklist of the areas to cover in a fuller psychiatric assessment, see Quick Guides.

The basic assessment described in this chapter is designed to obtain a clear account of the patient's main problem(s) and screen rapidly but systematically for evidence of common psychiatric disorders. If your basic assessment or other sources of information make you suspect a particular diagnosis, you should use the appropriate diagnosis-specific assessment(s) from Chapter 3, which cover *cognitive function, psychosis, mood disorders, anxiety disorders, eating disorders, substance misuse, somatic symptoms* and *the unresponsive patient*. Each assessment guide is designed to determine whether a disorder in that category is present and, if so, to establish the specific diagnosis and elicit the appropriate contextual information. Box 2.1 gives examples of how an assessment might proceed. Assessment of childhood disorders, learning disability, sleep and sexual functioning are covered in their respective chapters. Risk assessment is described in Chapter 4.

 Box 2.1 Using the basic assessment and diagnosis-specific assessments

Three examples show how an assessment may develop:

1 A woman complains of tiredness and feeling fed up. The basic assessment described in this chapter reveals evidence of depression and a recent increase in alcohol intake, but not of suicidal intent, psychosis or cognitive impairment. You proceed to the diagnosis-specific assessments for *mood* and *substance misuse* (Chapter 3). These assessments confirm the presence of a depressive disorder, but no significant alcohol problem.

Psychiatry Lecture Notes, Eleventh Edition. Gautam Gulati, Mary-Ellen Lynall and Kate Saunders. © 2014 John Wiley & Sons, Ltd. Published 2014 by John Wiley & Sons, Ltd.

2 A wife reports her 70-year-old husband is getting confused. Your initial suspicions are of dementia, so you do a diagnosis-specific assessment of his cognitive function. However, although his concentration is poor, he does not have typical memory loss or other symptoms of dementia. You decide to do a basic psychiatric assessment and you find evidence of depression, so you assess his mood, which leads you to a diagnosis of major depressive disorder.

3 A man is brought in having been found standing in the road naked, screaming at passers-by to stop irradiating him. You do not elicit any psychotic symptoms on the basic psychiatric assessment. Nonetheless, his presenting behaviour prompts you to do a diagnosis-specific assessment for psychosis. He may initially deny symptoms in case you are part of a conspiracy! Given that illicit drugs can produce this kind of behaviour, you also assess for substance misuse.

What is the mental state examination (MSE)?

All psychiatric assessments include a mental state examination (MSE) as well as the history. The scope of the MSE is a source of some confusion. Classically, the MSE is limited to those features present *at the time of the interview*, with everything else being in the history. Put another way, the MSE represents an objective cross-sectional description of the patient's presentation. Is the MSE the psychiatric equivalent of the physical examination? This is partly true: the MSE

is the occasion for the interviewer to note any signs of psychiatric disorder: for example, *'The patient keeps looking anxiously around'*. However, the MSE also includes formal descriptions of symptoms reported by the patient, for example, *'he described third party auditory hallucinations which were command in nature,'* and in this respect it overlaps with the history (Figure 2.1).

Components of the basic psychiatric assessment

The basic psychiatric assessment covers the areas shown in Table 2.1 and is outlined below. It consists of some pre-interview preparation, a history, a mental state examination, and possibly a physical examination. Variations on the structure presented here are common and often desirable: by responding flexibly to the direction the patient takes, rather than slavishly following a preconceived order of topics, you are likely to improve the history you obtain.

Before the interview

- **Location:** You will be discussing intimate, and sometimes distressing, topics. The room should be comfortable, and as soundproof as possible. This can be challenging, especially on medical wards.
- **Safety:** Occasionally patients may become disturbed or violent. Discuss with a senior member of staff – should you have a chaperone? Check local procedures – for example, are there panic buttons?

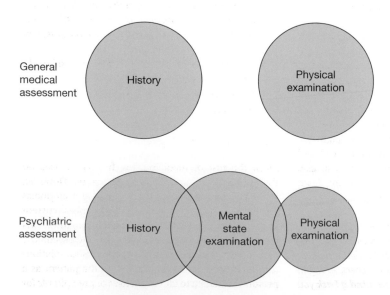

General medical assessment

History

Physical examination

Psychiatric assessment

History

Mental state examination

Physical examination

Figure 2.1 A comparison of medical and psychiatric assessments, showing the relationship of history, functional enquiry, mental state examination (MSE) and physical examination. Note the overlap between the components of the psychiatric assessment. For example, recent suicidal thoughts might be detected in the history or MSE; akathisia (restlessness) may be elicited as a symptom in the history or MSE or as a sign in the physical examination.

> **Table 2.1 The basic psychiatric assessment. See Appendices 1 and 2 for a fuller checklist of points to cover during the history and MSE**
>
> **Before you begin**
> - Information (referral letters, notes), location, safety
> - Introduction, consent, establish expectations
>
> **Basic details**
> - Method of referral
> - Age, marital status, occupation, current living arrangements
>
> **Basic history: current problems and background history**
> - Presenting complaint(s), and their history
> - Past psychiatric history
> - Family history
> - Personal history and premorbid personality
> - Social history (current circumstances)
> - Substance use: smoking, alcohol and illicit drugs
> - Forensic history
> - Past medical history and drug history
>
> **Basic mental state examination**
> - Appearance and behaviour
> - Speech
> - Mood
> - Thoughts
> - Perceptions
> - Cognition
> - Insight
>
> **Risk assessment**
>
> **Physical examination** if necessary
>
> **Corroborative history** if possible
>
> **Investigations** as necessary

Arrange seating so you are closer to the door than the patient. Safety is a particular issue for home visits.

- **Setting:** Chairs are best arranged at ninety degrees to each other. If a desk is required for making notes, this should not be directly between the patient and the interviewer. Sit in a relaxed and slightly forward posture. Arrange not to be interrupted – turn off mobile phones and pagers whenever possible.
- **Information:** Read any referral letter and previous notes. These may provide a preliminary diagnostic hypothesis, clarify the reason for the referral and suggest lines of questioning. The notes can also help you to identify a possible 'informant' from whom to gain a corroborative history.
- **Approach the patient:**
  - Introduce yourself, check the identity of the patient, describe what you are suggesting and obtain consent. For example: *'Hello, I'm a medical student and my name is X. Can I check that you are Y? … Thank you. Would you mind if I ask you some questions about what has happened to you? … Thank you. If it's okay with you, we'll go into an interview room to talk. This shouldn't take more than 20 minutes, and if you want to stop at any point, you can just say.'*
  - Emphasize confidentiality. If notes are to be taken, explain why.
  - Establish the patient's expectations for the interview.

The basic history

As in the rest of medicine, the history focuses on the problems the patient complains of. However, in the psychiatric history, there is a greater emphasis on the person's personality, life experiences, current circumstances and other contextual information. This 'background history' is a crucial part of the psychiatric assessment. It can enhance the therapeutic relationship by demonstrating an interest in the patient as a person. It can help to identify causes or precipitants for mental health problems such as bereavement, child-hood abuse or financial worries. It may also reveal personal factors that affect management, such as the presence of a supportive partner to supervise medication. How much background information you should seek depends on the nature of the patient's problems, and what is already known. For example, in general practice the patient's circumstances may be well known; for a woman newly referred to your out-patient clinic, more detailed questioning might be needed.

Some of the questions may feel invasive, to you or to the patient. Some tips ...

- Signpost: *'I'd like to ask about topics which are a bit more personal. Is that okay?'*
- Acknowledge embarrassment: *'I know these things are difficult to talk about ...'*
- Normalize: *'You've told me how ..., some people when they feel like that can ... Is that something you've felt?/Have you had any problems like that?'*
- Are you the right person at the right time to be asking these questions?

It can be hard to strike a balance between keeping control of the interview and allowing the patient sufficient time to answer questions fully and in their own way. As well as responding to what the patient says, be sensitive to non-verbal clues such as facial expression, posture and tone of voice.

Basic details

- Clarify the method of referral, if unclear from the notes.
- Clarify the patient's age, marital status, occupation and living arrangements.

Presenting complaint(s) and their history

- Start with open questions: *'What do you think is the main problem? How have you been feeling?'*
- Closed (but not leading) questions are used to clarify the responses: *'You say you're not sleeping well: can you tell me a bit more about that? What time do you wake?'*
- Encourage the patient to list their main problems and describe each in their own words. *'Do you have any other problems?'*
- Assess the nature, duration and progression of each of the symptom(s).
- Are there any precipitating and relieving factors?
- Assess the degree of functional impairment: effect on relationships, work, sleep, etc.
- How have others perceived the problems: *'What did your friends say about you when you were feeling like that?'*
- Treatments tried for the current problem.

 Box 2.2 Screening for alcohol problems

The FAST questions

1 How often do you have eight or more drinks on one occasion?

2 How often during the past year have you failed to do what was normally expected of you because of drinking?

3 How often during the past year have you been unable to remember what happened the night before because you had been drinking?

[For these questions, score 0 for never, 1 for less than monthly, 2 for monthly, 3 for weekly and 4 for daily or almost daily.]

4 Has a relative, friend, doctor or other health worker been concerned about your drinking or suggested you cut down?

[For this question, score 0 for never, 2 for yes but not in past year, 4 for yes, in the past year.]

The maximum score is 16, and a score of 3 or more indicates hazardous drinking. You may not need to ask all four questions: if you find out on Q1 that the patient drinks eight or more drinks at least weekly, she or he has already reached the threshold for hazardous drinking, so move straight to a full assessment of substance misuse (p. 35) and consider administering the AUDIT questionnaire (p. 36). Note that the FAST questions do not screen for alcohol *dependency*, which is better picked up by the CAGE questions.

The CAGE questions

The CAGE is an alternative and widely used alcohol screening tool. Its four questions are:

1 Have you ever felt you ought to **C**ut down on your drinking?

2 Have people **A**nnoyed you by criticizing your drinking?

3 Have you ever felt **G**uilty about your drinking?

4 Have you ever had a drink first thing in the morning (an '**E**ye-opener')?

If three or more yes answers are given, the likelihood ratio for problem drinking is 250.

Getting a list of the patient's problems allows you to start generating diagnostic hypotheses. Some problems will be symptoms (e.g. agitation); others will represent the patient's predicament (e.g. homelessness). The diagnostic importance of a particular symptom is affected by its characteristics (intensity, fluctuation, duration, etc.), associated features and functional impact. Knowing the relevant information to elicit comes rapidly with increasing knowledge and experience. A useful acronym is 'NOTEPAD': Nature, Onset, Triggers, Exacerbating/relieving, Progression, Associated symptoms, Disability. Get answers that are as precise as possible – for example, estimates of symptom duration. Finally, don't ignore 'medical' symptoms. A brief functional enquiry to elicit these should be included.

Past psychiatric history

- Nature of any previous psychiatric contact: *'Have you ever been an inpatient in a psychiatric hospital? Have you ever been in contact with the community mental health team? Were you given a diagnosis?'*
- Treatments used for previous episodes of psychiatric illness and their effects.
- Self-harm and harm to others: *'Have you ever harmed yourself or tried to kill yourself? Have you ever hurt anyone else?'*

About 50% of psychiatry referrals have had prior psychiatric contact. A previous diagnosis is best seen as a strong hypothesis to be tested. Keep an open mind – the new problem may be different, or the previous diagnosis might be wrong. Past history may also provide useful information about prognosis and the patient's attitude to their disorder and its management.

Family history

- Family tree – ask the ages, occupations and health of, at a minimum, parents, siblings and children. Draw out the tree.
- Quality of the family relationships: *'How do you get on with your family?'* Problems in family relationships are commonly associated with psychiatric disorder.
- Family psychiatric history: *'Has anyone in your family had problems like you're having now?'* Also ask about suicide, self-harm or substance misuse. A positive family psychiatric history is a risk factor for most psychiatric disorders, for both genetic and environmental reasons.
- Brief family medical history.
- Any recent events in the family.

Personal history and premorbid personality

- **Pregnancy, birth and childhood** – *'Are you aware of any problems around your birth or during your mother's pregnancy with you? Did you walk and talk at the right age, as far as you know?'*, childhood health problems, maltreatment.

- **Education** – did the patient enjoy school? bullying? finish school? special education classes?
- Occupations and reasons for changes, military service, job satisfaction.
- **Relationships** – number, duration, type, gender.
- **Traumatic events** – *'In your life, have you ever had a particularly horrible or frightening experience?'* Exposure to suicide or self-harm is worth exploring specifically as it is a risk factor for those behaviours in the patient.
- **'Premorbid personality'** – the patient's usual character, interests, belief and habits. *'How would your friends describe you? How do you cope in a difficult situation? Would you describe yourself as a loner or very sociable?'* (offering alternatives can be helpful) *'Do you believe there is something beyond us, like God? Is religion important to you?'*

Aspects of childhood can be associated with subsequent psychiatric disorder; for example, conduct disorder is associated with dissocial personality disorder, and childhood abuse is associated with all psychiatric disorders. The pattern of past relationships can give diagnostic clues, such as an absence of close relationships in schizoid personality disorder, or many turbulent ones in borderline personality disorder. The nature of employment may give clues to the patient's level of functioning. A deteriorating or disrupted work record may reflect a psychiatric disorder or a personality trait, respectively. The premorbid personality shapes the risk, type and prognosis of psychiatric disorder. Note that a patient's view of their personality and life may be distorted during psychiatric illness; for example, a depressed person will report themselves in an unduly negative light. Third party information may be useful in such cases. Questions on sexual history and functioning may be necessary at this stage, but detailed or especially sensitive discussion on this topic may better be deferred until a later stage.

Social history (current circumstances)

- **Current relationships:** *'Do you have a partner at the moment? Are they a man or a woman?'* (never assume gender).
- **Self-care and support:** *'Do you feel able to look after yourself at the moment?'* Who is there to support the patient, and who is dependent on the patient?
- **Current employment.**
- **Current worries** – finances, housing, relationship, etc.
- It can be helpful to ask the patient to describe a typical day.

Current relationships are important: they may contribute to the present disorder or have been damaged by it. Having a supportive partner improves outcome and assists management. Ongoing worries and stresses can perpetuate psychiatric disorder; their resolution is often part of management – for example, helping the patient sort out a housing problem. All patients with severe psychiatric disorder should have an assessment of needs (p. 84). Detailed information about the current circumstances is an essential component of this.

Alcohol and drug use

- *'Do you drink alcohol?'* Record the amount per week in units. If the patient drinks alcohol regularly, ask the four FAST or CAGE questions (Box 2.2). They take about 20 seconds.
- *'Have you ever used recreational drugs?'* If so, quantify the amount used: *'How much do you spend on X per week?'* can give a good guide and is often more accurate than asking the patient to estimate weights consumed. You can ask the CAGE questions for each recreational drug used.
- Impact on the patient's life: *'Has your drinking/drug use ever got you into trouble in your relationships? At work? With the law?'*

Alcohol and other drugs may be a cause, a component or a consequence of many psychiatric disorders, so should always be asked about. The recommended limits for alcohol intake are 21 units per week for men and 14 for women. One unit is half a pint of beer, a single measure of spirits, or a *small* glass of wine. Try out the NHS Choices Drinks Tracker free desktop and mobile app to calculate units per week.

Forensic history

- *'Have you ever had contact with the police? Were you charged? What happened?'*
- If there were incidents, did these relate to previous episodes of mental illness?

Having a 'forensic history' (i.e. a criminal record) may be directly related to a psychiatric disorder or be a coincidence. A history of violence will affect management regardless.

Past medical history and drug history

- *'Have you had any medical illnesses or operations?'*
- Current medication and adherence: *'Which ones do you usually take? Do they give you any side effects?'*
- Complementary therapies used.
- Allergies (important for the management plan).

The medical history is important because of the overlap between psychiatric and medical disorders.

Medical disorders can cause and be caused by psychiatric disorder, and the drugs used to treat psychiatric disorder may also cause medical problems. This co-dependence of mental and physical morbidity means that physical illness is common in people with psychiatric disorders, but it is often undiagnosed. Some patients forget that they have depot medication as it is administered by a nurse every few weeks. It is always worth asking specifically about injections.

The basic mental state examination (MSE)

The basic MSE described here concentrates on aspects of the recent mental state that are commonly affected by psychiatric disorder and that have diagnostic weight. Much of the MSE will have been covered in the history or from observations made in passing. However, the MSE is still useful to ensure (and to document) that you have checked for all important recent phenomena and provides a point of comparison over time. When you present your findings, you should clearly separate the history from the MSE. The headings of the basic MSE are:

1 **Appearance and behaviour** – an underestimated source of diagnostic information.
2 **Speech** – abnormal speech may be present in neurological, psychotic and mood disorders.
3 **Mood** – subjective and objective accounts of mood and its reactivity and congruency (terms explained below).
4 **Thoughts** – thought content, and the way thoughts flow, are affected in many psychiatric disorders. The nature of the abnormalities gives important diagnostic clues.
5 **Perceptions** – mainly affected in psychotic and organic disorders. Less florid alterations in sensory experiences also occur in anxiety disorders.
6 **Cognition** – cognitive impairment is characteristic of dementia and delirium, but can also occur in other disorders such as depression. If severe, it may make history-taking very difficult.
7 **Insight** – lack of awareness of illness is classically a sign of psychosis or 'organic' disorder. In all disorders, the patient's views as to the nature and significance of their problems are important, not least since they may affect their views about the need for (and choice of) treatment.

1) Appearance and behaviour

1 **Level of consciousness**: alert/hypervigilant/sleepy.
2 **Appearance**: dress, posture, self-care, apparent body mass index (BMI), self-harm/intravenous drug use, smell.

3 **Body language and movement**: overactivity, abnormal movements or gait, responding to hallucinations or talking to someone.
4 **Eye contact and rapport** with the interviewer: defensive, evasive, co-operative?

Many psychiatric disorders are accompanied by characteristic changes in manner, emotional expression or physical appearance. These often provide the first diagnostic clue. So, from the moment you meet, observe closely ... (see Box 2.3).

2) Speech

1 **Quantity and spontaneity**: does the patient speak spontaneously, or very little and only in response to questioning (poverty of speech)?
2 **Volume and rate**: pressure of speech (fast and difficult to interrupt)? slowed speech?
3 **Tone**: the emotional quality of speech – e.g. angry, sarcastic.
4 **Articulation/intelligibility**: is the patient's speech hard to understand? If so, is it because of articulation (dysarthria) or content (dysphasia)?

Quiet speech that tails off or is monosyllabic is typical of depression; the opposite occurs in mania. *Dysarthria* means a problem with articulation. It can manifest as slurred, strangled, staccato or nasal speech and suggests a neurological disorder (the differential is wide), intoxication or a side effect of antipsychotic drugs. *Dysphasia*, in which there is a problem understanding or communicating meaning, suggests a neurological disorder or thought disorder. The division between speech and thoughts is somewhat artificial, but abnormalities in the content or flow of what is said are usually recorded under 'thoughts'.

3) Mood

Disturbances of mood are usually in the depressive direction (low mood), but can also be manic (elevated mood). The direction of any alteration will usually be obvious, and questions can be focused accordingly.

1 **Subjective mood** (self-reported mood): '*How have you been feeling in yourself recently? How would you describe your mood just now? On a scale of 1 to 10? Have you been low in spirits or depressed? Can you still enjoy the things that you normally enjoy? Is life particularly good or more enjoyable at the moment? Have you been feeling more irritable than usual?*'
2 **Objective mood**: Record how the patient's mood appears to you – this may be different from subjective mood. You can describe:
   • the **mood itself** (elevated, depressed or unremarkable);
   • its **constancy** (flat, labile, reactive);
   • its **congruity** (congruous or incongruous).

The best screening questions for depression ask about persistent low mood and the loss of pleasure (anhedonia). *Constancy* describes how the mood shifts over the conversation: it is abnormal for mood not to shift at all. A *labile* mood showed marked fluctuation. *Congruity* describes how well the patient's mood fits with what they are thinking or perceiving. *Incongruity* of mood, for example no change in mood when describing a distressing experience, is a feature of schizophrenia. You should always screen for mood disorders. There is no evidence that asking about suicide increases the risk of it – probably the opposite. The mood section of the MSE can also reveal anxiety symptoms, although these are usually obvious from the patient's appearance, behaviour or thoughts.

 Box 2.3 The waiting room

You look into the waiting room and see a garishly dressed patient, pacing around and enthusiastically trying to engage other patients in conversation. Is he manic? Intoxicated? Disinhibited due to a frontal lobe tumour? The older patient in the corner is avoiding eye contact and with little facial expression – is he depressed? Is he parkinsonian? You notice he also has a tremor – that seems to support Parkinson's disease. Or could it be due to taking antipsychotic drugs or lithium? You call another patient in, and she starts talking to you, but keeps breaking off in mid-sentence and looking over her shoulder. Is she hearing voices? Does she think the room is bugged? Both could indicate paranoid schizophrenia.

 Box 2.4 Abnormal thoughts

Delusion: A false belief firmly held *despite contrary evidence* and out of keeping with the patient's cultural or religious background. For example, a patient is absolutely convinced that he is an assassin's target and so has locked himself in his flat and adopted a disguise. There may be one delusion or many, and they may be persistent or fleeting. Delusions carry special weight in the diagnosis of psychosis, so their recognition is an important skill.

An **overvalued idea** is a belief not held quite as strongly as a delusion, and is typically more 'understandable'. It is typified by the belief of a malnourished girl with anorexia nervosa that she is fat. There is a spectrum between delusions and over-valued ideas: thoughts which seem to fall near the boundary line ('partial delusions') are common during the development and treatment of psychosis.

Obsession: A recurrent thought, impulse or image that enters the subject's mind *despite resistance*. The patient realizes that it originates from their own mind and may not be true, but they cannot resist thinking it and often have to act upon it (a *compulsion*). For example, obsessional thoughts about having dirty hands may lead to the compulsion to wash repeatedly. These symptoms characterize obsessive-compulsive disorder and also occur in depression.

Formal thought disorder: Literally, this simply means disorder of the *form* of thought (rather than its content), and many conditions are associated with disordered thought. However, this term is often used to imply the disordered thought associated with psychosis.

Flight of ideas: Thoughts move rapidly from one idea to the next and are difficult to follow, but the links between the thoughts are understandable, if unusual (unlike in formal thought disorder).

4) Thoughts

1 **Form (or flow)**: Is the patient's train of thought difficult to follow? Try to describe how. Is there formal thought disorder or flight of ideas?

2 **Content**:
- **Over-valued ideas and delusions**: *'Do you feel that something strange is going on? Do you have any ideas your friends and family don't share? Is someone or something trying to control you? Is someone trying to interfere with your thoughts? Do you feel that people are against you or trying to harm you in some way?'*
- **Worries and obsessions:** *'Do you have particular things on your mind at the moment? Do you keep having the same thought going round and round in your mind? Do certain things keep coming into your mind, even though you try hard to keep them out? Do you worry about your health a lot?'*
- **Compulsions** (not strictly a thought, but useful to ask about this at the same time as obsessions): *'Do you ever find yourself doing the same thing over and over again, even though you've already done it well enough?'*
- **Phobias:** *'Do you have any special fears, like some people are afraid of spiders or mirrors?'*
- **Suicidal ideation:** Use cues from the patient to broach the subject. For example: *'It sounds as if*

life's a bit of a struggle at the moment. Do you feel like life isn't worth living? Do you have any plans to end your life?'
- **Morbid thoughts:** thoughts of harm to self or others: *'Have you thought of harming yourself in any way?'*

It is important to assess both the form and content of the thoughts. Giving the patient time to reply at length to an open question can highlight a problem with the form of thoughts – if you are finding the patient difficult to follow, this is a good indicator of thought disorder (or that they are brighter than you!). Write down a sample of what is said.

Abnormalities of thoughts and thought processes occur in many psychiatric disorders, and the precise form of the abnormality can be diagnostically important. See Box 2.4 for some important definitions. There are classic patterns of abnormal thought associated with schizophrenia (e.g. formal thought disorder, delusions, thought echo) and bipolar disorder (flight of ideas, grandiose delusions), which are discussed in more detail in other chapters. However, this section of the MSE could also pick up (for example) recurrent worries about physical health in hypochondriasis; a general theme of persecution in a delusional disorder; or a preoccupation with weight in an eating disorder.

5) Perceptions

- **Illusions and hallucinations**: *'Do you see or hear things that other people can't? Have you ever heard voices speaking when there was nobody there? Do things or people seem different from normal? When does this happen?'*
- **Derealization and depersonalization**: *'Do you ever feel detached from yourself, or from the rest of the world?'*

See Box 2.5 for some important symptom definitions and their significance.

 Box 2.5 Abnormal perceptions

A **hallucination** is a perception experienced as real *in the absence of a stimulus*. For example, hearing a voice in the corner of the room when no one is there. Like a delusion, the person is absolutely convinced (at the time) that the experience is real. They can occur in any sensory modality and are pathognomonic of psychosis. *Auditory hallucinations* are the most common and usually suggest an affective disorder, schizophrenia or acute drug intoxication. *Visual hallucinations* suggest an organic psychosis such as Lewy body dementia. *Olfactory hallucinations* occur in temporal lobe epilepsy. Hallucinations are common whilst falling asleep (hypnogogic) or waking up (hypnopompic), and are not abnormal.

An **illusion** is a misperception or misinterpretation *of an external stimulus*. For example, mistaking a shadow in the corner for a person when there is no one there. They have an 'as if' quality. They are common in the general population and in isolation have no diagnostic significance (and so must be distinguished clearly from hallucinations).

Depersonalization is a feeling of detachment *from the normal sense of self* – 'as if I am acting'. **Derealization** is a feeling of detachment *from the external world*. Both are a feature of anxiety disorders but can be mistaken for psychosis.

6) Cognition

- **Orientation**: Is the patient orientated in time, person and place?
- **Level of consciousness**: Is there 'clouding of consciousness' or is the patient alert?
- **Subjective report**: *'Are you having any problems thinking clearly?'*
- **Memory**: Show the patient three items (e.g. watch, pen, shoe) and ensure they have registered them; test for recall 2 minutes later.

Cognitive impairment is the hallmark of dementia and delirium. It can also occur as a feature of depression, especially in the elderly (sometimes called pseudodementia), and in schizophrenia (hence its former name of dementia praecox). In delirium there is *clouding of consciousness* (usually manifested as decreased responsiveness to, or awareness of, surroundings); in dementia there isn't. If significant cognitive abnormalities are detected, diagnosis-specific assessment of cognition (p. 19), physical examination and relevant investigations are essential.

7) Insight

- That they are ill: *'Do you think anything is wrong with you? What do you think is wrong?'*
- That their symptoms can be attributed to their illness: e.g. *'Do you think that your voices are real, or are they to do with your illness?'*
- That they need treatment: *'Do you need any treatment? What sort of treatment do you think you need?'*

Insight is not all or nothing, but a matter of degree, and it fluctuates according to the mental state. Moreover, insight is defined *with respect to something else*. It includes the person's ability to recognize abnormal mental experiences as abnormal; insight that they

are suffering from a psychiatric disorder; insight into the relationship between their symptoms and their illness; and insight into the need for and benefits of treatment. This last aspect has particular implications when considering compulsory treatment under the Mental Health Act. It is also very important to assess the capacity of the patient to accept or refuse treatment (see Chapter 19).

Ending the interview

As you come to the end of your interview:

1 Summarize what you have been told back to the patient. This helps ensure you have gained an accurate picture, and reinforces to the patient that you have been listening carefully.
2 *'Is there anything else that I haven't asked you, that you think I should know?'*
3 Give the patient an opportunity to ask questions.
4 Explain what you plan to do next.

When is a physical examination necessary?

The physical health of a psychiatric patient is important because:

- Medical conditions can present with psychological symptoms. For example, lethargy and low mood may signify anaemia, hypothyroidism or malignancy.
- Patients with psychiatric disorders have increased rates of medical illness for a number of reasons: there may be a common aetiology; the psychiatric disorder may have led them to neglect their health; or they may have medical side effects of the treatments used for psychiatric disorders.

So, in every assessment take account of the patient's physical appearance, as well as their age, symptoms, medical history, etc., and always consider what examination is required. This may include a brief examination of all systems. However, there is no pre-specified physical examination in the psychiatric assessment since it depends upon the setting, the patient, the disorder and the treatment.

- **The setting:** A full examination is performed on every psychiatric hospital admission because the psychiatrist takes medical responsibility whilst the patient is in hospital. A full examination should also be performed in any emergency assessment.
- **The patient:** A full examination should be performed if the patient has not been seen by a doctor recently, or if they are homeless, and hence at risk

of tuberculosis, malnutrition, etc. Relevant systems examinations should be performed if there is a known history of a medical disorder, or if functional enquiry reveals significant symptoms.

- **The disorder and its treatment:** For example, if alcohol misuse is suspected, examine for the physical signs that accompany it. Patients on long-term antipsychotic drugs should be examined for tardive dyskinesia.

For patients receiving psychiatric care in the community, the responsibility for the patient's physical health should be agreed between the psychiatrist and GP; usually it resides with the latter. This will include things such as monitoring of lithium levels, renal function and cardiovascular risk.

Basic investigations

Investigations should be used selectively to ensure that there is no underlying medical condition accounting for, or contributing to, the patient's psychiatric disorder, as well as baseline tests prior to commencing medication. For example:

- A urine drug screen in suspected drug-induced psychosis.
- Extensive biochemical, imaging and genetic investigations in a 30-year-old with dementia.
- A brain scan in someone with delirium and a history of a fall.
- Thyroid function tests in a patient with anxiety, palpitations and weight loss.
- Renal function prior to commencing lithium.

 Box 2.6 A 'one minute screen' for psychiatric disorder

There are occasions when only a moment can be spent on psychiatric assessment. Even this is worthwhile. The seven questions below screen rapidly for psychiatric disorders common in general practice and non-psychiatric inpatients. A positive response to any question should lead you to perform a fuller psychiatric assessment.

During the past month:

1 Have you felt low in spirits? (depression)
2 Do you enjoy things less than you usually do? (depression)
3 Have you been feeling generally anxious? (anxiety)
4 Are you worried about your health or other specific things? (health anxiety)

5 Has your eating felt out of control? (eating disorder)
6 Do you drink alcohol? If so, ask FAST or CAGE questions (Box 2.2)
7 Present three items and ask the patient to recall them after 2 minutes (dementia/delirium)

 FURTHER READING

Oyebode F, Sims ACP (2008) *Sims' Symptoms in the Mind: An Introduction to Descriptive Psychopathology*, 4th edn. Saunders/Elsevier, Edinburgh.

 KEYPOINTS

- The aim of psychiatric assessment is to gather sufficient information to make a diagnosis and set it in context.
- Most information comes from the history and mental state examination, although physical examination and investigations are sometimes important too.
- Diagnostic hypotheses should be made early in the assessment and then tested using more specific questioning.
- A flexible approach can be achieved by combining a basic assessment with diagnosis-specific assessments (Chapter 3), which are only used when the likelihood of a specific diagnosis is raised.
- Psychiatric disorder can and should be rapidly screened for in all medical settings (see Box 2.6).
- Interviewing skills allow you to gather information efficiently and form an effective alliance with the patient.

 SELF-ASSESSMENT

1 Which of the following is true?
   a The mental state examination is limited to features that the interviewer notices.
   b The 'FAST' questions serve as a screen for alcohol dependency.
   c Congruity describes how well the patient's mood fits with what they are thinking or perceiving.
   d Derealization is a feeling of detachment from the normal sense of self.
   e Delusions are disorders associated with schizophrenia.

Diagnosis-specific assessments

Learning objectives: how to assess ...

✓ cognitive function

✓ psychosis

✓ depression and mania

✓ anxiety disorders and somatoform disorders

✓ eating disorders

✓ sleep disorders

✓ alcohol and other substance misuse

✓ an unresponsive (or uncooperative) patient

When to use this chapter

The previous chapter described how to perform a basic assessment to screen for features *suggesting* a psychiatric disorder. In this chapter, we describe a number of in-depth assessments that help you come to a *particular diagnosis*. The assessments cover the commonest presentations and groups of diagnoses in psychiatry (listed above). Each section contains general advice about the areas to cover in your history and mental state examination (MSE), specific suggestions for questions to use, and definitions of key terms. You can think of these assessments as the 'extra bits' you need to do on top of the basic assessment if you suspect one of the associated diagnoses. Alternatively, possible diagnoses may occur to you at a later stage in the patient's care, leading you to assess for them more specifically. *We do not suggest reading this chapter in one go. Instead, read through a section as you come across a clinical problem requiring its use.*

The clinical features of psychiatric disorders are covered in later chapters, which you can refer to in conjunction with this chapter. Note that an adequate assessment often requires assessing more than one of the domains described below. The assessment of risk, sexual functioning, learning disability and children's problems are covered in other chapters.

How to assess cognitive function

'Cognitive function' is multi-faceted and includes domains such as attention, memory and language. We describe the approach to cognitive impairment first because it interferes with the psychiatric assessment, occasionally to the point that no useful history can be obtained from the patient. If the patient can't or won't engage in the assessment, see the section 'How to assess an unresponsive patient' (p. 37). If the impairment is life-long, consider learning disability.

Psychiatry Lecture Notes, Eleventh Edition. Gautam Gulati, Mary-Ellen Lynall and Kate Saunders. © 2014 John Wiley & Sons, Ltd. Published 2014 by John Wiley & Sons, Ltd.

What do you need to find out?

1 **Does the patient have significant cognitive impairment?**
2 **Is there a 'medical' cause?** E.g. intracranial tumour or other space-occupying lesion, meningitis, encephalitis ...
3 **If there is no obvious direct cause, is this *dementia, delirium or depression?*** Dementia and delirium are the two major causes of cognitive impairment, each with a range of specific causes that need to be investigated (see Chapter 13). In dementia, consciousness is unimpaired whereas the hallmark of delirium is '*clouding of consciousness*' – drowsiness, distractibility, fleeting delusions, and visual hallucinations. Dementia is chronic and progressive, while in delirium there is an acute onset and fluctuating course (Boxes 3.1 and 3.2). However, distinguishing between these differentials is often challenging in the acute setting, where you may have little information about the patient's usual level of cognitive function.

When do you need to assess cognition?

There are multiple reasons for assessing cognition, including:

- The patient has scored poorly on cognitive screening questions in the basic psychiatric assessment.
- The patient seems muddled ('query confused' on the triage slip in accident and emergency).
- The patient, often encouraged by their family, has come seeking help because of perceived forgetfulness.
- The patient is old (20% of the population over 80 years old have dementia).

> **Box 3.1 The differential diagnosis of confusion or memory loss**
>
> - Deafness or dysphasia can be misinterpreted as confusion – check that the person can hear; that any hearing aids used are working correctly; that they can understand; and that they can speak.
> - Dementia: Alzheimer's disease, vascular dementia and Lewy body dementia are the most common forms.
> - Depression, including pseudodementia.
> - Delirium – this is a clinical picture rather than a diagnosis and has multiple causes including CNS infection, sepsis, hypoxia, brain injury, drug toxicity, drug withdrawal syndromes and metabolic disturbance, to name but a few.

- Other psychiatric disorder, especially late-onset schizophrenia (paraphrenia), psychosis, mania, functional disorder.
- Transient global amnesia.
- Seizures – post-ictal state or temporal lobe epilepsy (i.e. complex partial seizure).
- Drugs, especially those with anticholinergic effects, can exacerbate any cognitive impairment.

Cognitive impairment: history and MSE

We will focus on an assessment of a stable patient in whom an acute medical cause such as hypoglycaemia has already been ruled out. In addition to the basic psychiatric assessment described in the previous chapter, you should focus on the aspects outlined below.

Check that the patient can hear and understand you

Talk to the informant first if the impairment is severe. Make it as easy as possible for the patient to hear and understand you: '*Do you have a good side?*'. Deafness is a classic, but hopefully rare, cause of a misdiagnosis of dementia.

> **Box 3.2 'Confusing' terminology**
>
> *Delirium, acute confusional state* and *encephalopathy* are all terms that refer to an acute or subacute change in cognition and the level of consciousness. They are often used synonymously, and while delirium is defined in DSM-IV, there is no widely accepted consensus about the distinction between these three terms.

Is there a perceived memory problem?

Ask whether the patient (or their informant) has noticed a problem with memory, and characterize this. While doing so, note the patient's understanding and use of language, and their ability to attend to the questions.

- '*Do you find yourself forgetting things? Can you give me some examples?*'
- '*When did it begin? Any idea what might have happened?*'
- '*What aspects of your life are affected?*' (e.g. work, cooking, shopping).
- '*Do you have any problems finding words, or understanding what people say to you?*'

Sometimes it is useful to ask the patient to describe the main events and chronology of their day (especially if you can corroborate the history). If they give an implausible story, consider *confabulation* (the fabrication of recent events to cover gaps in memory), which occurs in dementia and Wernicke–Korsakoff syndrome. Note that unawareness of self-identity is rare, even in severe dementia, and raises the possibility of a dissociative disorder (Chapter 10).

Look for features of delirium

- Is the person drowsy? Are they fully aware of their surroundings?
- Are they distractible? Irritable?
- Do they seem to be hallucinating?
- When did the problems start? (acute-onset supports delirium).
- Any obvious cause? (e.g. post-ictal, septic).

Memory tests

'I'm going to ask you some questions to test your memory.' This makes people anxious, so emphasize that it's not a pass or fail kind of test. Questions should test a range of memory domains. Note that none of the questions or tasks suggested below are wholly specific – they all rely on multiple cognitive domains, to differing degrees:

- **Orientation:** *'What day of the week is it? Which town are we in? What kind of place is this?'*
- **General knowledge:** e.g. *'Who is the Prime Minister?'*
- **Semantic knowledge:** e.g. point to objects and ask the patient to name them.
- **Working memory and attention:** ask the patient to spell a five-letter word backwards, or 'serial sevens' – take 7 from 100 and keep taking 7 away.
- **Comprehension:** can the patient respond to practical instructions? E.g. *'Pick up the pencil from the table and put it on the floor'*. If two-stage instructions are too difficult, try a simpler task: *'Close your eyes'*.
- **Recall** can be tested by asking the patient to recall the objects named, or the word spelt backwards, a few minutes later.
- **Executive function:** e.g. draw a circle and ask the patient to imagine it's a clock, and to put the numbers in and draw the hands pointing to a particular time (e.g. 9.30).
- Ask the patient to **write a simple sentence** of their own choice. This tests the ability both to generate and to write a sentence, so if this is difficult, you could dictate a sentence for the patient to write.
- **Abstract reasoning:** e.g. *'What's similar between a dog and a cat?'* or *'What does "a rolling stone gathers no moss" mean to you?'*

Ensure the patient has registered each question – don't be misled by sensory problems, and try to note any lack of attention or motivation. Memory can be tested more formally using various scales and screening tools, which comprise questions such as those listed here. The choice of scales and screens varies between clinicians and settings, but the most widely used scale (including by non-specialists) is the *Mini-Mental State Examination (MMSE)* – see Box 3.3.

 Box 3.3 The Mini-Mental State Examination (MMSE)

The MMSE is a test of cognitive function (not to be confused with the mental state examination!). It is used as a (fairly poor) screening test for dementia and to monitor changes in cognitive function over time. It is also used to determine which patients are eligible for cholinesterase inhibitor drugs for Alzheimer's disease, and to monitor the response to such treatment. The MMSE tests spatial and temporal orientation, short- and long-term memory, attention, language, calculation and visuo-spatial ability. It consists of 12 questions and is scored out of 30:

- 26–30 is a normal score
- 21–25 suggests dementia
- 20 or less is highly suggestive of dementia

Assess for depression

Depression can cause cognitive impairment, but may also be a consequence of it. Confusion has a wide differential (Box 3.1), but if neither delirium nor depression is present, the most likely diagnosis is dementia.

Appropriate 'medical' assessment

Do a careful physical examination. Look for evidence of vascular disease, thyroid status, alcohol abuse or infection. The neurological examination should include testing of cranial nerves and evaluation of cortical functions (e.g. apraxias, hemineglect, primitive reflexes).

What next?

If dementia is diagnosed, proceed to assess its likely cause, its effect on daily living and any associated problems. Delirium is due to a variety of medical conditions, many of which need urgent treatment.

How to assess psychosis

The cardinal features of psychosis (delusions, hallucinations and lack of insight) were defined in the basic assessment (Chapter 2) and relate mostly to the disorders covered in Chapter 12.

What do you need to find out?

1 **Is the person suffering from a psychosis?** Some people with strange ideas or strange behaviour may turn out to have an anxiety disorder, a personality disorder or no diagnosis at all. Similarly, some people can appear and behave entirely normally despite having a psychosis. Detection of a psychosis is therefore sometimes difficult, not least because people may be frightened of their experiences, or what will happen to them if they tell you.

2 **If so, what is the cause of the psychosis?** See Box 3.4 for the main differentials of psychotic symptoms.

 Box 3.4 The differential diagnosis of psychotic symptoms

Psychiatric disorders

- Schizophrenia
- Delusional disorders
- Psychotic depression
- Manic episode
- Schizoaffective disorder
- Schizotypal disorder
- Puerperal psychosis

'Organic' disorders

- Drug-induced psychosis
- Iatrogenic: L-dopa, methyldopa, steroids, antimalarials
- Complex partial epilepsy
- Delirium
- Dementia
- Huntington's disease
- Systemic lupus erythematosus
- Syphilis

An assessment of psychosis usually necessitates an in-depth assessment of mood and substance misuse (see the relevant sections of this chapter) because of the considerable overlap of these conditions. A risk assessment is needed as psychosis is associated with a risk of harm to self and, much less often, to others.

When do you need to assess for psychosis?

Psychosis may be suspected for diverse reasons, such as:

- Possible delusions elicited in the basic assessment.
- Bizarre or inexplicable behaviour.
- History of amphetamine use.
- A young adult found in a neglected state.
- A man heard talking to himself in a police cell.

Psychosis: history

You should start with the basic assessment as described in Chapter 2. The following have particular relevance:

- Ask about their current problems.
- Ask about complications of pregnancy or delivery, place of upbringing, academic achievements and social interests.
- Ask about family history of psychosis.
- Ask about past or current substance abuse. Alcohol and illicit drugs can induce psychosis.
- Ask about premorbid personality and level of functioning.
- Corroborate the history from an informant.
- Carry out a physical examination, concentrating on the neurological system.
- Consider laboratory investigations and magnetic resonance imaging (MRI) scan.

Family history, obstetric complications, an urban upbringing and problems at school are all associated with schizophrenia. A decline in level of functioning (intellectually and socially) is common before and during the onset of schizophrenia.

Psychosis: MSE

The diagnosis of schizophrenia and other psychoses relies on detailed evaluation of a number of symptoms and signs, especially concerning abnormalities of thought content and form, so the assessment is quite long. A set of symptoms called *first-rank symptoms* (Table 3.1) are accorded considerable significance in the diagnosis of schizophrenia, and it is

Table 3.1 First-rank symptoms of schizophrenia (for definitions, see Box 3.4)

Delusions
Delusional perception

Hallucinations
Thought echo
Third person auditory hallucinations
Running commentary

Thought flow and possession
Thought withdrawal
Thought insertion
Thought broadcasting

Passivity
Passivity of thought, feelings or actions

important to elicit them during the MSE, if possible. They are sometimes called Schneiderian symptoms after Kurt Schneider, the psychiatrist who described them. Listing and defining first-rank symptoms is a favourite exam question! However, there is little evidence of their diagnostic specificity or sensitivity first-rank symptoms occur in other psychoses, and not all people with schizophrenia have had one. The vocabulary used in psychiatry to describe the features of mental illness ('descriptive psychopathology') is particularly rich when it comes to describing psychosis – some key terms are defined in Box 3.5.

 Box 3.5 Describing psychosis

A *mannerism* is a repetitive movement or gesture that is complex and seemingly purposeful. A repeated simple and purposeless one is a *stereotypy*. Both occur in schizophrenia.

Catatonia describes a group of motor signs that are rare but characteristic of catatonic schizophrenia (a subtype of schizophrenia), although they can also occur in organic disorders or as an isolated 'catatonia syndrome':

- *Echopraxia/echolalia* – the patient imitates the interviewer's every action or word.
- *Automatic obedience* – compliance with all instructions regardless of consequence.
- *Ambitendency* – tentative movements back and forth, as if unsure what to do.
- *Posturing (catalepsy)* – the maintenance of inappropriate or bizarre postures.
- *Waxy flexibility* – limbs held in externally imposed positions, muscle tone is increased.
- *Negativism* – seemingly motiveless resistance to all instructions or attempts to be moved.

Flattened affect is a decrease in emotional responsivity and expression, even when emotionally charged topics are discussed. It is a negative symptom of schizophrenia, but needs to be distinguished from depression and parkinsonism. *Incongruous affect is* emotion not in keeping with the topic being talked about.

A *neologism* is a made-up word, usually invested with a personal meaning. Be sure the patient doesn't just have a larger vocabulary than you …

A *delusion* is a false belief. It is firmly held despite contrary evidence and is out of keeping with the patient's cultural or religious background. Different sorts of delusions are recognized:

- A *delusional perception* is a delusional interpretation of a normal perception. For example, a man saw a woman sneeze and knew this meant he must leave town. It is sometimes preceded by a sense of unease or perplexity that something strange is going on (*delusional mood*).
- In a *delusion of reference*, an event or message (often on TV) has a unique meaning for the person. An *idea of reference* is similar, but not delusional in intensity (and thus not a true psychotic symptom); it may occur in paranoid personality disorder.
- A *secondary delusion* is one that arises understandably from another mental state abnormality (e.g. delusions of guilt in depression); a *primary delusion* doesn't.
- Delusions may be classified by content. The most common are *persecutory delusions* (sometimes incorrectly called *paranoid delusions*), in which the person believes they are the victim of perceived injustice or conspiracy. *Grandiose* delusions are seen in mania, *nihilistic* ones in depression.

Thought disorder (also called *formal thought disorder*) occurs in schizophrenia. The connections between thoughts and ideas are obscure and there is a rambling quality. Descriptive terms include *knight's move thinking* and *loosening of associations* and, in rare severe cases, *word salad*. For example, in response to a question about what the person had been up to before the appointment: 'I got on the bus when I saw the man from the hostel, in the next street where I was. Like it was that dog again, you know? Still, doctor, what do you think? …'. A different type of thought disorder occurs in mania (flight of ideas).

In schizophrenia, abnormalities also occur in the perceived source, ownership and fate of thoughts and actions:

- **Thought insertion:** thoughts originate elsewhere and are put into the patient's head.
- **Thought withdrawal:** the experience of thoughts being removed from one's mind.
- **Thought broadcast:** the subject experiences his or her thoughts being available to and heard by others.
- **Thought block:** the flow of thoughts abruptly ends. Distinguish from thought withdrawal and from simple loss of concentration.
- **Passivity:** thoughts, feelings or actions are experienced as being under external control. For example, a person with schizophrenia who killed her son described being unable to resist carrying out this act because of the 'force' controlling her. Passivity phenomena are important in risk assessment (and in how resulting crimes are dealt with).

A *hallucination* is a perception experienced as real in the absence of a stimulus. The characteristic hallucinations of schizophrenia are *third person auditory hallucinations* (i.e. hearing the voice talking *about* you). Sometimes these take the form of a *running commentary* by two or more voices. Auditory hallucinations do occur in psychotic mood disorders, but are *mood congruent* – that is, critical and derogatory in severe depression; grandiose in mania. In schizophrenia, the hallucinations are usually incongruent.

Appearance and behaviour

- Note the patient's **manner**.
- **Movement:** are there *mannerisms* or *stereotypies*? Is the patient restless? Is there *catatonia*?
- **Dress:** is the patient dressed unusually? Is there evidence of self-neglect?

The patient may have a suspicious manner (you may be part of their conspiracy theory), be distracted (by hallucinations) or be distant and uninterested (negative symptoms of schizophrenia). Some people with schizophrenia may dress idiosyncratically. For example, a man wore a silver foil hat to prevent his thoughts being extracted. Motor abnormalities can occur as part of psychosis, but also as common side effects of antipsychotic drugs, especially the older 'typical' ones. The side-effects include *dystonia, parkinsonism, akathisia* and *tardive dyskinesia* (Chapter 7).

Mood

- Does the overall mood seem normal? Is it responsive? (*flattened affect*).
- Is the emotional expression appropriate to the topic being discussed? (*incongruous affect*).

Psychosis can occur as part of severe depression and in mania. In these cases, a mood abnormality is usually readily apparent.

Speech

Are made-up words (*neologisms*) used, or words and language used idiosyncratically? If the patient's sentences, or overall answers, don't quite make sense or seem puzzling or unexpected, it may signify thought disorder.

Thought content

- Is there any evidence of delusions?
- *'Is anything bothering you at the moment? Do you understand things differently from other people?'*
- *'Do people have a special interest in you? Are people against you? How do you know?'* (persecutory delusions).
- *'Is anything on the TV referring to you particularly?'* (delusions of reference).
- *'When did you first realize this* (delusional belief) *was true? How?'*

Because, by definition, a delusion is believed to be true, its detection requires you to be receptive to clues and sometimes to 'go along' with implausible statements in order to elicit more details. For example, a man matter-of-factly asks how you are affected by the Bulgarian mafia — the first hint of his psychosis. A non-committal reply leads him to elaborate and reveal his persecutory delusional system.

Flow and possession of thought

- Do the person's thoughts seem to flow normally? Is it difficult to follow the meaning of what the patient is saying? Write down a representative sample. Is there (*formal*) *thought disorder*?
- *'Do your thoughts sometimes stop suddenly?'* (thought block).
- *'Are your thoughts sometimes removed from your head?'* (thought withdrawal).
- Does the person feel in control of their thoughts and actions? *'Do your thoughts get put into your head from outside?'* (thought insertion). *'Can other people directly influence your thoughts or actions?'* (passivity; thought control). *'Are other people aware of your thoughts?'* (thought broadcasting).
- *'Do any of your thoughts get repeated in your mind like an echo?'* (thought echo).

Perceptions

- Does the person seem to be hearing things that are not there? *'Do you hear voices when there doesn't seem to be anyone present?'* (auditory hallucinations). *'Are the voices inside or outside your head?'*
- Content: *'What are they talking about? Do they comment on what you're doing?'* (running commentary). *'Do they want you to harm yourself or other people?'*
- *'Do they talk directly to you or about you?'* (second and third person hallucinations, respectively).
- Repeat similar questions for hallucinations in other modalities.

Cognition

- Is the patient disorientated?
- Is there cognitive impairment?

An acutely psychotic patient may be distracted by their experiences, or be worried that your questions are trying to trick or harm them, and therefore she or he may perform poorly on cognitive testing. Try and distinguish this from the perplexity of delirium. Although many people with schizophrenia are highly intelligent, the importance of cognitive impairment as an intrinsic part of schizophrenia is increasingly recognized. People with schizophrenia characteristically underestimate their age by several years, and perform worse than expected on most psychometric tests. This can be exacerbated by lack of motivation, and by some forms of medication.

Insight

- Insight about illness: *'Do you think you are ill in any way? Do others? Are the voices part of your illness?'*
- Insight about need for treatment: *'Do you need help? What sort?'*

Insight is characteristically lost in psychosis, but in practice it is affected to varying degrees (see Chapter 2). *Distorted awareness of reality* is a related term that conveys what is often apparent to the interviewer.

How to assess depression

There are separate assessments for lowered mood (depression) and for elevated mood (mania), described here in turn. However, in a patient presenting with depression, you *must* ask about past episodes of mania. Depression overlaps and coexists with so many diagnoses that many of the other assessments may also be necessary. The presence of mood disturbance requires risk assessment (mainly for suicide) as well.

What do you need to find out?

1 **Is the person depressed?** Depression must be distinguished from normal sadness or emotional distress (Box 3.6).
2 **If so, is the diagnosis a depressive disorder, or are the depressive symptoms part of another disorder?**
3 **If the diagnosis is a depressive disorder, what type is it?** Depression can be a single episode, recurrent or part of bipolar disorder. It may be classified as mild, moderate or severe, and it may include psychotic symptoms. At its most severe, patients may stop eating, drinking and even moving. *Depressive stupor* is life threatening and an indication for emergency electroconvulsive therapy (ECT). Depression is linked to many medical disorders and to drugs, both prescribed and illicit.

 Box 3.6 The differential diagnosis of depressive symptoms

- Normal low mood
- Disorder of low mood:
  - Current depressive episode
  - Recurrent depressive disorder, currently depressive episode
  - Persistent mood disorder, e.g. dysthymia
  - Seasonal affective disorder
- Bipolar disorder, currently depressive episode
- Depression secondary to another psychiatric disorder:
  - Anxiety disorder
  - Eating disorder
  - Schizophrenia, especially post-schizophrenic depression
- Reactive:
  - Acute stress reaction
  - Adjustment disorder (adaptation to a significant life change or stressful event)
  - Normal or abnormal bereavement reaction
- Substance misuse, especially harmful use of alcohol
- Depression associated with another medical condition:
  - Intracranial: any intracranial pathology including dementia, stroke, Parkinson's disease, multiple sclerosis, variant Creutzfeldt–Jakob disease (vCJD), head injury
  - Extracranial: hypothyroidism, hyperthyroidism, hyperparathyroidism, Addison's, Cushing's, hypercalcaemia, hypomagnesaemia, iron/B12/folate deficiency, glandular fever, hepatitis, HIV/AIDS
- Medications: antihypertensives, corticosteroids, H2R blockers, non-steroidal anti-inflammatory drugs (NSAIDs), anticonvulsants, combined oral contraceptive pill (OCP), chemotherapy agents, Roaccutane, benzodiazepines …

When do you need to assess for depression?

The following should alert you to possible depression:

- Detection of a depressive symptom or suicidal thought in the basic psychiatric assessment.
- Unexplained fatigue.
- Any chronic general medical condition, but especially neurological disease and chronic pain.

Depression: history

You should use the basic assessment as described in Chapter 2, but the following features have particular relevance if you suspect depression:

- Does the patient think they are depressed?
- Identify past and current stressors – marital strife, unemployment, etc.
- How has the patient tried to cope with the problems?
- Is there a past history of mood disorder? What has its course been? What treatment worked?
- Could this be bipolar disorder? *'In the past, have you had periods of better than usual mood, or boundless energy, or where you have behaved out of character?'*
- Does the person have depressive or anxious traits in their personality?
- Is there a family history of psychiatric disorder or suicide?

Severely depressed patients may deny that their mood is abnormal and decline treatment. Stressors (life events) can precipitate depression; identifying them helps make sense of the depression, and can be therapeutic. Many patients have had previous episodes of mood disorder: ask about their nature, treatment and outcome. It is important to identify a patient's usual coping strategies – these can be protective factors (e.g. seeking help from a supportive family), or they may lead to additional problems (e.g. use of alcohol). Depressive personality traits may affect the risk and outcome of depressive disorders: an informant is best placed to provide the personality information, untainted by the negative colouring of the patient's current low mood. A family history of depression is also a risk factor for depressive disorder and suicide.

Depression: MSE

Appearance and behaviour

- Does the patient look depressed? Does he or she exude a sense of gloom? Is he or she crying or agitated?
- Is there good eye contact?
- Is there a normal range of emotional expression?

In depression there is often decreased eye contact and a lack of expression and movement. This is called *psychomotor retardation*. Other depressed people are *agitated*, pacing to and fro or wringing their hands.

Speech

- Is the speech normal in speed, volume and amount?

In severe depression, speech is slow, quiet and sparse. Sentences tail off, as though the patient cannot summon the energy or concentration to continue.

Mood, including biological symptoms of depression

Questions here will cover many of the diagnostic criteria for depression:

- **Mood, interest and energy levels:** *'How have you been feeling in your spirits? Do you still enjoy the things that you usually do? … Can you give some examples? How is your energy level? Do you feel more tired or fatigued than usual? Do you easily get irritable?'*
- **Onset:** *'How long have you felt this way? Did anything seem to trigger it off?'*
- **Diurnal (daily) variation:** *'Is your mood lower at a particular time of day? How do you feel first thing? Do you often feel like crying?'*
- **Sleep:** *'How are you sleeping at the moment?'* If there is a problem: *'Do you have problems getting to sleep? Are you having difficulty sleeping through the night or do you wake early then can't get back to sleep? Or are you sleeping more than usual?'*
- **Appetite:** *'What is your appetite like? Do you enjoy your food? Have you lost weight?'*
- **Other somatic symptoms:** *'Are you constipated? Are your periods regular? Has your interest in sex changed recently?'*

The predominant subjective feeling in depression may be sadness, irritability, fatigue, lethargy or lack of energy. *Anhedonia*, the lack of pleasure from normally enjoyed activities, is a key symptom of moderate and severe depression. In severe depression, the normal *reactivity of mood* to circumstances is lost. Biological rhythms and drives are frequently impaired in depression. The presence of 'biological' or 'somatic' symptoms (relating to sleep, appetite, sex, gut function, etc.) is one way to define the boundary between mild depression and more severe cases. Sleep is affected in several ways. *Onset insomnia* (difficulty getting to sleep) is common when there is accompanying anxiety. Sleep is generally shallow and unrefreshing. *Early morning waking* is the most characteristic change, often occurring with diurnal variation of mood, so the patient is awake and at their most desperate when the rest of the world is asleep. Somewhat confusingly, *increased* sleep and sluggishness can also occur. Appetite tends to be reduced, contributing to constipation and weight loss. Irregular periods or amenorrhoea occur in women and there is a general loss of energy and libido.

Thoughts

- *'What things are on your mind at the moment? Anything particular bothering you?'*
- *'Do you see things getting better? What might improve things?'*
- *'Do you feel guilty about anything you have done?'*
- *'Do you feel that you are of value?'*
- *'Do you feel that people are getting at you? ... Is it justified?'*
- *'Do you have worries about your physical health?'*
- Make sure to ask in detail about suicidal thoughts and intent (Chapter 4).
- Are any of the thoughts obsessional in nature? *'Do you find yourself checking things repeatedly? Do you like things especially clean and tidy?'*
- Are any of the thoughts delusional?

In depression, prevailing thoughts (or 'cognitions') have a negative colouring (cognitive bias), centring upon perceived failures, worthlessness, low self-esteem, and so on. Hopelessness and guilt feelings are important, not only because they are distressing but also because they may lead to suicidal thoughts and intentions. Anxiety, health worries and physical symptoms are common in depression, as are obsessional thoughts and ruminations. However, if these are prominent, assess for anxiety and somatoform disorders ... and don't forget medical causes for physical symptoms! Delusions are rare in depression as a whole, but characterize psychotic depression. They tend to be *mood congruent* and *nihilistic*.

Perceptions

- Are there hallucinations? What are they like?

Hallucinations sometimes occur in psychotic depression. They are usually second person voices saying derogatory things, such as 'You are a horrible person'. Depressed people may also describe that sensations are less intense than usual and they feel isolated from the normal emotions and activities of the outside world.

Cognition

- Is concentration impaired? *'What is your concentration like? Can you read a paper or follow a TV programme?'*
- Is there objective evidence of cognitive impairment?

Depression, especially in older adults, can produce apparent cognitive impairment, sometimes called *pseudodementia*. This is a mixture of lack of motivation and poor concentration. It must be distinguished from dementia, as it responds to treatment of the depression.

How to assess mania

What do you need to find out?

1 **Is the person manic?** Mania is a pathological elevation of mood that causes substantial impairment in occupational and/or social functioning. Mania is the key syndrome in bipolar disorder but there are other differentials (Box 3.7). Milder manic symptoms do not necessarily cause impairment and are called *hypomania*. In hypomania, functioning may be improved but it can also precede a manic relapse.
2 **Has the person been manic in the past?** Even if the patient is currently depressed or euthymic (normal mood), a history of mania is important because of its diagnostic and therapeutic implications.
3 **Assess for depressive symptoms.** Most patients with an episode of mania will have had a history of depression, and some have current depressive symptoms (a *mixed affective state*).
4 **Assess for substance misuse.** Substance misuse is increasingly seen as a key component of bipolar disorder – its prevalence in patients with bipolar disorder is estimated at 35–60%.

A manic person may be unable to concentrate enough to give useful or consistent answers. If so, focus on observing and eliciting current symptoms and signs (but see Box 3.8). Take the rest of the history later, or from an informant. An informant usually paints a more dramatic picture of recent behaviour than does the patient. Gather evidence of specific dangerous or out-of-keeping behaviours, since they affect management – for example, whether the patient should be detained, or needs a pregnancy test.

 Box 3.7 The differential diagnosis of manic symptoms

- Mood disorder:
  - Manic episode (with or without psychotic symptoms)
  - Bipolar disorder, currently manic/hypomanic/mixed episode
  - Depressive episode (irritability mistaken for mania)
- Schizophrenia
- Anxiety/attention-deficit hyperactivity disorder (ADHD)
- Substance misuse: alcohol, amphetamines, cocaine, hallucinogens, opiates

- 'Organic':
  - Multiple sclerosis, frontal lobe tumour, hyperthyroidism
- Drugs: corticosteroids, withdrawal from benzodiazepines

When do you need to assess for mania?

This assessment may be triggered by:

- A hint of manic symptoms in the basic assessment or during assessment of depression.
- Recent grandiose, disinhibited or disorganized behaviour.
- A past history of bipolar disorder.
- A family history of bipolar disorder.

Mania: history

You should proceed with the basic assessment as described in Chapter 2, but the following points have particular relevance:

- Does the patient think they are unwell or need treatment?
- Corroborate recent history, especially with regard to unusual and inappropriate beliefs and actions.
- Assess the degree of dysfunction being caused by the symptoms. *'Are you having any problems in your job? And what about your relationships?'*
- Check recent use of illicit drugs or alcohol.
- Ask about sexual activity, particularly in a woman, due to the risk of unwanted pregnancy. E.g. *'Have you recently had a new sexual partner? Are you using any contraception? Could you be pregnant?'*
- Ask about past history of mania or depression.
- Has the patient ever been prescribed lithium or other mood stabilizer? Are they supposed to be taking it now? Have they been adherent?
- Ask about family history of mood disorders (bipolar disorder is strongly familial).
- Do a physical examination.

It is important to look for possible triggers of a manic episode, which can include amphetamines, steroids, alcohol and discontinuation of lithium therapy (lithium is a common long-term treatment for relapse prevention in bipolar disorder). Physical examination is indicated as mania can (rarely) be due to a medical disorder such as a frontal lobe tumour. A first episode of mania occurring above the age of 40 should prompt a thorough search for an underlying cause.

Mania: MSE

Appearance and behaviour

- **Manner:** is the patient elated, distractible, irritable?
- **Dress:** clothes and make-up may be bright and garish or dishevelled.
- **Movements:** look out for flamboyant or disinhibited gestures. The patient may try to hug you, snatch your notes or challenge your qualifications. Is the patient overactive?

Speech

- Is the speech fast? Excessive in amount? Loud? Hard to interrupt?

Speech in mania is fast, loud, expansive and hard to interrupt (*pressure of speech*). It reflects the underlying pressure of thoughts and the person's attempts to share their many wonderful ideas (Box 3.8).

 Box 3.8 'Sorry, I'm lost …'

It can be difficult to interview someone who is manic. If, reluctant to interrupt, you wait for a natural pause in the patient's flow before asking a further question, you may find it difficult to elicit the information you need. And you may find yourself tangled or lost in the many fast-thrown threads of their speech. One coping strategy is to interrupt each time you start to lose the thread to ask for clarification: *'Hang on a moment, I want to understand what you mean by …'* or *'Sorry, I know I'm being slow, but can you tell me again about …'* You may feel rude interrupting the patient frequently, but if it helps you to understand more of what they are trying to communicate, it is probably worthwhile.

Mood

- *'Have you noticed a change in your mood or energy level recently? Can you describe it? Do you feel happier or more confident than usual?'*
- *'Are you feeling full of energy?'*
- *'Have you been very irritable or impatient?'*
- *'How long has this been the case?'*
- *'How are you sleeping? More or less than usual?'*
- *'How is your appetite?'*
- *'Has your interest in sex, or other activities, changed?'*

An increase in energy level and drive to do things almost always occurs. However, the predominant emotion is not consistent – this can be euphoria and infectious gaiety, or sudden and extreme irritability. Some people with mania deny their mood is elevated, or are too busy to think about it. Mood can also be labile or *mixed* – simultaneous depressive and manic features. The duration of symptoms of elevated mood is important in making the diagnosis, and in the distinction of mania from hypomania (see Chapter 9). In mania, tiredness and the drive for sleep are decreased. A manic patient may stay up all night working or playing. Appetite may be increased, or the patient may be too busy to eat. Libido tends to be enhanced and sexual activity uninhibited.

Thought

- **Form**: Does the train of thought jump from one topic to another? (*flight of ideas*).
- **Content**: *'What's on your mind at the moment?'*
  - Are there grandiose delusions? Don't shy away from asking about this directly if you suspect mania: *'Do you have special powers or abilities? Can you do things which most people might find difficult or even impossible?'*
  - Is there any evidence of reckless or dangerous ideas? *'Have you got plans to buy anything? ... or any plans to travel?'*

Flight of ideas is a type of thought disorder characteristic of mania. Thoughts jump rapidly from one thing to another, with understandable, if unusual, connections between them. The links are often based on puns, rhymes and other associations – for example: 'I'm fine, a fine wine, whining and moaning like Jonah ... Jonah the whale ... in Wales ...'. Write down a snippet. The content of the thoughts is expansive and grandiose. There may be a single, preoccupying scheme (e.g. to build a football stadium in their garden), but usually there is a kaleidoscope of incomplete, jumbled ideas. In mania, the grandiose ideas may become delusional. Religious themes are common – for example, the patient knows he is the Messiah. Sometimes delusions are dangerous – the belief that one can drive excessively fast, or fly or borrow unrealistic amounts of money. Take these risks seriously: mania is unpredictable and these ideas may suddenly be acted upon.

Perceptions

- Is there any evidence of hallucinations?

Mood-congruent auditory and occasionally visual hallucinations occur. For example, voices telling the person what special powers they have and how they can save humanity.

Insight

Insight fluctuates in mania. A person may seem aware of their condition and agree the need for treatment one moment but not the next.

How to assess anxiety and stress-related disorders

Anxiety disorders, or 'neuroses' (see Box 3.9), are emotional disorders in which some form of anxiety is the central feature, manifesting as psychological, cognitive and physical (somatic) complaints. For various reasons, the anxiety disorders are classified together with *stress-related disorders* (where anxiety is attributed to a particular stressor) and *somatoform disorders* (where medically unexplained physical symptoms predominate). However, it is easier to divide them up here, so we start by covering anxiety and stress-related disorders. Somatoform disorders are covered in the next section. This is a notoriously confusing area, diagnostically speaking, and we suggest you read Chapter 10 in conjunction with these sections.

> **Box 3.9 Neuroses, neurotics and neuroticism**
>
> The anxiety disorders are sometimes referred to as *neuroses*. Strictly speaking, *neurotic symptoms* encompass psychological symptoms that are not classified as psychotic. However, in everyday use, 'neurotic' denotes a person who is excessively anxious, sensitive, tense or obsessive. Neurotic was also used in the Victorian and Edwardian eras to describe women who did not meet culturally imposed feminine standards. The folk memory of this derogatory usage and the discrepancy between the medical and lay interpretations of 'neurotic' mean that the term is perhaps best avoided. The term no longer exists in the DSM classification, but remains in ICD-10, so we have used it in this edition. The term *neuroticism*, on the other hand, has a different and well-characterized modern meaning: it is used in psychology to describe an individual's tendency to experience negative emotional states, and is a factor in personality assessment scales.

What do you need to find out?

1 **Does the person have pathological anxiety or anxiety-related symptoms?** A distinction must be made between pathological anxiety and worries and emotional distress that are within normal limits or are part of the person's personality. The presence of dysfunction is one criterion used in diagnosing an anxiety disorder, so assess the

symptoms' effects on, for example, relationships and work performance.

2 **Might the primary diagnosis be depression or a somatoform disorder?** Anxiety and related symptoms are common in other diagnostic categories. Anxiety often coexists with depression, so it will nearly always be necessary to assess depression at the same time. Substance misuse can be a cause of, or response to the symptoms, so this may need to be assessed. If the presentation is predominantly with somatic concerns (e.g. pain, fatigue), assess for a somatoform disorder.

3 **If an anxiety disorder is present, which one?** The differential diagnosis of anxiety is wide (see Box 3.10). Occasionally, but importantly, anxiety disorders can be due to a general medical condition such as hyperthyroidism.

 Box 3.10 The differential diagnosis of anxiety

- Normal anxiety
- Generalized anxiety disorder
- Obsessive compulsive disorder
- Panic disorder
- Stress reactions and adjustment disorders:
  ○ acute stress reaction
  ○ post-traumatic stress disorder
  ○ adjustment disorder
- Phobic anxiety disorders:
  ○ specific phobias (objects, animals, situations)
  ○ social phobia
  ○ agorophobia
- Hypochondriacal disorder
- Other psychiatric disorder: depressive disorders, eating disorders, dementia, delirium, psychosis
- Substance misuse
- Withdrawal from psychoactive medicines
- General medical conditions: hyperthyroidism, phaeochromocytoma, any cause of breathlessness (chronic obstructive pulmonary disease (COPD)/asthma) or palpitations (arrhythmias), poor pain control

When do you need to assess for anxiety disorders?

An assessment of anxiety might be triggered by:

- Someone who is preoccupied or clearly worried about something.
- A person distressed by a recent trauma.

- A patient who presents with depression.
- Someone who comes for help because anxiety prevents them from doing something they want or need to do – 'avoidance behaviour'.

Anxiety: history and MSE

In addition to the basic psychiatric assessment, you should focus on the aspects outlined below.

Characterizing the anxiety

Start with open questions:

- **Psychological symptoms:** *'Have you been worrying a lot about things recently? What about? Do you feel wound up or tense?'*
- **Timing, triggers and bodily symptoms:** *'Are the feelings there most of the time, or only in specific situations? … What things or situations make you anxious? Do you get sudden 'attacks' of anxiety? … How does your body feel then? Do you suffer from aches and pains?'*
- **Functional impact:** *'Can you put your worries out of your mind? Do you avoid doing things because of your worries? How do the symptoms interfere with your daily life?'*

Anxiety consists of *psychological* symptoms (e.g. tension, fear) and *bodily* symptoms (e.g. palpitations, sweating). Either can predominate. Anxiety is a state of arousal and may be apparent from the person's appearance and behaviour on MSE. With practice, it is usually possible to distinguish this from the agitation of depression. Anxiety has many forms: it is usually *situational* (*phobic*), occurring in response to a specific stimulus, but it can *generalized* or *free-floating*. Anxiety can also be paroxysmal – a *panic attack*. A panic attack is a discrete episode of severe anxiety that builds rapidly then gradually subsides over about an hour. People rapidly learn to *avoid* situations in which they feel anxious or uncomfortable. They may first present for help because of the practical problems that avoidance produces.

Obsessions and compulsions

- *'Do you get repeated unpleasant images or thoughts coming into your mind?'*
- *'Do you have to keep checking things, or keep things very clean and tidy? What do you do? How often?'*
- *'Do you try to resist the thoughts or the urge to respond to them? If you do, what happens?'*

Obsessions and *compulsions* are characteristic of obsessive-compulsive disorder (OCD) but also occur in depression, anankastic personality disorder, and as a rare side effect of treatment with dopamine agonists (e.g. in Parkinson's disease). Severe obsessions can, in practice, be difficult to distinguish from delusions.

Somatic symptoms

Enquire about somatic symptoms:

- *'How is your health generally?'*
- *'Do you suffer from severe tiredness or exhaustion?'*
- *'Have you ever lost your memory, sight or the use of part of your body?'*
- *'Have you felt detached or distant from yourself* (depersonalization) *or your surroundings* (derealization)?'

Unexplained physical symptoms are common in anxiety disorders, and in depression. If they are prominent and do not correspond to the 'biological' symptoms of depression, consider a somatoform disorder. Medically unexplained fatigue is the main feature of chronic fatigue syndrome (myalgic encephalopathy), but fatigue and lethargy also occur in depression. *Dissociative disorders* are rare psychiatric conditions in which there is loss of function (e.g. amnesia, paralysis, blindness). They are usually encountered in medical settings (e.g. after admission for neurological investigation). Feelings of detachment from self (*depersonalization*) or surroundings (*derealization*) are common symptoms of anxiety disorders, may occur in healthy people when tired, and are occasionally a diagnosis in their own right. Such feelings are hard to describe (e.g. *'It's as if there is glass between me and the world'*) and must be distinguished from psychotic symptoms.

Other important questions

- *'When did the symptoms start?'*
- *'Did they seem related to recent events? Have there been major events or difficulties in your life recently? Have you ever had a particularly horrible or frightening experience? How has it affected you?'*
- How has the person coped with their symptoms? (alcohol, drugs, family support) Have they had any treatment?
- Is there a family history of anxiety?

Many people have had anxiety symptoms for years before seeking help. If similar symptoms have been present since adolescence, consider personality disorder. Whilst all anxiety disorders are made worse by stress, sometimes the symptoms are best understood as a response to a major stress or life change – a *stress-related disorder*. If the stress was within the past few days, then consider an *acute stress reaction*. If the stressor was weeks or months ago, the category is *adjustment reaction. Post-traumatic stress disorder* (*PTSD*) is a form of stress-related disorder in which a *significant* event (e.g. rape, serious accident) is followed by reliving of the trauma in flashbacks or nightmares, and avoidance of similar situations. In many anxiety disorders, substance misuse can be a prominent feature – people turn to alcohol and other maladaptive strategies (e.g. avoidance) to cope with their symptoms. These responses may exacerbate the situation and should be dealt with as part of the treatment. It is also important to elicit the family history: while the genetic contribution to anxiety is modest, there may also be relevant learned behaviours from anxious relatives.

How to assess somatic symptoms and somatoform disorders

Somatic (bodily) symptoms and concerns about health can of course be a presentation of a medical condition and should be assessed accordingly. They may also occur in any psychiatric disorder, particularly anxiety disorders, depression and eating disorders. *Somatoform disorders* really apply to patients where the somatic symptoms are most prominent, and none of these other categories seems applicable. See Chapter 10 for more detail on somatoform disorders.

What do you need to find out?

1 **Are the patient's somatic symptoms medically unexplained?**
2 **If so, is the diagnosis a somatoform disorder**, or are the symptoms part of another disorder?
3 **If the diagnosis is a somatoform disorder, what type is it?** (Box 3.11) Somatoform disorders can manifest predominantly with somatic symptoms, or predominantly with concerns about health or appearance.
4 **What does the patient want done?** A frequent medical attender and 'thick notes' suggest a chronic somatization disorder. Many patients want medical rather than psychiatric treatment. They may want treatment that you consider inappropriate (e.g. a further surgical referral) and decline treatment you do recommend (e.g. psychological therapy). They may also minimize their distress to lessen the probability of a psychiatric diagnosis.

The assessment usually proceeds more smoothly if you pay due attention to and make it clear that you accept their somatic symptoms before asking about psychological ones. For some patients, treatment isn't their priority: they may seek validation that they are ill; others want you to complete insurance claims. The potential for conflict can be reduced if you ask what they want, without necessarily acquiescing to it.

 Box 3.11 The differential diagnosis of somatic symptoms

- General medical problem
- Associated with another psychiatric disorder, especially depression or anxiety
- Hypochondriacal disorder
- Body dysmorphic disorder
- Somatization disorder
- Persistent somatoform pain disorder
- Somatoform autonomic dysfunction

When do you need to assess for a somatoform disorder?

An assessment for a somatoform disorder might be triggered by:

- Detection of somatic symptoms that appear unexplained by a medical condition.
- Preoccupation with health or disease.
- Repeated and excessive seeking of medical assessment or treatment.

Somatoform disorders: history and MSE

In addition to the basic psychiatric assessment, the following features have particular relevance if you suspect a somatoform disorder:

- Are they unduly preoccupied with their health?
- Are they repeatedly seeking reassurance from you that they do not have a particular disease? (suggests *hypochondriasis*)
- Is there evidence of depressed or anxious mood?
- *'How is your health?'*
  - Does the patient emphasize somatic complaints?
  - *'Do you have many aches and pains, or other bodily symptoms?'*
  - *'Do you take regular painkillers?'*
  - *'Do you have medical problems your doctor can't explain?'*

- *'What do you think causes your symptoms? Are you fearful that you have a particular medical condition?'*
- *'What do you think about your appearance?'*
  - Do they hide aspects of their body or appearance? (suggests *body dysmorphic disorder* or an eating disorder).
- What is the nature and quantity of the medical history?
  - Do they have evidence of many previous operations?
  - Is there evidence that they have deliberately made themselves ill (e.g. omitting their insulin)?
- Will the patient cooperate with a psychiatric assessment?
- *'What do you think should be done about your symptoms?'*

Patients with somatoform disorder typically perceive their health as poor even when it is objectively good. They will often want extensive investigation, and may not be reassured by negative results. Many bodily concerns and symptoms may be reported. The more somatic symptoms they have, the less likely they are to have a medical condition: the presence of many chronic symptoms suggests somatization disorder. Depressed mood or anxiety are often apparent or suspected, but may be denied by the patient. If you conclude either is present and significant, then the somatic symptoms will usually be viewed as symptoms of a depressive or anxiety disorder, and treated as such.

A strong fear of a particular medical condition is typical of *hypochondriasis*. Patients may have unlikely theories about what causes their symptoms, but these should not be delusional – if so, the patient has a psychosis of some kind.

Chronic pain (including persistent somatoform pain disorder) is not simply either 'medical' or 'psychological'. All pain is a subjective experience, with a complex relationship to inciting sensory stimuli, influenced by both peripheral and central nervous system (including psychological) mechanisms. Chronic pain seems to be due to rewiring of the circuits used to process sensory stimuli, and is reflected by changes in the structure and function of these circuits, as detected by neuroimaging. It can be difficult to manage: analgesia may not bring much relief, and long-term analgesia use can itself be harmful.

Rarely, patients deliberately make themselves ill (or apparently so). This may be for *unconscious gain*, such as a need to take on the sick role i.e. a *factitious disorder*, or it may be in order to gain some *more understandable advantage* (e.g. money) – this is *malingering*.

How to assess eating disorders

What do you need to find out?

1 **Does the patient have an eating disorder?** The core feature is an over-evaluation of shape and weight. The disorders must be distinguished from problems of weight, shape or diet occurring in other psychiatric disorders or secondary to a medical disorder (Box 3.12).

2 **If so, is it anorexia nervosa or bulimia nervosa?** The former is characterized by low body weight, the latter by repeated binges which punctuate the purgative behaviours such as dietary restriction. However, many patients with an eating disorder do not fit into either of these classic categories, or shift between them.

3 **Is their physical health in danger?** Physical complications of anorexia nervosa are serious and can be life-threatening.

4 **Is there evidence of depression or anxiety disorder?** Depression and anxiety are often comorbid with eating disorders. Risk assessment is important since deliberate and accidental self-harm can occur.

5 **A corroborative history:** People with eating disorders can be difficult to engage and tend to minimize their problems, so take the opportunity (and the time) to form a good relationship, and plan to corroborate the history.

 Box 3.12 The differential diagnosis of eating disorders

- Anorexia nervosa
- Bulimia nervosa
- Other eating disorder
- Depression
- Body dysmorphic disorder
- Rarely, a general medical condition:
  - inflammatory bowel disease
  - hypopituitarism
  - malignancy

When do you need to assess for an eating disorder?

Assessment for an eating disorder may be triggered by:

- A patient saying she has problems controlling her eating.
- Medically unexplained weight loss.
- A teenage girl with fatigue or amenorrhoea (but remember that these disorders do occur in men).
- A patient who looks thin or is wearing several layers of clothes on a hot day.

Eating disorders: history

In addition to the basic psychiatric assessment described in the previous chapter, you should focus on the aspects outlined below.

Methods of weight control: eating and purging behaviour

- **Diet:** *'Describe a typical day's food intake. Are you on a diet? If so, what sort? How strict?'*
- **Binges:** *'Do you ever feel out of control and eat a large amount of food rapidly? If so, what do you eat in a binge? Afterwards, how do you feel? What do you do?'*
- **Vomiting:** *'Do you ever make yourself sick?'*
- **Exercise:** *'What exercise do you do? How often?'*
- **Purgatives and appetite suppressants:** *'Do you use laxatives, diuretics or slimming pills? Do you drink large amounts of coffee? Have you tried any other ways of losing weight?'*
- *'Have you been overweight in the past?'*

A description of a typical day's intake is an informative way of discovering the patient's eating patterns and the quantity and type of food being consumed. But, as with alcohol histories, interpret with caution. A person's response to being asked about their diet or current weight can itself give clues. Bingeing followed by induced vomiting is the main feature of bulimia nervosa. Note that misuse of diuretics increases the risk of hypokalaemia, which is one of the causes of death in eating disorders.

Body image disturbance: attitude to weight and shape

- *'What is your current weight? How often do you weigh yourself?'*
- *'Have you ever been very overweight or underweight?'* (a past history of obesity is common).
- *'Do you think you are fat? How much would you like to weigh?'*
- *'How do you feel about your body? How would you like it to be?'*
- *'Do other people say you're too thin? Do you believe them?'*
- *'How would you feel if you were a size bigger?'*

Preoccupation with weight and diet and *distortion of body image* are key diagnostic features, so explore fully the patient's views on the subject. A patient may be convinced she is overweight despite being demonstrably underweight (an overvalued idea, or delusion). A low body weight is seen as an accomplishment, not a problem, to a person with anorexia nervosa.

Physical symptoms of weight loss

- *'Are you taking the oral contraceptive, or any other hormonal contraceptive? Do you get periods?'*
- *'Are your periods regular? When was your last period? When did your periods begin?'*
- *'Have you been more tired or weaker than usual?'*

Amenorrhoea (or scanty, irregular periods) is a feature of anorexia nervosa. If the disorder began in the patient's early teens, menarche may never have occurred. Fatigue, lethargy and weakness are consequences of starvation and should alert the doctor to the need for physical examination and investigation.

Psychosocial risk factors

- What is the attitude of other family members and friends to food?
- **Perfectionism** (a common personality trait, especially in anorexia nervosa): ask about academic and other achievements and intentions.
- **Activities**: ballet dancing, modelling, athletics and other activities where thinness and fitness are valued are risk factors.

Physical examination and investigations

- Weigh the patient and measure them, in their underwear if possible – a patient may use heavy clothing to mask their weight.
- Calculate the body mass index (BMI), which is weight (kg)/[height (m)]^2. BMI should be 18–25. In anorexia nervosa, the BMI is below 17.5 – sometimes well below.
- Are they wearing baggy clothes?
- Is there lanugo hair (fine, downy hair on the arms, back and face)?
- Are there scars suggestive of self-cutting?
- Are there calluses on the hands? Poor state of teeth? (from self-induced vomiting)
- Cardiovascular exam: bradycardia and peripheral oedema are common in anorexia nervosa, and hypokalaemia can give rise to arrhythmias.
- Note secondary sexual characteristics.
- Perform relevant investigations to rule out other causes of anorexia and weight loss and to check for *complications* of weight loss.

How to assess sleep

Key components of a sleep assessment include:

1 **How is their sleep and sleep hygiene?** The mnemonic 'BEARS' (outlined below) ensures you cover the important aspects of sleep-wake cycles.
2 **Could medications or another psychiatric disorder underlie their problems?**
3 **Corroborative history from a bed partner, if possible.**
4 **Physical exam and investigations**, including rating scales, sleep diary, electroencephalography (EEG).

When do you need to assess sleep? (Box 3.13)

Clues to disordered sleep include:

- Sleeping <5 or >10 hours per night.
- Weekend 'catch-up' sleep, although common, indicates sleep curtailment.
- Multiple jobs or children.
- Shift work.
- High alcohol or caffeine intake.
- Psychiatric or neurological illness.

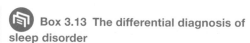 **Box 3.13 The differential diagnosis of sleep disorder**

- Poor sleep hygiene
- Substance-related: alcohol, caffeine and medication
- As part of or secondary to psychiatric disorder, especially mood disorder
- Neurological: restless leg syndrome, periodic limb movement disorder, dementia
- General medical condition: obstructive sleep apnoea, reflux, asthma, chronic pain
- Circadian: shift-work, jet-lag

Sleep history

Start with 'BEARS':

1 **Bedtime and sleep hygiene**
- *'How long does it take you to fall asleep? What stops you falling asleep?'*
- *'What do you do just before you go to bed? Do you use a computer just before you go to bed?'*
- Alcohol/smoking/caffeine before bed? (caffeine half-life is approx. 6 h).
- *'Do you have a bed partner? Do they stop you getting to sleep?'*

2 Excessive daytime sleepiness
- *'Do you fall asleep when you don't want to?'*
- *'Do you fall asleep when watching TV? During conversations? While driving?'* (subsequent questions indicate progressively worse sleepiness).

3 Awakening
- At night: *'Are you having difficulty sleeping through the night? What awakens you? How long are you awake for? What keeps you from falling back asleep?'*
- Early-morning wakening: *'Are you having any difficulty sleeping until the morning? What is your mood like in the morning?'*

4 Regularity and duration
- *'Do you usually go to sleep at the same time? What time do you typically fall asleep? And what time do you wake? What's the earliest you go to sleep? And the latest?'*
- *'Do you work odd hours or shifts?'*
- *'Do you give yourself restrictions on how much you let yourself sleep?'*

5 Snoring: *'Have you or anyone else noticed you snore loudly/stop breathing in your sleep?'*

Other important questions:
- Quantify and discuss their caffeine and alcohol intake. Many patients do not appreciate the extent to which coffee and stimulant drinks can affect sleep quality.
- Prescribed and over-the-counter medications.
- Past psychiatric history and a psychiatric screening assessment.
- Medical conditions.
- Corroborative history from a bed partner, if possible.

Further assessment

The physical exam should include BMI, blood pressure, neck circumference, examination of the oral cavity, pupils (for stimulant use), assessment of thyroid status and a neurological exam (if suspicious of restless leg syndrome or periodic limb movement disorder).

Questionnaires used to assess sleepiness include the *Epworth Sleepiness Scale* and the *Stanford Sleepiness Scale*. Typical questions present everyday scenarios; for example, having a conversation, and asking respondents to rate their likelihood of dozing. *Sleep quality* can be assessed using tools such as the *Pittsburgh Sleep Quality Index*.

More complex tests are available, although these are rarely used outside of the research context or specialist sleep clinics. In *actigraphy*, the patient wears a watch-like accelerometer device on their wrist. The gold standard test is *monitored polysomnography*, which includes EEG, electro-oculography (EOG), chin and neck electromyography, oximetry and ECG. In the *multiple sleep latency test*, patients are given opportunities to nap at 2-hourly intervals, and the time from the lights going out until sleep onset is recorded. A healthy sleeper would take 5–15 minutes to fall asleep and wouldn't go into REM sleep during the 20-minute nap period.

How to assess alcohol and other substance misuse

Use of alcohol and illicit drugs is common. Substance misuse can be a diagnosis and a problem in its own right, as well as contributing to the cause and persistence of many other psychiatric disorders. Note that where an intoxicated person lacks capacity, you may treat them without their consent under the Mental Capacity Act. However, intoxication with alcohol or any other substance is not grounds for detention under the Mental Health Act.

What do you need to find out?

- **Which substance(s) are misused and in what way?** This includes establishing the duration, quantity and pattern of use.
- **Is the person dependent on the drug?** Physical dependence is the most serious form of substance misuse.
- **What are the complications of the misuse?** Substance misuse produces diverse medical, psychiatric and social harms.
- **Is there any psychiatric comorbidity?** Given the diagnoses that arise from or coexist with substance misuse, it is also important to assess for psychosis, mood disorder and cognitive function. A full psychiatric assessment is best deferred until the person is sober.
- **Risk assessment** is also necessary as substance users have high rates of deliberate and accidental self-harm.

When do you need to assess for substance misuse?

Clues that could prompt an assessment include:

- Identification of significant alcohol intake during a psychiatric screening assessment.
- Insomnia in a stressed and depressed executive.

- Acute psychotic symptoms in a young person.
- Unexplained recurrent episodes of irritability or low mood.
- Perinasal inflammation.
- Needle marks.

Assessment of alcohol misuse

In addition to the basic psychiatric assessment described in the previous chapter, you should focus on the aspects outlined below.

The quantity and the pattern of consumption

- *'Can you describe what drinks you have in a typical day?'*
- *'Do you drink every day?'*
- *'Do you sometimes drink much more than that?/Do you binge?'*
- *'How long have you been drinking at this level?'* (Regular drinking that began in early adolescence is common amongst alcohol misusers).

Self-reports of consumption are underestimates (by half, as an unproven rule of thumb). The description of a typical day can be more revealing and accurate than asking about weekly intake. Check the type of drink: a pint of standard beer/lager/cider is 2 units, but stronger versions are 3 units. Also ask about the associated behaviours and feelings. Use the AUDIT screening questionnaire (Box 3.14). It takes about 2 minutes. Note that the FAST questions asked in the basic assessment (Chapter 2) are modified and extracted from the AUDIT.

> **Box 3.14 Alcohol Use Disorders Identification Test (AUDIT)**
>
> 1 *How often do you have a drink containing alcohol?*
>
>   (0) never. (1) monthly or less. (2) 2–4 times a month. (3) 2–3 times a week. (4) 4 or more times a week.
>
> 2 *How many drinks containing alcohol do you have on a typical day when you are drinking?*
>
>   (0) 1 or 2. (1) 3 or 4. (2) 5 or 6. (3) 7–9. (4) 10 or more.
>
> 3 *How often do you have six or more drinks on one occasion?*
>
>   (0) never. (1) less than monthly. (2) monthly. (3) weekly. (4) daily or almost daily.
>
> 4 *How often during the past year have you found that you were not able to stop drinking once you had started?*
>
>   (0) never. (1) less than monthly. (2) monthly. (3) weekly. (4) daily or almost daily.
>
> 5 *How often during the past year have you failed to do what was normally expected of you because of drinking?*
>
>   (0) never. (1) less than monthly. (2) monthly. (3) weekly. (4) daily or almost daily.
>
> 6 *How often during the past year have you needed a first drink in the morning to get yourself going after a heavy drinking session?*
>
>   (0) never. (1) less than monthly. (2) monthly. (3) weekly. (4) daily or almost daily.
>
> 7 *How often during the past year have you had a feeling of guilt or remorse after drinking?*
>
>   (0) never. (1) less than monthly. (2) monthly. (3) weekly. (4) daily or almost daily.
>
> 8 *How often during the past year have you been unable to remember what happened the night before because you had been drinking?*
>
>   (0) never. (1) less than monthly. (2) monthly. (3) weekly. (4) daily or almost daily.
>
> 9 *Have you or has someone else been injured as a result of your drinking?*
>
>   (0) no. (2) yes, but not in the past year. (4) yes, during the last year.
>
> 10 *Has a relative, friend, doctor or other health worker been concerned about your drinking or suggested that you cut down?*
>
>   (0) no. (2) yes, but not in the past year. (4) yes, during the last year.
>
> AUDIT scoring and interpretation: numbers in parentheses are scores for each question, so maximum score is 40. A score of 8 or more indicates a strong likelihood of hazardous or harmful alcohol consumption; 20 or more suggests dependence.

Dependence and withdrawal

- *'Do you have to drink more than you used to in order to get the same effect?'*
- *'Have you tried to cut down the amount you drink? What happened?'*
- *'Do you feel that you have lost control over your drinking?'*
- *'Do you drink more than you intend to?'*
- *'Do you ever have a drink in the morning to get you going?'*
- Ask the patient to rate the importance of drinking compared with other activities.
- Identify if the patient continues to drink despite awareness that it is harmful.

Dependence describes a cluster of physiological, behavioural and cognitive features arising from sustained use of alcohol, opioids, amphetamines and some other drugs. Its features include a *compulsion* to take the substance, *tolerance* (the need for increasing doses of the substance to achieve the same subjective effect) and *withdrawal symptoms*. Dependence is associated with serious medical and psychiatric complications. Withdrawal symptoms are a physiological reaction to a lack of the dependent substance. They can arise from some prescribed drugs, including benzodiazepines and some antidepressants. The features of alcohol withdrawal include tremor, retching, sweating and muscle cramps. If severe, it is called *delirium tremens*.

Psychosocial complications

Ask whether drinking has caused any psychological or social problems.

- *'Have you ever got into trouble due to your drinking?'*
- *'Have you got into financial problems due to your drinking?'*
- *'Have you ever missed work or lost a job due to your drinking?'*
- *'Has drinking interfered with your relationships?'*
- *'Have you ever been in trouble with the police (e.g. drink driving) due to your drinking?'*

Psychiatric and medical complications

- *'Has drinking affected your physical health? For example, jaundice, shakes, hepatitis?'*
- *'Have you ever had blackouts while drinking?'*
- Ask about the patient's medical and psychiatric history. Psychiatric disorders associated with alcohol misuse include depression, psychosis, delirium and dementia, as well as suicide and sexual dysfunction.

Physical examination

Examine the patient for the stigmata of alcohol dependence (Chapter 14). A physical examination, focusing on liver disease and neurological signs, is essential because of the many effects of alcohol on the body. Medical problems suggested by the history or physical examination need investigation and may require liaison with the GP or a physician.

Investigations

Many may be indicated – for example, breath or blood alcohol, full blood count (FBC), liver function tests (LFTs), urine or hair analyses. The mean corpuscular volume (MCV) and hepatic γ-glutamyl transpeptidase (GGT) are raised in 60–70% of patients with alcohol misuse. If other causes of their elevation are excluded, they are useful markers of alcohol misuse and for monitoring progress.

Use of other substances

The same sort of questions should be repeated for each class of misused drug as for alcohol (above). Many people who misuse one drug misuse at least one other. Patients may need reassurance about confidentiality when discussing illegal drug use. But remember that not all misused drugs are illegal – for example, analgesics. For illegal drugs, estimates of money spent are usually the best guide to intake: *'How much do you spend a week on heroin/crack?'* Remember to ask about the route of administration: *'Have you ever used needles? Have you ever shared? Have you been tested for hepatitis or HIV?'* Urine screens pick up some drugs or their metabolites, for varying lengths of time after use. Hair analyses are more sensitive (and cover a longer time frame) but are not widely available. In intravenous drug users (IVDU), consider testing for hepatitis B and C, and human immunodeficiency virus (HIV).

How to assess an unresponsive patient

By unresponsive, we mean a person who does not participate in the assessment, rather than an unconscious patient. Such people may be seen in a psychiatric clinic or ward, or when a psychiatric consult is requested in a general hospital or other medical setting. This could be a patient found standing rigidly in the street staring at the sky; a patient who does not speak; or an aggressive patient who does not reply to any questions and demands to leave.

What do you need to find out?

Why is the person unresponsive? Lack of cooperation with the assessment, due to inability or unwillingness, is uncommon but causes obvious problems. When communication is limited, you will need to focus on clues from the patient's appearance, behaviour and physical examination, and any corroborative history.

The main diagnostic questions are:

1 **Is there clouding of consciousness?** If so, consider delirium, stupor and their various causes.
2 **If not, is there evidence of psychosis, severe mood disorder or dissociative disorder?**

These disorders can all present with unresponsiveness.

3 **Is the person intentionally uncooperative?** This may be a sign of malingering or simply a belief that they are better off keeping quiet.

Complete the basic psychiatric assessment when the patient becomes responsive. An assessment of *cognitive function* and *psychosis* will almost certainly be needed.

 Box 3.15 The differential diagnosis of unresponsiveness

Stupor describes a condition in which the patient does not speak, move or respond, but appears fully conscious. Amongst psychiatric in patients, the main causes of stupor are:

- Catatonic schizophrenia
- Severe depression
- Psychomotor slowing in advanced dementia
- Drug-induced states, e.g. sedatives, neuroleptic-malignant syndrome
- Akinetic mutism
- Dissociative disorder
- Feigned unresponsiveness
- Hypoactive delirium
- Rarely: parkinsonism (decompensated due to e.g. an infection, missed medication), locked-in syndrome, epilepsy, encephalitis

  In other populations (e.g. neurology wards, hospital inpatients) the proportions are different.

The unresponsive patient: history and MSE (Box 3.15)

Background information

Is there an informant? Your problems are largely solved by a good informant or past records. For example, the patient may be known to have catatonic schizophrenia, a recent head injury, or be wanted by the police. Get as many details as possible, covering:

- Onset, course and duration of current episode.
- Past medical and psychiatric history.
- Medication, drug and alcohol history.
- Check the person's pockets and possessions for other clues.
- Check hospital and GP records in case there is a past history.

Level of consciousness

- Is the patient responsive to her surroundings? Is she paying attention to what is going on?
- Ask her to nod or open her eyes.
- Does she move? Do her eyes follow a moving object?

Establishing if there is clouding of consciousness is crucial since it indicates delirium and the need for urgent medical treatment.

Facial expression and communication

- Does his expression change?
- Does he seem afraid, depressed, preoccupied or hostile?
- Does he speak spontaneously or in response to questions?
- Can he communicate in other ways – for example, by writing or hand signals?

Facial expression and behavioural responses give diagnostic clues. For example, the characteristic appearance of a severely depressed patient; perplexity and fear in someone with psychosis or delirium; the hostility of someone with a personality disorder who does not want to be interviewed. In *elective mutism*, usually seen in children, the unresponsiveness is limited to speaking: other forms of communication are intact.

Physical examination

Unresponsive patients can be aggressive, and any physical examination will be without their consent. So, ensure the environment is safe and be accompanied – you may need a witness to confirm what took place.

- What is the patient's attitude to being examined?
- Is posture abnormal? Is it awkward or bizarre?
- Are there spontaneous movements, including stereotyped movements or mannerisms?
- Is muscle tone normal? Is there resistance when you try to make a movement?
- Examine the neurological system in as much detail as possible (cranial nerves, reflexes). Consider asking for an urgent neurological or general medical consultation if no clear psychiatric cause for the unresponsiveness is found.
- Do a general physical examination for signs of recent hygiene, trauma, intoxication, etc.

The motor exam is mainly aimed at detecting *catatonia* (see Box 3.5), which usually occurs in catatonic schizophrenia but is also caused by some rare neurological syndromes. The classic combination of increased muscle tone, decreased consciousness and hyperthermia suggests neuroleptic malignant syndrome. Surreptitious observation may reveal that patients behave differently when unaware they are being observed, indicating feigned unresponsiveness.

 FURTHER READING

Cowen P, Harrison P, Burns T (eds) (2012) *Shorter Oxford Textbook of Psychiatry*, 6th edn. Oxford University Press, New York.

 KEYPOINTS

- Thorough assessment allows the suspicion of a psychiatric disorder to be confirmed or dispelled.
- Relevant contextual information is also needed to help explain the causes and correlates of the disorder.
- Many patients will need assessment of several different domains.

 SELF-ASSESSMENT

1 Which of the following is not a first-rank symptom of schizophrenia?
   a Thought disorder
   b Thought insertion
   c Thought echo
   d Thought withdrawal
   e Thought broadcasting

2 Which of the following is true of obsessions?
   a They are not always perceived as intrusive.
   b They are diagnostic of obsessive-compulsive disorder.
   c They are also known as overvalued ideas.
   d They are often secondary to compulsive behaviours.
   e They may be a medication side effect.

3 Which of the following is true of hallucinations?
   a They can occur in severe depression.
   b They are misperceptions of external stimuli.
   c If they are visual, this suggests schizophrenia.
   d Voices talking to the person are characteristic of schizophrenia.
   e Hallucinations that occur on falling asleep are called 'hypnopompic'.

4

Risk: harm, self-harm and suicide

Learning objectives

✓ To understand the relevance of risk assessment in psychiatry

✓ To develop a framework for the clinical assessment and management of the risk of suicide and self-harm

✓ To be able to describe the relevance and key issues in the management of the risk that individuals with a mental disorder may pose to others

---

Risk in psychiatry

In psychiatry, *risk* refers to the probability that an adverse event such as self-harm, suicide or harm to others will occur. Public and professional concern about such events makes *risk assessment* and *risk management* an important part of psychiatric practice. A brief evaluation of risk, especially of suicide, is always part of the core assessment, but often a more detailed risk assessment is required. For example, in someone with:

- current suicidal intent;
- a history of mood disorder, psychosis or substance abuse;
- a history of self-harm or violence to others.

This chapter covers the assessment and management of risk in general, and self-harm, suicide and danger to others in particular. Harmful outcomes can never be eliminated. However, competent risk assessment and management can decrease their likelihood.

Risk assessment

When assessing the risk of harm to self or others, look for features associated with an increased risk. Try to gather the information from different sources – patient, informants, medical records, social services, police, etc.

In the *history*:

- Previous harm to self or others – the past is the best predictor of the future.
- Recent actions suggestive of impending harm (e.g. buying a rope, stockpiling medications, making a will).
- Recent major stresses or losses.
- Depressive disorder, psychosis, substance abuse or personality disorder.

In the *mental state*:

- Suicidal or violent thoughts.
- Significant mood disturbance.
- Psychotic symptoms, especially passivity or persecutory delusions.

In the *context*:

- Demographic factors (Table 4.1).
- Abuse of drugs or alcohol.
- Social restlessness – for example, few relationships, frequent changes of address.
- Exposure to suicide or self-harm among friends or family.
- Easy access to potential weapons or victims.

Psychiatry Lecture Notes, Eleventh Edition. Gautam Gulati, Mary-Ellen Lynall and Kate Saunders. © 2014 John Wiley & Sons, Ltd. Published 2014 by John Wiley & Sons, Ltd.

Formulation of risk

After completing the risk assessment, document the findings:

- What potential harmful outcome, if any, has been identified?
- How immediate and long lasting is the risk?
- What factors may increase or decrease the risk? These can be thought of as static (e.g. male gender) or dynamic (e.g. mental state, alcohol use).
- What can be done to reduce the risk?

Formal quantification of risk is not advised as there are no validated assessment tools, and given the individual nature of any particular patient such approaches can both amplify and downplay the actual risk.

 Clinical scenario

Mr J is referred for a psychiatric opinion because he has threatened to kill his wife and himself. He has convictions for grievous bodily harm and theft. You find no evidence of depressive disorder, psychosis or violent thoughts. However, he admits to drinking heavily at weekends, whereupon he becomes threatening and low in mood. His wife and the police (with his permission) corroborate the history. Your preliminary conclusion is of an alcohol-related problem and possibly personality disorder. His risk of harm or self-harm is low when sober but quite high when intoxicated or stressed. This fluctuating pattern of risk will continue as long as his drinking problem does. Marital strife is the other factor increasing risk.

Risk management

Risk management aims to:

- Reduce the level of immediate risk.
- Maintain it at the lowest level that is achievable.
- Set up a process for ongoing review of risk.

Table 4.1 Risk factors for suicide

Factor	Comment
Demographic factors	
Male	There are exceptions, such as in China where rates are higher in women
Increasing age	
Living alone	
Unemployed	
Recent life crisis	
Previous self-harm	Increases suicide rates 60-fold
Occupation	High rate in vets, doctors, nurses, pharmacists, farmers – this may reflect access to means
Exposure to suicide	Suicide in the family or among friends. Also exposure in the media or on social media
Illness-related factors	
Chronic medical problems	
Psychiatric disorder:	Present in 90% of those who die by suicide, usually depression
Depressive disorder	15% suicide rate in severe depression
Schizophrenia	>10% commit suicide
Substance misuse	Especially alcohol and opioid dependence
Personality disorder	Higher suicide rate, especially cluster B
Being in psychiatric care	75% of suicides have been in psychiatric treatment
In-patient	5% of suicides
Recent discharge from psychiatric hospital	
Mental state factors	
Depressed mood	
Expressed wish to be dead	
Detailed suicide plans	
Hopelessness	
Lack of reason to go on living	e.g. bereavement

Risk management strategies can be divided into immediate and longer term interventions. *Immediate interventions* may include:

- Psychiatric admission, if necessary under the Mental Health Act.
- Acute sedation.
- Ensuring adequate community support.
- Lowering of tension and the provision of reassurance as a result of the assessment.
- Making the family and significant others aware of the risk.
- Removing access to means (e.g. disposing of stockpiled medication).
- Notifying the police.

Longer term interventions include:

- Effectively treating psychiatric disorder.
- Implementing the Care Programme Approach.
- Alleviating social stresses.
- Enhancing positive coping strategies.

In all cases, ensure that:

- The management plan is documented and communicated to all others involved in managing the case.
- A date is set for reviewing the case and the plan – this may be within hours for an acutely suicidal in-patient, or every year for a stable patient in the community.

 Clinical scenario *(continued)*

You discuss Mr J with your colleagues and draw up a risk management plan. A copy is also given to Mr J, his wife and his GP. Mr J is given advice to help him cut down his drinking. The couple refer themselves to Relate to try to reduce conflicts between them. It is made clear to Mr J that he will be held responsible should he harm his wife. He agrees to record his alcohol intake and to return in 6 weeks.

Suicide and self-harm

Definitions

Suicide is a deliberate act performed in the expectation of death, where the outcome is fatal. Although suicide is clearly defined by death, establishing intent retrospectively is often difficult – some suicides are acts of self-harm in association with distress, which go tragically wrong.

There is no international consensus regarding the nomenclature for acts that do not result in death, which can lead to some confusion. Common terms include:

- *Self-harm (SH)* is the umbrella term for self-inflicted non-fatal harm regardless of whether the person expressed a wish to die. Self-cutting is the most common in the community, though self-poisoning accounts for 90% of medical presentations of SH.
- *Attempted suicide* is a term that may be used where there was a definite attempt by the individual to take his or her life; and *parasuicide* can be used when the degree of suicidal intent associated with the act is not clear, although this term is not frequently used.

Non suicidal self-injury (NSSI) is a relatively new term that is used extensively in the United States. It is used to describe self-injurious behaviour that is not suicidal in nature. However, it is not clear who determines intent (patient or clinician) and given that intent varies as well as the elevated risk of suicide associated with NSSI many clinicians believe the term to be unhelpful.

Self-harm

Self-harm is important because:

- *It is common.* There are about 150 000 presentations to general hospitals in the United Kingdom with SH each year. SH accounts for 10% of all acute medical admissions. It is the most common reason for acute admission of women, and the second most common for men. It is particularly common in young women, and rates among adolescents of both genders have been increasing.
- *It is a risk factor for further acts of SH and for suicide.* About 20% present with further acts of SH, and 1–2% will die by suicide in the following year.
- *It can be the presenting feature of serious psychiatric disorder.* Depression, anxiety disorders, substance misuse disorders and/or a cluster B personality disorder are common.

Motivations for SH are various and mixed. Only a minority have clear and sustained suicidal intent. Many acts are an impulsive response to what is perceived as an intolerable situation, or an attempt to influence the behaviour of others. SH often occurs under the influence of alcohol.

- SH can also represent a failed outcome of a determined attempt at suicide. Though rare, recognition of this small group is important.

Suicide

Though not a common cause of death, suicide is the third biggest cause of lost years of life because it often affects young adults. It is also the most common cause of death in girls aged 15–19 years worldwide. People who commit suicide are often depressed, and perceive the future as both intolerable and hopeless. Occasionally, this perception may be shared by others (e.g. in cases of terminal cancer), but usually it is strongly biased by depressed mood. Suicides are often planned. The risk factors for suicide are shown in Table 4.1.

- There is an increased risk of suicide in the weeks after discharge from a psychiatric hospital. This should be taken into account when planning management over this period.
- Suicide rates in young men increased in the United Kingdom in the 1980s and 1990s, before plateauing. The reason is unknown.
- In depressed patients, suicide may occur during the initial recovery phase – some people are so depressed that, until then, they lack the motivation to kill themselves despite a wish to be dead. In schizophrenia suicide tends to occur early in the illness. Therefore, suicide risk assessments and interventions to reduce risk should not stop when clinical improvement has begun.

Assessment of suicide risk

Assessing suicide risk is part of the core psychiatric assessment. If present, a full assessment is then essential. This follows the general principles of risk assessment, taking into account the risk factors for suicide (Table 4.1). Particular attention is paid to:

- The person's expressed intent.
- Their mental state.
- Recent acts of SH.
- Access to lethal means.

Never omit to assess suicide risk because you think (a) it might precipitate suicide or (b) someone really planning to kill themselves will deny it. Neither is true – the evidence is that recognition and active management may prevent suicide. Many people who kill themselves have been in contact with a doctor in the days before the fatal act. This is particularly relevant for primary care as only 25% of those who die by suicide in the United Kingdom are known to psychiatric services at the time of their death.

Assessment following SH

All patients who have self-harmed should have a psychosocial assessment, even if only briefly, to determine their risk of a repeat attempt and to identify the presence of a significant psychiatric disorder. Rating scales have limited utility and are not recommended. Certain characteristics of the act of SH predict a higher suicidal intent, and a higher risk of subsequent suicide:

- The attempt was planned.
- Affairs were put in order beforehand.
- The person took precautions to avoid discovery.
- They did not seek help afterwards.
- They used a method that they believed to be dangerous.
- They left a suicide note.
- They have an active mental illness.

Management after SH

General management

The number of patients seen because of an act of SH is large, and their management presents a challenge to medical and psychiatric services, especially if these are not well integrated (Chapter 18).

- For many cases, no specialist care is indicated, and the patient is discharged to their GP. It is therefore important to ensure the GP receives clear and prompt communication about the outcome of the assessment (Chapter 5).

 Clinical scenario

Ms S was seen in A&E having taken 20 paracetamol tablets earlier that night. She had been drinking and had taken them after a row with her boyfriend. She had not planned to kill herself and now felt foolish about her behaviour. She was unaware that paracetamol could be lethal. She was offered an appointment for out-patient counselling but declined, preferring to see her GP.

- A minority of patients are found to be at acute risk of suicide and require immediate and intensive management. The priority is to keep the person safe. This may be achieved by psychiatric admission, sometimes under the Mental Health Act. Serious suicidal intent may be sufficient grounds for admission under the Act, even if the presence of a psychiatric disorder has yet to be established. If admission is not used, it is important to ensure that relatives are aware of the severity of the situation and know how to contact services urgently if necessary.

 Clinical scenario

Mr P was found in his fume-filled car in an isolated field. After being resuscitated he expressed anger at being saved and said that he still wanted to die. He was found to be suffering from psychotic depression and had previously taken a serious overdose. He was admitted to hospital under the Mental Health Act and treated with ECT.

- Recognizing and treating depression effectively is a priority, given the importance of depression as a factor in suicide.
- Many SH patients have personal, relationship or social problems for which they may be offered help – for example, by counselling or problem-solving therapy, or by referral to community mental health psychology services.

Management of patients who repeatedly self-harm

A small number of people, mostly young women, present repeatedly with SH by taking overdoses or cutting. A diagnosis of personality disorder (dramatic cluster; see Table 15.1) is often made, and a history of childhood sexual abuse or other trauma may emerge. Management includes:

- Providing psychological support that is not contingent on acts of SH.
- Checking for emergent depressive disorder.
- Dialectical behaviour therapy (DBT; see Chapter 7) has been found to be effective in reducing frequency of self-harm.

Suicide as a public health problem

Prevention of suicide in the population has been a priority for health policy, but it is difficult to achieve, in part because social and political factors, and not just medical ones, are important (Table 4.2).

Clusters and contagion

- Clusters are groups of suicides that occur more closely in time or place than might be expected.
- These are a true phenomenon.
- Adolescents are particularly vulnerable.
- Exposure to real or fictionalized accounts (e.g. TV) of suicide increase risk.
- Celebrity status increases the risk.

Table 4.2 Prevention of suicide

Individual interventions
Better detection and management of:
    suicidal intent in patients attending medical services
    depressive disorder
    substance misuse

Population interventions
Public education and discussion
Education of doctors and others (e.g. teachers)
Easy, rapid access to psychiatric care or support
    groups (e.g. Samaritans)
Make it harder to attempt suicide, e.g. by:
    limiting access to paracetamol – smaller bottles,
      blister packs
    withdrawal of the analgesic coproxamol – especially
      dangerous in overdose
    make it harder to fix a hose over exhaust pipes
    safety nets around high buildings and bridges
Decreasing societal stressors – unemployment,
    domestic violence, etc.
Reducing substance misuse

Psychopharmacology and suicidal behaviour

No psychotropic drugs are licensed for the prevention of suicidal behaviour; however, a number are associated with reduction in suicide risk, and in recent years there has been concern that certain drugs may increase individual risk.

- *Antidepressants* – while antidepressant prescribing reduces suicide at a population level there have been some reports of increases in suicidal ideation and behaviour in the first 10–14 days of treatment. This is particularly true in those under the age of 25. This is not a reason to avoid prescribing but patients and relatives should be advised of this and patients should be more closely monitored during this period.
- *Lithium* is the drug with the most evidence in reducing completed suicide and suicide attempts, independent of its effect on mood symptoms. However, concerns regarding its lethality in overdose mean that this is not used in clinical practice solely for suicide reduction.
- *Clozapine* is also associated with a reduction in suicidal behaviour, which is likely to be secondary to its greater effectiveness as an antipsychotic drug.
- *Tricyclic antidepressants (TCAs)* and *monoamine oxidase inhibitors (MAOIs)* should always be prescribed cautiously in those with suicidal ideation because of their toxicity in overdose.

Risks to others

Despite the public perception, psychiatric patients are more likely to be victims than perpetrators of violence, and the vast majority of aggressive acts are committed by people in the absence of a psychiatric disorder. Nevertheless, knowing when and how to assess and manage potential harm to others is an important aspect of psychiatric practice.

Assessment of risk to others

The psychiatric disorders most associated with increased risk of violence are substance abuse and personality disorders (especially dissocial personality disorder). Schizophrenia and mania have also been linked to an increased risk. These disorders act cumulatively – so the risk is greater in a person with more than one of these diagnoses.

- Harmful acts are occasionally *directly* due to the disorder. For example, passivity experiences or persecutory delusions in schizophrenia, or nihilistic delusions in psychotic depression, may lead to harm to others. More commonly, violence results *indirectly* from the same combination of frustrations and personality that determine such acts in anybody. The disorder merely decreases the threshold (and perhaps increases the chances that the aggressor is caught).
- As with most behaviour, the strongest predictor of future violent behaviour is previous violent behaviour.

Management of risk to others

After identifying a risk to others, the clinician should do all they reasonably can to prevent the harmful outcome.

- Check access to weapons and whether there are specific plans or identified victims.
- Warn a potential target – the risk to others can override patient confidentiality – for example, in cases of *morbid jealousy*.
- Discuss the risk with a forensic psychiatrist.
- If there is known or suspected psychiatric disorder, consider admission, if necessary to a secure unit.
- Conversely, if psychiatric assessment reveals no evidence of psychiatric disorder, this conclusion should be clearly recorded.

Clear documentation and effective communication of the risk assessment and management plan are crucial. In the United Kingdom, there are Multi Agency Public Protection Panels (MAPPPs) where statutory agencies can refer and discuss individuals who are concerning in terms of their risk to others. For example, it may be necessary to involve social services where there is a concern about a child being at risk, or liaise with police or probation services as individuals may already be known to them, if there is concern about a serious risk to others.

FURTHER READING

NICE (2004) CG16: The short-term physical and psychological management and secondary prevention of self-harm in primary and secondary care. Access at: http://www.nice.org.uk/CG16

NICE (2011) CG133: The longer term treatment of self-harm. Access at: http://guidance.nice.org.uk/CG133

Davison SE (2005) The management of violence in general psychiatry. *Advances in Psychiatric Treatment*, 11, 362–370. Access at: http://apt.rcpsych.org/content/11/5/362.full

KEYPOINTS

- Risk in psychiatry refers to the risk of self-harm, suicide and the risk of harm by the patient to others.
- Assessment of suicide risk should be included in every psychiatric assessment.
- Detection of risk should lead to active management of the risk.
- Self-harm is very common. All patients who have recently self-harmed should be screened for suicidal risk and for psychiatric disorder.
- The majority of people committing suicide have depressive disorder or other chronic psychiatric disorder. However, suicide also occurs in people with no known psychiatric history, especially in young men.
- Most psychiatric patients are not violent. Most violent crimes is not perpetrated by psychiatric patients.
- Substance misuse, personality disorder, schizophrenia and mania are all associated with increased risk of harm to others, especially if they coexist.

> **?** **SELF-ASSESSMENT**
>
> 1 A 15-year-old girl attends A&E with multiple lacerations to her arms. Staff notice that she has multiple healed wounds on her arms and legs. How would you classify her risk?
>   a At risk of subsequent suicide.
>   b At risk of further self-harm.
>   c At no increased risk as she will 'grow out' of this behaviour.
>   d At increased risk of further self-harm and subsequent suicide.
>
> 2 A 26-year-old man has become manic and is being commenced on an antipsychotic medication and a mood stabilizer. He works as a delivery van driver. What should you advise him?
>   a Not to drive until the medication regimen is settled.
>   b To contact the Driver and Vehicle Licensing Agency (DVLA) and inform them about what has happened.
>   c He can continue driving as long as he doesn't feel too drowsy.
>   d You are going to contact his insurer and the DVLA to inform them he should not be driving.

5

Completing and communicating the assessment

Learning objectives

✓ How to make a *differential diagnosis*

✓ How to identify *causative (aetiological) factors* that have contributed to the disorder

✓ How to plan your initial *management*, and think about the longer term management

✓ How to think about the *prognosis*

✓ How to *summarize and present the case*, in a variety of formats

---

How to use this chapter

The process of psychiatric assessment described in Chapters 2–4 provides diagnostic information and an understanding of the patient in their context. This evidence is now combined to allow you to make a diagnosis, identify the causative factors, plan your management and consider the patient's prognosis. This chapter covers these points in turn, and an overview of this process is given in Figure 5.1. Through the chapter, we follow a single clinical case, which provides concrete examples of the approach described. To read the start of the case, turn to Box 5.1.

Diagnosis

Your history and mental state examination will suggest a number of possible diagnoses and rule out others. Sometimes, the diagnosis will be clear-cut, but usually there is a differential that requires further investigation. Either way, draw up a list of the key features in favour of, and against, each plausible diagnostic possibility. Weighing the diagnostic evidence helps clarify your own thoughts about the case. It is also useful to others who may refer back to your assessment if there is a subsequent review of the diagnosis. Remember that making a psychiatric diagnosis is an important step with consequences – it has drawbacks (e.g. stigmatization) as well as benefits (e.g. effective treatment). Differential diagnoses for common presenting symptoms are covered in the boxes in Chapter 3.

 Box 5.1 Mr K – a case of attempted suicide

Mr K, 55, was referred after a suicide attempt. You have elicited many depressive symptoms, some anxiety symptoms and an alcohol intake of 40 units/week. There are no features suggestive of psychosis or personality disorder, nor of imminent suicide risk. Your provisional diagnosis is a depressive disorder (moderate severity), plus alcohol misuse.

Psychiatry Lecture Notes, Eleventh Edition. Gautam Gulati, Mary-Ellen Lynall and Kate Saunders. © 2014 John Wiley & Sons, Ltd. Published 2014 by John Wiley & Sons, Ltd.

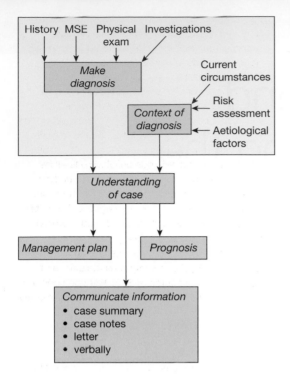

Figure 5.1 Overview of assessment and management. MSE, mental state examination.

Aetiology (see Chapter 6)

Having made a provisional diagnosis, you should consider the contextual information collected during your assessment, particularly those factors that appear to help explain the origins and evolution of the disorder. When considering causative factors in psychiatry, the two key variables are:

1 The *type* of factor – usually divided into biological, psychological and social.
2 The *time* at which the factor operates. A useful mnemonic for this is 'the four Ps': predisposing, precipitating, perpetuating and protective.

Types of causes: biological, psychological and social

The development of psychiatric disorders is influenced by biological (genetic and environmental), psychological and social factors. Sometimes one predominates; sometimes another, but all three always contribute something. Hence the *biopsychosocial model* of psychiatry, which requires that due attention is paid to all three areas, and which encourages an equally eclectic approach to treatment. The biopsychosocial model may seem obvious. However,

psychiatry has at times been guilty of focusing too closely on one or other of its components.

Timing of causes: predisposing, precipitating, perpetuating and protective (the four 'P's)

In terms of timing, causal factors can be:

1 **Predisposing:** factors that exert a long-term or distant causal effect, such as family history and early childhood experiences.
2 **Precipitating:** factors that explain why the disorder has occurred *now*. They include recent life events, injuries, new medical conditions, and discontinuation of medication.
3 **Perpetuating (or maintaining):** factors affecting the course of a disorder. Common ones include ongoing marital problems, social problems, and non-adherence with treatment. The nature of the disorder itself is also relevant: for example, Alzheimer's disease, being a progressive condition, requires no external perpetuating factors.
4 **Protective:** factors that protect against the development of psychiatric disease, or aid its resolution, e.g. strong social support networks.

A strength of the four 'P's approach is that it helps you to organize your thoughts in a way that relates not only to your management, but also to common patient questions: *'Why has this happened to me?'* (predisposing factors); *'Why has this happened now?'* (precipitating factors); and *'How can I get better?'* (in part, by tackling maintaining factors, and by drawing on strengths). In practice, a useful tip is to combine the 'type' and 'timing' approaches to causative factors in a 3 × 4 table, as in Box 5.2. This provides a template that can be filled in as details of the case emerge.

Another way to clarify the role of causal factors and the interplay between them is to create a **life chart**. This is most useful when the history is long and complex, to show whether illness episodes, or recovery from them, are related to specific factors, and whether there is any pattern of treatment response. A life chart can be time consuming to compile, but is usually worthwhile. Table 5.1 shows a life chart for Mr K.

Management

Having made a diagnosis and investigated the causative factors, move on to consider the management and the prognosis. These will follow directly from your current understanding of the case, and will need to be mentioned in the summary, letter or phone call that will follow the assessment. Management in

Box 5.2 Causative factors in Mr K

Clinical scenario

Mr K was made redundant 6 months ago. He is gay and his long-term partner left him around the same time, after which he had several casual sexual encounters. He has no close friends or relatives. Mr K had a stroke 2 years ago, which left him with a mild hemiparesis. He has had two past depressive episodes. His father committed suicide when Mr K was 5.

Based on our knowledge of the origins of mood disorders (see Chapters 6 and 9), several causative factors can be proposed. Not all factors may be relevant, and some may be not be 'provable' facts, but all merit consideration. Note that the same factor (in this case alcohol) can fit into multiple boxes.

Having hypothesized the causal factors, try to substantiate them. In this case, you should find out more about his alcohol misuse, discover his views on his sexuality and investigate how he feels about the redundancy, and its financial consequences. You should examine for neurological deficits and consider an HIV test. You find that Mr K has only minimal physical impairment from his stroke, but does have mild hypertension and a carotid bruit. He has misused alcohol intermittently for many years; the recent increase in consumption seems to have been a response to his low mood. His sexuality conflicts with his religious beliefs. He feels he was made redundant unfairly because he had taken sick leave, and has been left with serious financial problems. He is HIV negative. His notes reveal a similar clinical picture during previous depressive episodes, with a good response to antidepressants. In one episode, he also developed psychotic symptoms (delusions of guilt) and had a course of ECT. You conclude that he has a recurrent moderate to severe depressive disorder.

	Predisposing	Precipitating	Perpetuating	Protective
Biological	Genetic predisposition Cerebrovascular disease Alcohol misuse	Recent increase in alcohol consumption	Alcohol misuse	
Psychological	Psychological effects of father's suicide Stress related to sexual issues (difficulties arising from secrecy about orientation?) Past history of depression	Recent breakdown in a serious relationship	Stressors continue	Good insight into need for treatment
Social		Social isolation (has his stroke stopped him from driving?) Being made redundant	Social isolation continues Unemployment affecting his self-esteem or causing financial worries	

psychiatry involves making a number of decisions, which may need to be made rapidly:

- **Is treatment indicated?** Some assessments produce no evidence of psychiatric disorder, or no indication for treatment, other than reassurance and a clear statement of your conclusions.
- **How urgent is the problem?** Acute psychosis and severe mood disorders generally need immediate treatment. Serious risk of self-harm or harm to others is a major determinant of urgency. Is the patient sufficiently ill or at risk to need compulsory treatment?
- **Where should treatment take place, and who should give it?** Most psychiatric disorders are treated by GPs; some will be referred to psychiatrists; a very few need admission. The role of each party in implementing a management plan should be clear.

Table 5.1 A life chart for Mr K

Age	Events	Psychiatric disorder	Treatments
0	Complicated delivery		
5	Father commits suicide		
10	Mother remarries		
17	Turbulent home life	Depression, moderate	Amitriptyline 150 mg, 6 months
20	Joined navy; binge drinking		
25	'Came out'; left navy		
30	Met current partner		
35	Became storeman	Depression, severe	ECT × 6; fluoxetine 20 mg, 12 months
40	Mother dies		
45		Intermittent heavy drinking	Counselling
50	Hypertension		Beta-blocker started, use continues
53	Mild stroke		Physiotherapy
54	Made redundant		
55	Relationship ends	Current depressive episode	

Treatment decisions depend primarily on the diagnosis. However, they are also affected by the context – another reason why contextual information was collected in the assessment. For example, is the patient motivated enough for a psychological treatment? Does their job mean that sedative antidepressants should be avoided? What drug did they respond to last time?

Prognosis

Once you have a diagnosis and a reasonable understanding of the context, a provisional judgement about prognosis should be possible. Together with the diagnosis, it is the prognosis that is of most concern to the patient, their relatives and the referrer. *Short-term prognosis* depends mainly on the natural history of the disorder and, particularly, the treatment response. It is usually possible to give a rough estimate of the likelihood of improvement and its timing. *Long-term prognosis* is much more difficult to predict, and opinion on this issue may be deferred. It may be easier to estimate after an initial response to treatment has been observed. While each condition has its own prognostic indicators, some indicators of poor prognosis are common to all psychiatric conditions:

- Insidious onset.
- Longer duration of disorder prior to treatment.

- Comorbid personality disorder.
- Comorbid substance misuse.
- Lack of close relationships.
- History of non-adherence to treatment.

Summarizing and communicating cases

If it is to be useful, the understanding of the case that you have obtained must be communicated effectively to others. Below, we outline four different types of communication – an oral presentation of a case, a written case summary, a problem list and a GP letter. When planning this communication, ask yourself:

- **What does the recipient want and need to know?** This can vary from a detailed discharge summary for the psychiatric case notes, to a brief letter informing a GP that the dose of a drug has been changed. Avoid unnecessary information – it obscures the important messages. On the other hand, always include important negatives (e.g. 'He is not suicidal', 'She is not psychotic', 'Medication is not indicated'), and it is usually helpful to state the diagnosis and the current treatment in any letter. Similar rules apply to oral presentations.

- **What does the recipient know already?** If you are summarizing a person's tenth admission, information about the previous nine is likely to be available to and known by everyone, and may not need to be repeated. Conversely, a psychiatric court report should be written assuming that the recipient knows nothing about the person and nothing about psychiatry (or psychiatric terminology).
- **What does the patient need to know?** Informing the patient (and family) of the outcome of the assessment is the beginning of effective management. Patients are entitled to know what is written about them; indeed, as a rule, consider copying all correspondence to the patient unless you have clinical reasons not to do so. This has many potential benefits, but may be particularly challenging in psychiatry because of the nature of the patient's illness or the content of the letter (e.g. in an acute psychosis, or if there is a potential risk to others). In such circumstances, and when there is an urgent issue, you may prefer to convey the information to others by phone.

Written and oral case summaries

A case summary or 'formulation' is a concise, informative way of summarizing a psychiatric assessment. It is also educational for the creator since it involves weighing up the evidence and showing how you came to your conclusions. Example case presentations for Mr K are given – the presentation can either be oral (as in Box 5.3) or written (as in Box 5.4). The areas that should be covered are provided as a checklist in Quick Guide 1.

 Box 5.3 An oral case presentation of Mr K

Mr K is a 55-year-old unemployed storeman, seen in clinic last week following an overdose and admitted voluntarily because of suicidal intent and many depressive symptoms. Relevant factors included recent redundancy, relationship break-up and alcohol abuse.

On the history, Mr K complained of 6 months of low mood with poor sleep and loss of appetite. Over the last 2 months, he has engaged in self-harm, culminating in a suicide attempt last week. He had intended to kill himself and was found by chance. He now states that he does not wish to die. Mr K also describes anxiety symptoms including worrying about his health, feeling tense, socially phobic and that he lies awake worrying. He has a past psychiatric history of two depressive

episodes when aged 17 and 35, one of which required ECT. He suffered a mild hemiparetic stroke 2 years ago.

There is a family history of depressive disorder, and Mr K's father committed suicide when Mr K was 5 years old. Mr K's partner left him 3 months ago and at present he has no close friends or family. He was made redundant 6 months ago. He currently drinks over 40 units per week on a background of a long history of harmful intake.

On mental state examination (MSE), Mr K was visibly upset and made little eye contact. His speech was slow and quiet. His mood was subjectively and objectively low and he described feelings of worthlessness and guilt. He did not report any current suicidal thoughts. There were no abnormal perceptions and he had good insight into his illness and need for treatment, both psychological and pharmacological. There were no features suggestive of psychosis, personality disorder or previous manic episodes on the history or MSE, nor of imminent suicide risk.

My differential diagnosis comprises a depressive disorder, an anxiety disorder, alcohol misuse, and mood disorder associated with his stroke. A depressive disorder seems the most likely diagnosis, given the prominence and severity of the depressive symptoms, including biological symptoms of depression. Moreover, his depression predated the anxiety symptoms, the recent increase in alcohol consumption and the stroke. The severity of the stroke seems insufficient to explain his symptoms. My provisional diagnosis is thus of recurrent depressive disorder, current episode severe.

Turning to the aetiology, Mr K has a number of predisposing factors for a depressive disorder including his father's suicide, alcohol misuse, guilt about his sexuality, a stroke 2 years ago and two prior depressive episodes. The factors that may have precipitated the current episode are his redundancy 6 months ago, the breakup of his long-term relationship 3 months ago, and his recent increased alcohol intake. Perpetuating factors include his current social isolation, feelings of guilt about recent casual homosexual affairs, continued alcohol intake and financial worries. A key protective factor is his good insight into his illness and need for treatment.

As for the management, I plan to treat Mr K as a voluntary inpatient. In the short term, I will repeat the LFTs, suggest an HIV test, review his old notes and phone the GP for background, as well as seeking an opinion regarding treatment of his hypertension. I suggest that his mental state is monitored at least daily, with close nursing observations while he remains actively suicidal. He should also be monitored for signs of alcohol withdrawal. As for drug treatment, I suggest starting an SSRI antidepressant, with benzodiazepine as required for sleep or sedation. When his mental state settles, I will perform a further assessment of his current stressors. Longer term, he will need continuing support, so I suggest that we begin the Care Programme Approach assessment.

Regarding the prognosis, his history predicts a good response to antidepressants. However, if stressors continue, recovery will be compromised and he will be vulnerable to relapse.

 Box 5.4 A written case summary for Mr K

Opening statement

Mr K is a 55-year-old unemployed storeman, seen in clinic last week following an overdose and admitted voluntarily because of suicidal intent and many depressive symptoms. Relevant factors included recent redundancy, relationship break-up and alcohol abuse.

Differential diagnosis:

1 *Depressive disorder*

   For: subjectively and objectively low mood, suicidal ideation, recent self-harm, poor sleep, loss of appetite, feelings of guilt and worthlessness; two prior depressive episodes.

   Against: his depressive symptoms could be secondary to diagnoses 2–4.

2 *Anxiety disorder*

   For: worrying about his health, feeling tense, socially phobic and lies awake worrying.

   Against: the depressive symptoms began first, and are clearly more prominent.

3 *Alcohol misuse*

   For: drinking 40 plus units/week; long history of harmful intake; describes withdrawal symptoms when in the navy (30 years ago).

   Against: intake over past few years has averaged 25 units/week; recent increase postdated onset of symptoms; normal LFTs and MCV.

4 *Mood disorder associated with stroke*

   For: stroke 2 years ago.

   Against: first episode preceded the stroke; severity of stroke seems insufficient to explain his symptoms.

Diagnosis

Recurrent depressive disorder, current episode severe.

Context and cause

- *Predisposing:* father committed suicide when Mr K was aged 5 years. Alcohol misuse. Guilt about his sexuality. Stroke 2 years ago. Two other depressive episodes (at age 17 and 35), one requiring ECT.
- *Precipitating:* partner left him 3 months ago after 25 years. Increased alcohol intake. Made redundant 6 months ago.
- *Perpetuating:* social isolation – no close friends or family. Feeling guilty about recent casual homosexual affairs. Continuing high alcohol intake. Financial worries.
- *Protective:* good insight into his illness and need for psychological or pharmacological treatment.

Management plan

1 Further investigations: repeat LFTs and HIV test (last done 10 years ago); get old notes; phone GP for background. Needs a medical opinion regarding hypertension and its treatment.

2 Monitor mental state daily. Continue nursing observations whilst actively suicidal.

3 Observe for signs of alcohol withdrawal.

4 Start antidepressant (citalopram 20 mg). Benzodiazepine if required for sleep or sedation.

5 As mental state settles, assess further the current stressors – employment, finance, sexuality.

6 Longer term will need continuing support – begin Care Programme Approach assessment.

Prognosis

His history predicts a good response to antidepressants. However, if stressors continue, recovery will be compromised and he will be vulnerable to relapse.

Problem lists

Once the background to a case is familiar, the emphasis usually switches to current problems and their solution. Problem lists ensure that the key issues are identified and dealt with. A problem list for Mr K is shown in Table 5.2.

Table 5.2 A problem list for Mr K

Problem	Action	Agent	Review
Suicide risk	Close observation	Nursing staff	Daily
Depression	Start citalopram 20 mg once daily	Psychiatrist	One week–plan to increase dose
Insomnia	Sleep hygiene; hypnotics	Psychiatrist	One week
Social isolation	Investigate supports	Social worker	One week
Sexual guilt	Get contact number of local gay groups	Social worker	One week
HIV status	Consider HIV test	GUM clinic for advice	Two weeks
Alcohol misuse	Counselling	Specialist nurse	Unspecified

Letters between psychiatrists and GPs

Letters from psychiatrists to GPs should be as concise as possible. Remember you are usually offering the GP advice, not giving instructions. Also bear in mind that the GP will often know more than you about the person's history and circumstances. Take into account the purpose of the referral: was it for an opinion or for continuing care? Has the GP asked a specific question or requested a particular intervention? Generally the GP is most interested in:

- The diagnosis.
- A specific management plan, including the date of review and what he or she is expected to do.
- What the patient/relative has been told, and whether they have been copied into the correspondence, as mentioned above.
- What the patient and GP should do if matters unexpectedly deteriorate (or improve).

As a final visit to Mr K's case, Box 5.5 is a letter to his GP, a year later.

  Box 5.5 Psychiatric discharge letter to GP

Dear Dr Hall,
Re: Mr J.K., d.o.b 1.1.58, 24 Easy Street, Anytown
Diagnosis: recurrent depressive disorder, currently in remission

Course and current situation

Mr K has made a good recovery from his illness as detailed in the summary sent to you on his discharge from the ward 6 months ago, although as you know, he required augmentation with lithium for full recovery. At review in clinic today he was entirely free of symptoms.

Management and prognosis

Thank you for prescribing his medication (citalopram 60 mg o.d.; lithium carbonate 800 mg nocte), which he has taken as prescribed. His lithium level should continue to be checked every 6 weeks and maintained at 0.5–0.8 mmol/L; it was stable at 0.72 mmol/L last week. He should continue on the medication for at least another 6 months. At that time he intends to stop it, but he is aware that his risk of relapse will be lower if he remains on citalopram. When he does decide to stop, it should be tailed off gradually, over several weeks.

Mr K is fully aware of the diagnosis and our analysis of its causes (especially the relationship break-up, and his alcohol intake). We have addressed these issues, and they appear largely resolved. His drinking is now within normal limits, and he has begun a new relationship, which is going well. His financial worries have evaporated having been left money in an aunt's will.

We have not arranged to see him again. Please get in touch if you wish to discuss his case further, or if problems recur.

Yours etc.
cc Mr J.K.

Letters from GPs to psychiatrists should follow the same principles. The psychiatrist wants to know:

- The presenting complaint(s), the chronology and the GP's provisional diagnosis.
- What is the reason for the referral: for a diagnostic opinion, treatment advice or ongoing care?
- Is there an acute crisis? If not, why refer now?

- Past psychiatric and medical history.
- Key personal and social details (e.g. recent stressors, drug misuse).
- Any specific issues to be aware of (e.g. language difficulties, history of violence, vulnerable dependants).

 KEYPOINTS

- Completing the psychiatric assessment involves using the information you have collected to make a diagnosis, understand its likely causes, plan management and estimate prognosis.
- When thinking about why the disorder has arisen, divide the factors according to type (biological, psychological and social) and timing (predisposing, precipitating, perpetuating and protective).

- A written case summary comprises an introductory statement, the diagnoses and evidence for and against each differential diagnosis, the causative factors, the management plan and the prognosis. As well as communicating information to colleagues, it is also a good intellectual exercise when developing skills or practising for an examination.
- Tailor the content and format of any communication to the needs of the recipient. Be concise, structured and emphasize the points relevant to diagnostic and management decisions.

6

What causes mental health problems?

Learning objectives

✓ How to conceptualize aetiology in psychiatry

✓ To be able to think through *epidemiological*, *psychological*, *social* and *biological* aspects around causation in psychiatric disorders

Thinking about aetiology in psychiatry

Psychiatric disorders, like all illnesses, are caused by multiple and diverse influences – some known, many unknown. A corollary of this is that very few 'causes' are either necessary or sufficient; rather, each factor acts to alter the risk of disorder. The contribution of specific 'causes' differs from patient to patient, but as a rule each of the major psychiatric disorders is characterized by a well-established set of risk factors. For example, we might hypothesize that a teenager's eating disorder arises from any or all of:

- Inheritance of a genetic predisposition.
- Childhood obesity.
- Wanting to be a ballerina.
- Peer and media pressure to be thin.
- Disturbed 5-HT (5-hydroxytryptamine) neurotransmission.
- A hypothalamic tumour.

Aetiological conclusions should be just as evidence based as therapeutic and diagnostic ones, but the complex aetiology of psychiatric disorders can frustrate efforts to elucidate their pathophysiology. Rare familial single-gene dementias aside, almost all psychiatric disorders have multiple causes, and a given causal factor often contributes to several different disorders. The methods used to elucidate the causes of psychiatric disorder are correspondingly varied (Table 6.1). In this chapter, we describe how different methods can and have been used to tease apart the causes of mental health problems.

Epidemiology

Epidemiological methods can be applied to social, psychological or biological studies. They have contributed in two main ways to psychiatry. Firstly, population surveys have provided good information about the *prevalence* and *incidence* of the major psychiatric disorders, their sex and age distribution, and so on. This basic demographic information underpins most other kinds of aetiological research. Secondly, cohort and case-control studies have identified *risk factors* for psychiatric disorders, ranging from urban birth to autoimmune diseases to viral infection and drug side effects. An example is the finding that head injury increases the risk of dementia. Sometimes, as in this example, the causality of an epidemiological finding is fairly clear, but often it is not (e.g. the association of unemployment with depression), and further studies must be carried out to see which way the causal arrows point. Longitudinal, prospective studies, starting with healthy but 'at-risk' individuals and following them up until illness develops in some, are a powerful design, where feasible. Crucially, they help distinguish 'state'

Psychiatry Lecture Notes, Eleventh Edition. Gautam Gulati, Mary-Ellen Lynall and Kate Saunders. © 2014 John Wiley & Sons, Ltd. Published 2014 by John Wiley & Sons, Ltd.

Table 6.1 Methodologies used to study the causes of psychiatric disorders

Field	Approaches
Epidemiology	Prevalence and incidence studies Risk factor studies
Sociology	Life events Family influences Cultural factors Illness behaviour
Psychology	Behavioural theories Cognitive theories Psychodynamic theories Personality theories Neuropsychology
Biology	Genetics Biochemistry, pharmacology and immunology Brain imaging Neuropathology Animal models

abnormalities (associated with the 'state' of having the disorder) from 'trait' abnormalities (a permanent individual characteristic, which may be a risk factor for development of the disorder)

Sociology

Social factors are important in both the cause and shaping of psychiatric disorder. They can operate at different levels:

- *The immediate environment.* One's surroundings act as non-specific risk factors for illness. For example, psychiatric disorders are twice as common in those living in deprived conditions as in those living in affluent conditions. Many mechanisms are probably involved, including social conflict, substance misuse, noise and overcrowding; there may also be underlying factors that contribute independently to poverty and psychiatric disorder. In addition, having a psychiatric disorder may make it harder for the person to improve their circumstances and make continuing poverty more likely.
- *Life events (specific external stressors).* These include marriage, bereavement, unemployment and moving house. Life events, especially negative ones, lead to an increased risk of psychiatric disorder, notably depression, in succeeding months. The hypothalamo-pituitary-adrenal (HPA) axis is often implicated to explain this relationship,

since the HPA axis, including cortisol production, is integral to the stress response, both normal and abnormal. If a recent life event is the predominant, understandable trigger for a psychiatric disorder, the diagnostic category of *stress reaction* or *adjustment reaction* may be appropriate.

- *The social and family group.* Parents, siblings and others close to us are important influences on our development and functioning – for better and worse. For example, childhood emotional deprivation predisposes to later depression, whereas being in a close relationship protects against the effect of stressors.
- *The wider environment.* Environment in a broader sense is also relevant. For example, societal attitudes contribute to the prevalence of eating disorders, whilst political decisions affect the types and quantities of substances misused. Sociologists have also investigated transcultural differences in the occurrence of psychiatric disorders – many are universal, but some are much more common in particular populations.
- Some of these apparently 'social' influences actually involve genes too, because genes and environment interact. In other words, it is 'nature plus nurture', not 'nature versus nurture'.

Sociological research by Brown and Harris, working in London in the 1970s, had an enormous impact on our understanding of depression. They asked why depression was particularly common in women of low socio-economic status, and why some women did not get depressed despite similar circumstances. They identified several factors (examples of the 'four Ps' approach to causation introduced in Chapter 5):

- Women who as children had suffered a life stressor such as emotional deprivation or death of a parent were at greater risk of depression (*predisposing factor*).
- In the women who had one or more of the predisposing factors, depressive disorder was *precipitated* by a single major life event or by an accumulation of minor stressors.
- Women who had a *protective factor* such as social support from an intimate relationship in their life were less likely to become depressed after a major adverse life event.
- Continuing stress and lack of support acted as *perpetuating* factors.

Family theories

Family theories view psychiatric disorder in one member as reflecting an abnormality in the whole family. They are applied particularly to childhood psychiatric disorders, where the theories have inspired a treatment approach – *family therapy*. However, it has been hard to confirm the aetiological role of the family. Recent research shows that resemblances between family members are influenced by genes at least as much as by the family environment. An example where family factors (in a sociological sense) were wrongly invoked is autism, which was attributed to parents being aloof or obsessional ('refrigerator mothers'), whereas in fact it is highly genetic. In the 1950s, schizophrenia was explained in terms of parenting styles (the 'schizophrenogenic mother') and patterns of family communication ('double bind', 'schism and skew'). Such abnormalities, if they occur, seem more likely to be the result, not the cause, of having a son or daughter with schizophrenia in the house.

The sick role and illness behaviour

The *sick role* describes four processes that occur when someone is ill:

- Exemption from normal obligations (such as earning a living).
- A right to receive care.
- An obligation to cooperate with care.
- A desire to recover.

Illness behaviour refers to the behaviour of the person in the sick role. Both the sick role and illness behaviour are sociological concepts that describe normal processes. They can also be excessive or maladaptive, and then are relevant to understanding the presentation and persistence of psychiatric (and medical) disorders. People differ markedly in their response to symptoms – that is, they vary in their illness behaviour and readiness to adopt the sick role. Some are stoical and are reluctant to complain, while others dramatize symptoms and have a low threshold for medical consultation. These individual differences are compounded by society's views about psychiatric disorder – including stigma and ignorance about their nature and treatability. As a result, psychiatric patients may have more difficulty than medical patients in negotiating a sick role. A patient's relationship to the sick role can be pathological: patients with medical complaints who appear to adopt the sick role unnecessarily or excessively (i.e. have *abnormal illness behaviour*) may have depression or a somatoform disorder. The benefits of the sick role (sometimes called *secondary gain*) play an especially important role in dissociative and somatoform disorders (Chapter 10).

Antipsychiatry

Some sociologists, and some psychiatrists, have argued that psychiatric disorders are not medical illnesses, but merely social constructs to label and deal with deviant behaviour. This thesis – *antipsychiatry* – was particularly influential in the counter-culture environment of the 1960s, with Thomas Szasz, an American psychotherapist, being a leading figure. A related stance (*'critical psychiatry'*) is currently advocated in some quarters. Antipsychiatry sees psychiatric disorders as predominantly social in origin and requiring psychosocial interventions. It is influenced by particular philosophical beliefs, and marked by scepticism as to the importance of medical and neuroscientific aspects of causation and management. Many current and ex-service users are also critical of psychiatric interventions, as implied by the name of the 'Psychiatric Survivors Movement'. As medical practitioners, we should engage with concerns about patient rights and the patient experience. However, whilst antipsychiatry was and is important in drawing attention to the limitations of psychiatric knowledge and the dangers of stigmatization and institutionalization, there is little evidence to support its tenets regarding the causes of mental distress. A denial of the biological component of psychiatric disorders is not helpful to ill patients.

Psychological factors

There are various psychological models of psychiatric disorder, differing in their theoretical background and experimental support, but sharing two features:

- They are extensions of theories of normal psychological processes.
- The theory is complemented by a psychological treatment that arises from it.

Behavioural theories

Many of our actions are explicable in terms of learned behaviours or *conditioning*. There are two types of conditioning, *classical* and *operant*. These underlie contemporary *behavioural theories* of normal and abnormal behaviours. Behavioural theories gave rise to *behavioural therapy*, which is an effective intervention in its own right for several childhood disorders and anxiety disorders.

In *classical conditioning*, we unconsciously associate two stimuli that regularly occur together. In Pavlov's classic experiments, dogs were given food when a bell was rung. After a while the dogs began to salivate when the bell rang, even if no food was there. This conditioning gradually wears off (*extinction*). People are classically conditioned in many ways – for example, a person may become aroused at the sight of lingerie if they have come to associate it with impending sexual gratification. Conditioning is important in the development of some psychiatric disorders. For example, agoraphobia developing in a person who was assaulted twice in the street; she associates leaving the house with the fear of attack, which she avoids by staying at home.

Operant conditioning describes how a behaviour will occur more frequently if it is rewarded (*positive reinforcement*), and decreases if it is not (*negative reinforcement*) or if it has unpleasant consequences (*punishment*). Rats learn to press a lever if it gives them food but not to press it if it doesn't, or if they receive a painful shock. Children will shout and scream if they learn that this behaviour gets them an ice cream; on the other hand they learn to be polite if that is effective in obtaining one. Adults, though they may not like to admit it, are equally susceptible to conditioning. *Learned helplessness* is an example of operant conditioning. Animals subjected to a period of inescapable stresses (electric shocks) eventually give up trying to avoid them because such behaviour is never rewarded. A similar mechanism is proposed to explain why childhood adversity predisposes to depression in adulthood.

Cognitive theories

The core assumption of cognitive theories is that cognitions (thoughts, patterns of thinking and ways of processing information) influence our mood, behaviour and physiology, and that inaccurate or distorted cognitions can lead to inappropriate or abnormal mood and behaviour. Cognitive theories of behaviour developed partly in reaction to the behaviourist approach that predominated in the early twentieth century, which placed little value on internal representations or psychological mental states. Cognitive theories of depression and anxiety disorders are especially well developed. A cognitive model explaining how panic disorder develops is summarized in Box 6.1. Cognitive theories are well validated and are clinically important because they have led to an effective and widely used form of psychotherapy – *cognitive therapy*.

 Box 6.1 A cognitive model of a panic attack

A woman gets a twinge of chest pain whilst reaching for a tin of beans in the supermarket. She has the thought that it might be a heart attack, even though in fact it's a muscle strain from overdoing it

at the gym that morning. Having had the thought, she becomes more anxious about the possibility of a heart attack, and all that entails, and beings to experience the physiological changes associated with anxiety – such as palpitations, sweating … and chest tightness. She interprets these sensations as confirming that she is having a heart attack, the anxiety increases and she has a panic attack. Although it passes, the next time she is in the supermarket she recalls the episode, becomes hypervigilant for bodily sensations and a second panic attack occurs more readily than before. As the cycle continues, her cognitions and the associated symptoms are repeated until she has established panic disorder.

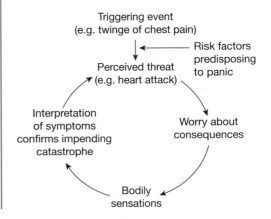

Cognitive distortions can arise for different reasons. For example, the woman in Box 6.1 may be concerned about a heart attack because of an episode of childhood myocarditis, the recent death of a relative from a heart attack or from watching an item on the news on heart disease in women.

Psychodynamic theories

Psychoanalysis, associated with Sigmund Freud and his followers, is a complex theory of psychological processes and the origins of psychiatric disorders, especially anxiety disorders. It also refers to the therapy inextricably linked to the theory. Psychoanalysis has changed a lot since the time of Freud, and the generic term *psychodynamic* is usually used to describe theories that combine Freudian elements with later ideas. Psychoanalytic theory holds that the mind is partitioned; some is conscious but much is unconscious. In Freud's final model, the components of the mind were the *ego*, *superego* and *id*: the ego is the part of us in contact with reality; the superego is like our conscience;

and the id is our instinctive drives and desires. The energy of the id is called *libido*, which is primarily sexual in nature. Feelings and memories of which we are unaware, especially those arising from very early in life, shape our current thoughts, feelings and actions. We use unconscious *defence mechanisms* to reduce tensions that exist between our conflicting desires (Table 6.2). These mechanisms may be healthy or dysfunctional. Anxiety disorders (neuroses) result from a failure to progress through normal stages of mental development and develop adaptive defence mechanisms.

Psychodynamic theories have been influential but are much less prominent or important in modern psychiatry. This is partly because they are not true scientific theories, in the sense of being empirically testable or refutable. When elements of the theories have been tested, they have not been well supported by evidence. Moreover, psychodynamic psychotherapies are still of unproven efficacy. They are now of very limited availability in most healthcare systems, but are still available as NHS treatments for some patients in some regions.

Nevertheless, psychodynamic insights are clinically useful in emphasizing that early experiences, and unconscious processes, can affect our feelings and actions, whatever the mechanisms involved. The defence mechanisms described have intuitive validity and the associated vocabulary permeates present-day descriptions and conceptualization of mental processing. Moreover, identification of the transference and counter-transference inherent to the doctor-patient relationship can improve our practice, both in psychiatry and in general medicine.

The role of personality

Personality describes our persistent pattern of thoughts, attitudes and behaviours. As such, it is critical to psychiatric disorder, but the very fact that the two are so intertwined makes it hard to identify the specific aetiological relationships between them. It is clear, though, that:

- Different personality types predispose to different psychiatric disorders.
- Personality affects the clinical picture of psychiatric disorder.
- Personality affects the prognosis of psychiatric disorders.

Personality can itself be abnormal (*personality disorder*), and interact with and coexist with psychiatric disorders. These issues are discussed in Chapter 15.

Biological models

Genetics

Evidence from various sources can suggest a genetic basis for a given psychiatric disorder:

1 **Familial clustering and twin studies:** Familial aggregation can be shown to reflect shared genes not shared environment if twin studies show a higher concordance rate in monozygotic (MZ; identical) than dizygotic (DZ; non-identical) twin pairs, because MZ twins have essentially identical genomes, but DZ twins share only 50% of genes. These studies establish the *heritability* of a disorder (or trait) – see below.

Table 6.2 Defence mechanisms

Defence mechanism	Definition
Repression	Suppressing desires and memories from consciousness
Denial	Behaving as though genuinely unaware of external reality
Projection	Attributing your own feelings to someone else
Displacement	Shifting emotions from the appropriate object or person to a more acceptable target, e.g. kicking the dog rather than your father
Reaction formation	Behaving in a way opposite to your (unacceptable) instincts
Regression	Returning to an earlier pattern of behaviour, e.g. to become more dependent on others
Sublimation	Finding a socially acceptable alternative outlet for emotions
Intellectualization	Thinking about your emotions rather than feeling them

2 **Adoption studies:** The incidence of the disorder remains increased in adopted-away children (though this doesn't control for prenatal environment – which is relevant for some disorders, including schizophrenia).

3 **Associated genetic abnormality:** E.g. a known chromosomal (*cytogenetic*) aberration – for example, Down's syndrome or fragile X syndrome. Where the genetic changes are more subtle, or present to a degree in healthy individuals – e.g. DNA copy number variation (CNV) – the role of these genetic differences is less clear.

4 **A known pathological or biochemical abnormality:** The underlying gene is a *candidate gene* for the disorder. For example, in Alzheimer's disease, the β-amyloid protein in senile plaques led to the discovery of amyloid gene mutations. The lack of definitive lesions in most psychiatric disorders means there are few convincing candidate genes.

Apart from a few dementias (e.g. Huntington's disease) and developmental disorders (e.g. tuberous sclerosis), psychiatric disorders are not caused by gene mutations following mendelian inheritance patterns. Instead, there are genetic variants (*polymorphisms*) that act as risk factors, significantly but slightly increasing susceptibility to the disorder.

Heritability refers to the size of the genetic predisposition; it describes the proportion of the disorder in the population that is attributable to genes. It is best measured in large-scale twin studies. Note that heritability is a population average figure: any given individual's disorder may be much more or less 'genetic'. Heritability estimates for psychiatric disorders (for which good data are available) are shown in Table 6.3. The rest of the 100% not explained by heritability denotes the environmental contribution, including individual-specific and shared environmental factors.

Although there is a substantial heritability for many psychiatric disorders, it is proving difficult to locate the chromosomal loci and susceptibility genes driving this heritability (the next step in Figure 6.1). There are several possible reasons for this:

- There are many genes, each conferring individually only a small amount of the risk for a psychiatric disorder.
- The genes interact with each other (*epistasis*), and with environmental factors (gene × environment, or GE), in ways that are very hard to detect and measure.
- The disorder may be caused in different people by different genes (*genetic heterogeneity*) or different variants of the same gene (*allelic heterogeneity*).
- The causative genes may not map onto the currently defined clinical syndromes – that is, the wrong patients, genetically speaking, are being grouped together.

Table 6.3 Recent heritability estimates for psychiatric disorders

Disorder	Heritability (%)
Bipolar disorder	85
Schizophrenia	81
Alzheimer's disease	75
Anorexia nervosa	60
Alcohol dependence	56
Major depressive disorder	37
Autism	37
Generalized anxiety disorder	28

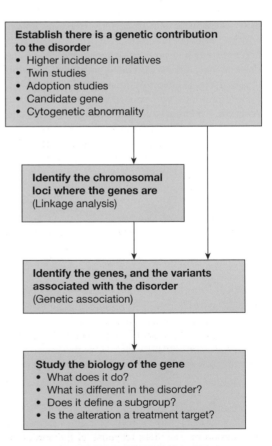

Figure 6.1 Finding genes for psychiatric disorders.

Nevertheless, the search is worth pursuing since identification of genes gives clues as to the core biological basis for an illness, and potentially for its effective treatment (e.g. several current treatment trials to correct the β-amyloid abnormality of Alzheimer's disease).

Biochemistry and pharmacology

Biochemical theories propose that psychiatric disorders are caused by a biochemical abnormality, usually affecting the level or activity of a neurotransmitter, or the enzymes that metabolize it, or the receptors to which it binds, or the transporters that regulate its levels in the synapse. For example, the 5-HT (serotonin) theory of depression variously implicates 5-HT_{1A} receptors, 5-HT transporters and tryptophan hydroxylase. Many of these theories were based originally on the mechanisms by which psychotropic drugs work. For example, antipsychotics treat schizophrenia and were found to block dopamine receptors; this observation led to the dopamine hypothesis of schizophrenia. Forty years later, there is now evidence it is true, to some degree, but the line of reasoning (from treatment target to pathophysiology) is flawed: diuretics treat heart failure, but heart failure is not usually due to renal disease.

Peripheral markers

The brain is relatively inaccessible, so many biochemical measurements have been made in cerebrospinal fluid (CSF), blood or urine. A robust finding is that people who are impulsive and aggressive have low CSF levels of the metabolite of 5-HT, suggesting impaired functioning of the central 5-HT system. However, it is often unclear whether peripheral markers reflect the situation in the brain.

In a *neuroendocrine challenge test*, a substance known to produce a change in the plasma level of a hormone is administered. The size of the change reflects the sensitivity of the neural control system that mediates the response. For example, in the *dexamethasone suppression test*, plasma cortisol is measured after a dose of dexamethasone, to assess HPA axis function. Many people with severe depression fail to suppress cortisol, which led to the 'steroid hypothesis' of depression.

The study of body fluids in psychiatry is of renewed interest in the current search for *biomarkers*: that is, biological indices (such as levels of gene expression, or of metabolites) that can help predict the onset, progression or treatment response of a disorder, or help in its differential diagnosis.

Neuropathology

Biochemical studies of the brain after death were crucial in the understanding of Alzheimer's disease; in particular, the discovery of cholinergic deficits and the β-amyloid protein. Similar approaches have revealed abnormalities in other psychiatric disorders, including schizophrenia, mood disorders and autism, though no comparably clear picture has emerged. Part of the problem is that studies of postmortem brains have many limitations, such as the effects of dying, death and a bias towards old, medicated and chronically ill cases. This makes it difficult to establish whether alterations occurred early or late in the disease, and findings may simply reflect the effects of treatment, or the effects on the brain of the consequences of psychiatric disorders, such as institutionalization, interpersonal difficulties, unemployment or substance misuse.

Structural and functional neuroimaging

A range of neuroimaging techniques are now available that allow the living brain to be studied. By using first-episode and unmedicated subjects, the confounders mentioned above can be avoided.

Computed tomography (CT) and structural magnetic resonance imaging (MRI) allow brain *structure* to be investigated in vivo. For example, they show that patients with schizophrenia have enlarged lateral ventricles, and that the hippocampus is smaller in those with recurrent depressive disorder. Longitudinal MRI studies are increasingly used. For example, they show that some differences in brain structure long precede the onset of symptoms in schizophrenia, whilst others develop as the illness does. Structural MRI methods such as diffusion tensor imaging (DTI) can now also identify the white matter pathways that connect one part of the brain with another – many people think the anatomical basis of psychiatric disorders is not to be found in any one place, but in how the brain is wired up, in both a structural and a functional sense.

A variety of neuroimaging techniques can also be used to obtain information that reflects real-time neuronal activity. Functional MRI (fMRI) measures regional brain metabolism; electroencephalography (EEG) measures electrical activity; and magnetoencephalography (MEG) measures the weak magnetic fields produced by neuronal currents. Positron emission tomography (PET) and single photon emission computed tomography (SPECT) use radioactive ligands to measure brain receptors or metabolites.

They have shown, for example, that people with schizophrenia do not have elevated dopamine D_2 receptors (as one version of the dopamine hypothesis had proposed). The methods are limited by the radioactivity involved, and a lack of suitable ligands for many molecules of interest (e.g. glutamate receptors).

Information from neuroimaging techniques points to the specific brain regions and receptors that may be involved in the pathophysiology of a disorder, or in its response to treatment. Imaging phenotypes, like peripheral blood measurements, could also serve as biomarkers. While neuroimaging currently remains a research tool in psychiatry, it could soon provide meaningful information to clinicians at the level of individual patients, allowing more tailored treatment decisions, or providing better information on prognosis, for example following a first episode of psychosis.

Animal models

No one would suggest that a rat can get schizophrenia – and how would we know if it did? However, animal studies have contributed to psychiatric research in various ways and they continue to be of use:

- To assess the effects of an experimental intervention (e.g. in utero inflammation, maternal separation, neonatal hippocampal damage) upon relevant behaviours (e.g. cognitive performance, social interactions) and biology (e.g. receptor sensitivity).
- *Transgenic* animals (with DNA from another species artificially inserted) allow the role of specific genes in brain function and dysfunction to be investigated. For example, mice containing a mutated human amyloid precursor protein gene develop cognitive impairment and histological features of Alzheimer's disease; mice without a prion protein gene are resistant to prion disease.
- Animals, usually rats, are still widely used to test potential psychotropic drugs.

 KEYPOINTS

- The cause of most psychiatric disorders is multifactorial, involving biological, psychological and social contributors.
- There is a genetic predisposition to most disorders, and sometimes a large genetic contribution. However, the number and identity of the genes involved in most disorders remain unknown.
- Other biological aetiological factors are diverse and include head injury, infections, and drug side effects.
- Important psychological factors are early experience, cognitive style and conditioning.
- Social influences include childhood deprivation, relationship problems, family structure and unemployment.

 FURTHER READING

Cowen P, Harrison P, Burns T (eds) (2012) *Shorter Oxford Textbook of Psychiatry*, 6th edn. Oxford University Press, New York.

 SELF-ASSESSMENT

1 Which of the following is true, concerning the heritability of psychiatric disorders:
   a Heritability refers to the penetrance of a gene.
   b Heritability is measured using genome-wide association studies.
   c The heritability of schizophrenia is about 40%.
   d The heritability of depression is about 40%.
   e The heritability of anxiety disorders is less than 10%.

2 Which of the following is true, concerning research tools in psychiatry:
   a Functional MRI (fMRI) is a non-invasive imaging technique that measures neuronal activity.
   b Positron emission tomography (PET) uses radioactive ligands to measure brain receptors or metabolites.
   c Biomarkers are molecules that can help predict the onset, progression or treatment response of a disorder, or help in its differential diagnosis.
   d In adoption studies, an increased incidence of the disorder in adopted-away children proves that there is a genetic component to the disorder.

Treatment

Learning objectives

✓ To be able to demonstrate a working knowledge of the uses, side effects and mechanisms of action of commonly prescribed psychiatric drugs and of electroconvulsive therapy

✓ To be able to describe common modalities of psychotherapy

✓ To understand the relevance of social interventions in psychiatry

Psychiatric treatments may be categorized as *biological* – drugs and electroconvulsive therapy (ECT); *psychological* – the psychotherapies; and *social*. A combination of approaches is usually used. Sometimes *compulsory* treatment is given. Chapter 8 considers how treatments are delivered and services organized.

Drug treatments

The study of psychiatric drugs – their mechanisms, uses, effects and side effects – constitutes *psychopharmacology*.

Principles and practice of prescribing

Drugs used in psychiatry can be grouped into eight main categories (Table 7.1).

- Consult a more detailed text for complete information about individual drugs, doses, side effects, drug interactions and contraindications.
- Always check the British National Formulary or similar before prescribing any drug with which you are not wholly familiar.
- Box 7.1 summarizes the important principles that govern the prescription of all psychiatric drugs.

Bear these in mind as you read on, and try to put them into practice.

- Many patients – maybe even the majority – do not take their drugs regularly. This is by no means unique to psychiatric patients but is complicated in psychiatry by the fact that many patients will refuse medication because of the nature of their illness: for example, a psychotic patient who refuses medication because he believes you are trying to poison him. This issue is variously called *compliance, adherence* or *concordance*, and the lack of it is a major reason for apparent non-response to medication. Box 7.2 lists the main reasons for the problem and how to minimize it.

> **Box 7.1 Principles of psychiatric prescribing**
>
> - *Choose the right drug.* This requires an adequate assessment, accurate diagnosis and consideration of other factors such as comorbid medical conditions and suicidal ideation.
> - *Give the right dose.* Antidepressant doses are often inadequate, antipsychotic doses excessive. Each poses risks: lack of efficacy and unnecessary side effects, respectively.

Psychiatry Lecture Notes, Eleventh Edition. Gautam Gulati, Mary-Ellen Lynall and Kate Saunders. © 2014 John Wiley & Sons, Ltd. Published 2014 by John Wiley & Sons, Ltd.

Table 7.1 **Drug treatments in psychiatry**

Type	Example	Main indications
Antidepressants		Depression, anxiety disorders
SSRIs	Fluoxetine, sertraline	
TCAs	Amitriptyline	
MAOIs	Phenelzine	
SNRIs	Venlafaxine	
Other	Mirtazapine	
Mood stabilizers		Bipolar disorder
Lithium		
Valproate		
Lamotrigine		
Carbamazepine		
Hypnotics and anxiolytics		Anxiety, insomnia
Benzodiazepines	Diazepam	
Antipsychotics		Schizophrenia, other psychoses
First-generation ('typical') antipsychotics	Haloperidol	
Second-generation ('atypical') antipsychotics	Clozapine, olanzapine	
Anticholinergics	Procyclidine	Extrapyramidal side effects of antipsychotics
Stimulants	Methylphenidate	Attention deficit disorder
Drugs for dementia		Alzheimer's disease (moderate to severe)
Cholinesterase inhibitors	Donepezil	
NMDA receptor antagonist	Memantine	
Drugs used in substance dependence		Detoxification, abstinence
Alcohol	Disulfiram, acamprosate	
Smoking	Bupropion	
Opiates	Methadone, buprenorphine	

SSRIs: selective serotonin reuptake inhibitors; TCAs: tricyclic antidepressants; MAOIs: monoamine oxidase inhibitors, SNRIs: selective serotonin and noradrenaline reuptake inhibitors; NMDA: *N*-methyl-d-aspartate.

- *Give the drug for the right duration.* Antidepressants tend to be given for too short a period and anxiolytics for too long. Again, the trade-off is between incomplete response and adverse effects, including the potential for dependence.
- *The efficacy and side effects of drugs within a class may differ.* The choice of drug is determined largely by previous experience in any specific patient, side effects (e.g. sedative profile), strength of evidence. Drugs with solid evidence of efficacy and known safety should be used preferentially. A family history of drug response can be informative, particularly in bipolar disorder.
- *Avoid combinations of drugs from the same class.* There is no evidence for greater efficacy, and often more side effects.

- *Psychiatric drugs are better than placebo ... but not always by much.* Due humility is essential, along with a clear grasp of how and when to prescribe appropriately – and an awareness of, and willingness to use, alternative strategies.

 Box 7.2 **Non-compliance in psychiatry**

Major causes are:

- Reluctance to accept the need for treatment.
- Lack of belief in drug efficacy.
- Concern about drug side effects, including worry about becoming 'addicted'.
- Stigma.
- Forgetfulness.
- Expense.

- As an effect of the disorder being treated – for example, a severely depressed person may feel they do not deserve to recover.

Improve compliance with medication by:

- Establishing a good therapeutic relationship.
- Explore the patient's views about their illness and its treatment. Correct any misapprehensions, but respect their views if they disagree with yours.
- Sharing of information about the evidence for (and against) the drug. Give simple, clear advice and figures – for example, 'You have a 60% chance of being a lot better after a month'. Give the patient a chance to ask questions or dispute the evidence. And ensure you discuss the risks and benefits of *not* taking the treatment. Written information about their treatment should routinely be offered to patients.

Antidepressants

Antidepressants are effective, readily available and a first-line treatment for depressive disorders. Some are also used to treat other disorders such as obsessive-compulsive disorder (OCD). The major classes are shown in Table 7.1. Selective serotonin reuptake inhibitors (SSRIs) and tricyclic antidepressants (TCAs) have similar efficacy, with about 60% of patients responding after 6 weeks. Over the same period, 30–40% respond to placebo.

- Patients often want to stop antidepressants too soon. Antidepressants usually produce some reduction in symptoms by 4–6 weeks, but it may take many months for the patient to recover fully. Continued treatment maintains the improvement in the medium term (6–9 months after getting better). Prolonged use halves the chances of relapse in those at risk.
- All antidepressants are thought to work by enhancing activity of the monoamine neurotransmitters noradrenaline (NA) and/or serotonin (5-HT; Figure 7.1a,b).
- The focus here is on the drugs; see other chapters for discussion about their use in management. Chapter 9 discusses the treatment of depression, including combination therapies and treatment resistance.

Selective serotonin reuptake inhibitors (SSRIs)

SSRIs are the usual first-line antidepressant.

- **Mode of action**. Selectively inhibit synaptic 5-HT reuptake transporters, thereby increasing synaptic 5-HT concentration (Figure 7.1a).

- **Practical usage**. Start at full dosage, once daily with breakfast. Onset of antidepressant action becomes evident in 7–14 days. However, side effects (see below) occur in the first few days – remember to warn the patient of this. Consider giving a hypnotic for the first few weeks to aid sleep. Always withdraw an SSRI slowly at the end of treatment.
- **Individual SSRIs**. There are some modest differences in properties between SSRIs. A good first choice is *sertraline* (50–100 mg/day), which is effective, well tolerated, has few interactions with other drugs, and maybe is associated with a lower incidence of sexual dysfunction. *Escitalopram* (10 mg/day) is also well tolerated although not available generically and therefore more expensive. *Fluoxetine* (20–40 mg/day) has a long half-life, so is useful if compliance is poor, and withdrawal reactions are rare (but drug interactions persist longer).
- **Side effects**. Usually well tolerated, though 15% have nausea, abdominal discomfort, diarrhoea, insomnia and agitation, mainly in the early stages. Sexual dysfunction (lack of libido, anorgasmia) is common in women and also occurs in men. SSRIs may increase the risk of upper gastrointestinal bleeding and hyponatraemia. Some people experience discontinuation symptoms (insomnia, nausea, dizziness, agitation) when stopping the drug; hence withdraw over a few weeks.
- **SSRIs and suicide**. There have been concerns that SSRIs are associated with an increase in suicidal thoughts and behaviour in the early stages of treatment, particularly in younger adults and children. Patients should always be monitored for suicide risk carefully at this time. However, this must be set against the reduction in suicide risk associated with the effective treatment of depression.
- **Overdose**. Few effects; rarely if ever fatal. Citalopram is significantly more toxic in overdose than other SSRIs.
- **Cautions and contraindications**. Few. May increase seizures in epilepsy. Coadministration with serotonergic drugs (including monoamine oxidase inhibitors (MAOIs), L-tryptophan, lithium and St John's wort) may lead to *serotonin syndrome*, a potentially life-threatening condition that includes tachycardia, shivering, sweating, hyperthermia and hyperreflexia, progressing to shock and renal failure.

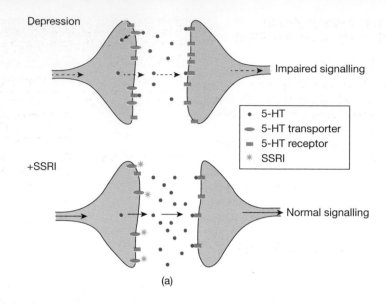

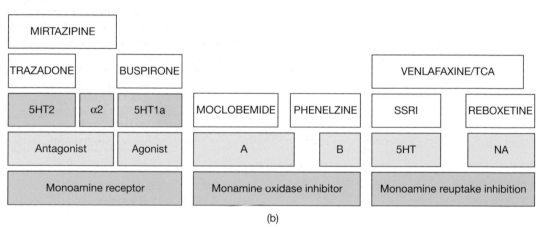

Figure 7.1 (a) A highly simplified schema for the proposed mechanism of action of selective serotonin reuptake inhibitors (SSRIs). In depression, there is thought to be a relative 5-HT deficiency, and upregulation of 5-HT receptors. The net effect is abnormal signalling and functioning of the postsynaptic neuron. SSRIs block the 5-HT transporter, and increase 5-HT in the synapse. The antidepressant effect takes several days to occur, because other adaptive changes also have to occur (to restore normal firing of the neuron, downregulate receptors, and other secondary effects). Tricyclic antidepressants (TCAs) work similarly, but act upon presynaptic receptors and noradrenergic synapses too. (b) An aide-memoire for the mechanism of action of various antidepressants. The receptors on which the antidepressants work often also give an indication of what side effects to expect.

Selective serotonin and noradrenaline reuptake inhibitors (SNRIs)

Venlafaxine (75–375 mg/day) and *duloxetine* (60 mg/day) are the only members of this group.

- **Mode of action**. SNRIs potently block 5-HT and NA reuptake but do not block cholinergic receptors.

- **Practical usage**. Venlafaxine (but not duloxetine) is slightly more effective than SSRIs. Its main indication is for SSRI non-response. Give twice daily, though a long-acting (once daily) form is available.
- **Side effects**. Resemble those of SSRIs, but may be worse. At high doses, hypertension may occur and should be monitored. Not sedative. Avoid MAOIs.

Noradrenaline and serotonin specific antidepressant (NASSA)

Mirtazapine (15–45 mg nocte).

- **Mode of action**. Increases activity in the NA and 5-HT systems by blocking the negative feedback of NA on presynaptic alpha-2 receptors. Alpha-2 blockade also enhances 5-HT release.
- **Practical usage**. Often used as a second-line treatment, and in combination with SSRIs as a third-line treatment.
- **Side effects**. Relatively sedating although this is not dose dependent. Less sexual dysfunction or nausea than SSRIs. Associated with weight gain.

Tricyclic antidepressants (TCAs)

TCAs are predominantly used for people who are intolerant of, or unresponsive to, SSRIs. They may also have slightly greater efficacy in severe depression and in chronic pain.

- **Mode of action**. Inhibit presynaptic NA and 5-HT transporters. Some TCAs are more selective for one monoamine than another – e.g. clomipramine mainly acts on 5-HT; desipramine on NA. Unlike SSRIs, TCAs block various receptors, contributing to their side-effect profile (Table 7.2).

- **Practical usage**. Usually given at night (due to their sedative action) or in divided doses. Delayed onset of action as for SSRIs. Reduction in anxiety (anxiolysis) and sedation occur rapidly. To minimize initial side effects, start at a low dose and increase over 10 days.
- **Side effects**. See Tables 7.2 and 7.3. The ability to drive and use machinery may be impaired due to drowsiness.

Table 7.2 Receptor blockade by tricyclic antidepressants (TCAs) and their associated side effects

Receptor blocked	Side effect produced
Muscarinic cholinergic	Dry mouth, urinary retention, constipation, blurred vision, glaucoma, tachycardia, delirium, sexual dysfunction
Alpha-1 adrenergic	Postural hypotension, drowsiness, sexual dysfunction
Histamine H_1	Drowsiness, weight gain
Other or unknown	Arrhythmias, seizures

Table 7.3 Side effects of conventional antipsychotics

Side effects	Comments
Common	
Extrapyramidal (EPS)	See text. Related to dopamine D_2 receptor blockade in basal ganglia
Acute dystonia	
Parkinsonism	
Akathisia	
Tardive dyskinesias	
Hyperprolactinaemia	Due to D_2 receptor blockade in the pituitary. May lead to osteoporosis in women
Galactorrhoea	
Amenorrhoea	
Sexual dysfunction	
Anticholinergic	As for TCAs, see Table 7.2
Anti-adrenergic	As for TCAs, see Table 7.2
Weight gain	Due to histamine H_1 or $5-HT_{2C}$ receptor antagonism
Rare or idiosyncratic, but severe	
Neuroleptic malignant syndrome	Dangerous, see text
Photosensitivity	Especially chlorpromazine
Cholestatic jaundice	Especially chlorpromazine
Retinal pigmentation	
Blood dyscrasias	
Seizures	
Tachyarrhythmias	
Hypothermia	

- **Individual TCAs.** *Lofepramine* is an effective TCA and generally well tolerated. *Amitriptyline* is very sedating and anxiolytic and is used at low doses for analgesia and insomnia.
- **Overdose.** Dangerous in overdose, causing tachyarrhythmias, seizures, coma and death.
- **Cautions and contraindications.** Avoid in glaucoma, prostatism, recent myocardial infarction, cardiac failure, and porphyria. Increase seizure frequency, so caution in epilepsy. Avoid combining with MAOIs.

Monoamine oxidase inhibitors (MAOIs)

MAOIs (e.g. *phenelzine* (15–90 mg/day), *tranylcypromine* (10–30 mg/day)) are third-line antidepressants; their use is limited by toxicity and inferior efficacy compared with TCAs and SSRIs.

- **Mode of action.** Prevent breakdown of monoamines in presynaptic terminals by the enzyme MAO, thereby increasing transmitter availability.
- **Uses of MAOIs.** The main indication is atypical depression (Chapter 9). Also used in treatment-resistant depression, either alone or in combination.
- **Practical usage.** Ensure the patient is aware of the necessary dietary restrictions and drug interactions (see below). Wait 2 weeks after stopping a TCA and up to 5 weeks after an SSRI (depending on the half life of the SSRI). Prescribe in divided doses.
- **Side effects.** Postural hypotension, insomnia, ankle oedema, dry mouth, dizziness, agitation and headache.
- **Overdose.** Hypertension, delirium, coma and death.
- **Cautions and contraindications.** Prescribe with caution. MAO also metabolizes tyramine, so eating tyramine-containing foods (e.g. cheese, red wine, broad beans, pickled herrings, game and Marmite) whilst on MAOIs can cause a hypertensive crisis (*'the cheese reaction'*) – headache, palpitations, fever, convulsions and coma. Such foods should be avoided. There are also dangerous interactions with many drugs, including opiates, insulin, cold remedies, antiepileptics, SSRIs and some TCAs. Avoid MAOIs in cardiac or hepatic failure or porphyria.
- **Reversible MAOIs.** Unlike classical MAOIs, *moclobemide* (300–900 mg/day) is virtually free from the cheese reaction and associated risks (because it only inhibits one form of MAO-A, and does so reversibly). It is sometimes known as a RIMA – reversible inhibitor of MAO-A.

Other antidepressants

Other antidepressants are available that do not fall readily into a specific class. None is more effective than SSRIs or TCAs, and none is widely used.

- Low-dose *trazodone* (50–100 mg at night) is a useful (non-addictive) hypnotic.
- *Reboxetine* is a selective NA reuptake inhibitor. It is non-sedating and may improve social functioning. It appears to be less effective *and* less well tolerated than SSRIs. It is often experienced as quite activating.
- *Agomelatine* is a new antidepressant: a melatonin MT_1 and MT_2 receptor agonist and $5-HT_{2C}$ receptor antagonist. Initial efficacy and tolerability data are encouraging, but its position in clinical practice remains unclear.
- *St John's wort* is an extract of the plant *Hypericum perforatum*, available without prescription and tried by many patients. It is an effective but weak antidepressant. Though a 'natural' remedy, it has side effects and drug interactions, and there are reports of toxicity. It is also an enzyme inducer and can interfere with the metabolism of other medications, e.g. the oral contraceptive pill.

Mood stabilizers

Not a pharmacological class, *mood stabilizer* is a term describing a drug used to prevent relapse in bipolar disorder. Some are also useful in the treatment of acute mood episodes. Lithium was the first and remains the standard therapy. Other mood stabilizers include antiepileptic drugs (e.g. valproate, carbamazepine and lamotrigine) and antipsychotics (e.g. olanzapine and quetiapine).

Lithium

- **Mode of action.** Uncertain, but probably acts on second messenger systems via the phosphatidylinositol and glycogen synthetase kinase 3 (GSK3) pathways.
- **Uses.** Usually given as lithium carbonate. Primary indication is relapse prevention in bipolar disorder; effective against both manic and depressive relapses; reduces risk of relapse by about 40%. Needs to be given for at least 18 months for the benefit to be clear. Also effective in acute mania (though antipsychotics work faster) and as an adjunctive treatment for depression (Chapter 9). Family history of bipolar disorder responsive to lithium predicts a good response. It is also associated with reductions in suicidal behaviour but is not indicated for specific use in this way due to its toxicity in overdose.

- **Side effects**. At therapeutic levels (0.5–1.0 mmol/L): fine tremor, metallic taste, dry mouth, thirst, mild polyuria, nausea and weight gain. Hypothyroidism occurs in 20% of women (although thyroid problems are associated with bipolar disorder independent of treatment); rarer in men. Renal impairment occasionally occurs following prolonged use.
- **Overdose**. Toxic symptoms occur above 1.5 mmol/L: coarse tremor, agitation, twitching, thirst and polyuria. Above 2.5 mmol/L: polyuric renal failure, seizures, coma and death. Toxic levels can result from mild dehydration, or with low-salt diets. Fatalities after overdose are not uncommon; survivors may be left with renal failure or brain damage.
- **Practical usage**. Before prescribing, a detailed discussion about the commitment and potential dangers is necessary. Do a physical examination, measure electrolytes, creatinine clearance, thyroid function and also perform an ECG if indicated. During treatment measure lithium levels regularly (weekly at first, then 3-monthly once stable). Titrate dose (usually 400–1200 mg/day) to keep the plasma level at 0.5–1.0 mmol/L. Test thyroid and renal function every 6 months. Withdraw gradually, in order to avoid rebound mania.
- **Cautions and contraindications**. Many. Avoid if adherence is likely to be variable or short lived. Avoid in renal failure and pregnancy. Do not combine with diuretics, angiotensin-converting enzyme (ACE) inhibitors or high-dose antipsychotics. Use cautiously with NSAIDs (non-steroidal anti-inflammatory drugs).

Valproic acid

Valproic acid (prescribed as sodium valproate or valproate semisodium) is commonly used but is less effective, and has a weaker evidence base, than lithium. It has a place when lithium is not tolerated, contraindicated or ineffective. The combination of lithium plus valproate is more effective than valproate monotherapy and, possibly, than lithium monotherapy.

- **Mode of action**. In epilepsy, works by blocking sodium channels and increasing GABA (γ-aminobutyric acid) turnover.
- **Practical usage**. Dose depends on the drug formulation. Valproate semisodium is started at 250–500 mg/day and titrated upwards every few days, depending on adverse effects. The usual maintenance dose is 750–1250 mg/day. Plasma levels can be measured, but no therapeutic range for mood stabilization has been established.

- **Side effects**. Sedation, tiredness, tremor and gastrointestinal disturbance may occur. Reversible hair loss occurs in 10% of patients. May cause thrombocytopenia.
- **Cautions and contraindications**. May increase plasma levels of other protein-bound drugs (e.g. other antiepileptics). Associated with neural tube defects – avoid in pregnancy, and use with caution in women of childbearing potential.

Carbamazepine

Carbamazepine is probably less effective than lithium or valproic acid, but may be used when these are contraindicated, ineffective or not tolerated.

- **Mode of action**. In epilepsy, works by blocking sodium channels.
- **Practical usage**. Start at low dose (200 mg twice daily (b.d.)) and build up to 600 mg b.d. Measure plasma levels if signs of toxicity (ataxia, confusion, blurred vision) emerge. Check white cell count after a week.
- **Side effects**. If erythematous rash or leucopenia occur, stop the drug. Other side effects are nausea, dizziness, drowsiness and hyponatraemia.
- **Cautions and contraindications**. Carbamazepine is a potent enzyme inducer, so other drugs will be metabolized faster – for example, the contraceptive pill. Avoid MAOIs or if there is evidence of hepatic failure, arrhythmias or pregnancy.

Lamotrigine

Lamotrigine is also an antiepileptic drug. It prevents depressive episodes. It is also probably effective in acute depressive episodes in bipolar disorder, although its use as monotherapy is limited because of the slow titration required.

- **Mode of action**. In epilepsy, blocks sodium and calcium channels, and decreases glutamate release.
- **Practical usage**. Start very gradually, initially 25 mg daily for 2 weeks then 50 g daily for 2 weeks. The usual dose in bipolar disorder is 100–300 mg daily.
- **Side effects**. A rash occurs in 3–5% of patients, requiring that the drug be stopped. The risk is reduced by a gradual increase in dose. Other side effects include nausea, headache, tremor and dizziness.
- **Cautions and contraindications**. Plasma levels are increased by valproate (so use 50% of dose). A combination of lamotrigine and carbamazepine may cause neurotoxicity.

Anxiolytics

These drugs are also known as *hypnotics* and *sedatives* if being used to help sleep. Benzodiazepines are the main class, and in the 1960s and 1970s were very widely prescribed. With increased awareness of their potential for dependency and withdrawal problems (Chapter 14), benzodiazepines have been replaced by SSRIs or TCAs as the usual drugs for anxiety. However, anxiolytics are still used as a short-term treatment.

Benzodiazepines

The former popularity of benzodiazepines is understandable: they are highly effective and relatively free of unpleasant side effects.

- **Mode of action**. Potentiate inhibitory transmission via the benzodiazepine-binding site of the GABA$_A$ receptor.
- **Uses in psychiatry**. Relief of acute anxiety and treatment of panic disorder, phobic anxiety and insomnia. Also used for delirium tremens, and to augment antipsychotics for sedation in acute psychosis.
- **Practical usage**. *Diazepam* (2–5 mg once or twice daily) is the standard anxiolytic. For intramuscular or intravenous administration use lorazepam (1–4 mg 4 hourly). *Temazepam* (20 mg) is shorter acting and used for insomnia. In the USA, *alprazolam* (250 µg three times a day) is widely used for panic disorder.
- **Side effects**. Drowsiness, 'hangover effects', headache, nausea, ataxia, dysarthria and delirium. Occasionally, disinhibition or aggression. Should not normally be prescribed for longer than 4 weeks, to prevent dependency. Withdrawal symptoms include rebound anxiety, insomnia, visual and auditory hallucinations and seizures. This is managed by switching from short-acting benzodiazepines to diazepam, and by tapering the dose over several weeks or longer.
- **Overdose**. Very rarely fatal in healthy people. *Flumazenil* can be used acutely to reverse the effects.
- **Cautions and contraindications**. The sedative effect may interfere with driving ability, especially if combined with alcohol.

Other anxiolytics

- *Propranolol* reduces the somatic symptoms of anxiety (tachycardia, tremor) but its role is limited to use in performance anxiety. Avoid in asthmatics as it can cause bronchospasm.

- *Buspirone* is a non-sedating anxiolytic, used in generalized anxiety disorder. It is said not to be addictive, and takes several days to work.
- The 'z-drugs' (*zolpidem, zopiclone* and *zaleplon*) enhance GABA transmission and are used mainly as hypnotics, claimed to produce fewer hangover effects and less tolerance than benzodiazepines, although the evidence that there are any worthwhile clinical benefits is limited. Zaleplon has a particularly short half-life.
- Low-dose TCAs also have anxiolytic and hypnotic effects – for example, *amitriptyline* (25 mg) or *trazodone* (50 mg) – and are not addictive.

Antipsychotics

Antipsychotics (also called *neuroleptics* or *major tranquillizers*) are the mainstay of treatment for schizophrenia and other psychoses.

A more important classification is into two main groups: the older, *conventional* (typical) antipsychotics, and the newer second generation (atypical) ones (Box 7.3). There are differences between them (see below) but the fundamental properties are the same for all antipsychotics:

- All antipsychotics work primarily by blocking D$_2$ dopamine receptors. This reverses the excessive dopamine activity in the mesolimbic system thought to cause the symptoms of psychosis. D$_2$ receptor blockade also contributes, along with antagonism at other receptors, to their side effects.
- Antipsychotics are effective against positive psychotic symptoms regardless of diagnosis, in about 70% of patients within 6 weeks. *Clozapine* is the only antipsychotic with a greater efficacy (see below). Onset of action is gradual, over 1–2 weeks. Antipsychotics are also used in prevention of relapse of psychosis, in delirium and in severe depression.
- There are several serious side effects (see below). Knowing how and when to explain the potential side effects is difficult if a patient is acutely psychotic. It should be done as soon as the mental state permits.
- Avoid prescribing above recommended limits, either for non-response or to produce sedation. There is no evidence of greater efficacy, no pharmacological rationale and good evidence of harm.

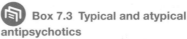 **Box 7.3 Typical and atypical antipsychotics**

The term 'atypical' was applied to *clozapine* (see below), the first antipsychotic that did not produce extrapyramidal side effects (EPS). This is the correct usage of the term: an antipsychotic that does not produce EPS at clinical doses. Since clozapine, many other antipsychotics have been marketed as atypical. However, the terminology is confusing because:

- Atypical is sometimes wrongly thought to imply greater efficacy, because clozapine also proved to be more effective than other antipsychotics. This property is not shared by other atypical antipsychotics.
- Alternative terms – which are also unsatisfactory – include '*second generation*' and '*novel*'.
- Several mechanisms have been proposed to explain 'atypicality'. One is that the drugs block D_2 receptors transiently and are sensitive to endogenous dopamine levels; another is that they also block $5\text{-}HT_{2A}$ receptors.

Side effects of conventional antipsychotics

These are many and serious (Table 7.3). Their prevalence and severity vary from one drug to another, depending on their pharmacological profile. The main features of two widely used typical antipsychotics, *haloperidol* and *chlorpromazine*, are summarized in Table 7.4.

Extrapyramidal side effects (EPS) are a major problem. EPS are motor abnormalities related to the dopaminergic receptor blockade in the basal ganglia. There are four types:

1 *Acute dystonia* – painful contractions of muscles in the neck, jaw or eyes. Young men given high doses are particularly vulnerable. Onset is within hours or days. They are treated with intramuscular or intravenous anticholinergic agents.
2 *Parkinsonism* – decreased facial movements, shuffling gait, stiffness and sometimes tremor. Common in early weeks of treatment. Managed by reducing the dose or temporarily adding an anticholinergic. Easily mistaken for depression or negative symptoms in schizophrenia.
3 *Akathisia* – a feeling of restlessness and a need to walk around. It is very unpleasant and occurs in the first months of treatment. May be mistaken for psychotic behaviour. Treat by lowering the dose or temporarily giving propranolol.
4 *Tardive dyskinesia (TD)* – uncontrollable grimacing movements of face, tongue or upper body. This is both distressing and disabling. TD occurs in about 5% of patients taking long-term antipsychotics every year. There is no way of predicting who will develop it. Neither is there any reliable treatment, and it can be irreversible.

Two other rare but life-threatening adverse effects to note are:

- *Neuroleptic malignant syndrome* (NMS). The features are pyrexia, stiffness, autonomic instability (e.g. tachycardia, fluctuating blood pressure) and seizures, leading to coma. Raised serum creatine kinase, metabolic acidosis and leucocytosis are characteristic. The incidence is about 1 in 500. It is fatal in about 10% of cases and requires urgent medical care. If a patient on an antipsychotic develops a fever without a clear cause, stop the drug temporarily and monitor. NMS can occur with any antipsychotic, especially the high potency ones (e.g. haloperidol), and following a dose increase. After an episode of NMS, restart treatment gradually, using an atypical antipsychotic, and with careful monitoring.
- Prolongation of the QTc interval on the ECG, which predisposes to a serious arrhythmia called *torsade de pointes*, has been associated with some antipsychotics, probably related to inhibition of specific cardiac potassium channels. It may explain the low but increased incidence of sudden death reportedly associated with antipsychotics.

Table 7.4 Side-effect profile of selected antipsychotics

	Typical dose (mg/day)	EPS	Prolactin elevation	Anticholinergic side effects	Sedation	Weight gain
Conventional						
Haloperidol	2–12	+++	+++	+	+	–
Chlorpromazine	50–400	++	++	++	++	++
Atypical						
Risperidone	2–8	+	++	–	–	++
Olanzapine	5–20	–	–	–	+++	+++
Clozapine	300–900	–	–	+	+++	+++

EPS, extrapyramidal side effects.

Atypical antipsychotics

Atypical antipsychotics are widely used as first-line agents instead of the conventional drugs (Table 7.5) compares to two classes of antipsychotics. Side-effect profiles that differentiate three widely used atypical antipsychotics are shown in Table 7.4.

- There is no good evidence that, as a group, atypical antipsychotics are more effective than conventional antipsychotics.
- *Risperidone* has the best long-term evidence for efficacy and, unlike other atypical antipsychotics, is available as a depot injection.
- *Olanzapine* has the next largest body of evidence for its effectiveness and may be slightly more effective than atypical agents other than clozapine; its sedative effects can be useful. Equally, it probably has a greater propensity to cause metabolic syndrome (see below).
- *Amisulpride* may have some efficacy against negative symptoms.
- *Quetiapine* is very sedating and has an increasing evidence base in the treatment of bipolar depression.
- *Aripiprazole* has a different mode of action, it is a dopamine partial agonist. This means it 'stabilizes' dopamine – antagonizing it when levels are high and mimicking it when dopamine is low.

However, atypical antipsychotics also have potential disadvantages (Table 7.5):

- *Weight gain.* This varies between drugs, and also occurs with some typical antipsychotics. Clozapine and olanzapine are the worst, with mean weight gains of about 5 kg over 6 months. A genetic polymorphism in the 5-HT$_{2C}$ receptor may contribute to individual vulnerability to weight gain.
- *Hyperglycaemia and type 2 diabetes.* There is an increased incidence of type 2 diabetes in patients with schizophrenia, their relatives, and in people taking antipsychotics. It is now known that atypical drugs (particularly olanzapine and clozapine) can induce hyperglycaemia and insulin resistance.
- The above two elements are part of *metabolic syndrome,* which also comprises dyslipidaemia and hypertension. It markedly increases risk of death from cardiovascular disease, and should be screened for before and during treatment with any antipsychotic. Various monitoring guidelines have been produced; one is summarized in Table 7.6, along with the principles of management.
- *Stroke.* Atypical antipsychotics should not be used routinely in dementia because of some

---

Table 7.5 Atypical compared with conventional antipsychotics

Advantages of atypical antipsychotics
Fewer EPS (definite)
Greater overall tolerability (probable)
Lower risk of tardive dyskinesia (probable)
Greater overall efficacy (unlikely)
More efficacy against cognitive symptoms (possible)
More efficacy against depressive symptoms (possible)
More efficacy against negative symptoms (unlikely)

Disadvantages of atypical antipsychotics
Metabolic syndrome more likely (probable)
Weight gain more likely (probable)
Type 2 diabetes mellitus more likely (possible)
Stroke more likely in the elderly (possible)

Specific advantages of clozapine
Efficacy in treatment-resistant schizophrenia (definite)
Reduced risk of suicide in schizophrenia (probable)

Specific disadvantages of clozapine
Risk of agranulocytosis
Need for regular blood tests

EPS, extrapyramidal side effects.

Table 7.6 Metabolic syndrome: monitoring and management in patients taking antipsychotics

Before treatment
History of hypertension, cardiovascular disease, diabetes, obesity
Blood pressure and pulse
Weight and height (to calculate BMI)
Waist and hip circumference (and the ratio)
Glucose and lipid levels (do not need to be fasting)
Glycosylated haemoglobin
Agree responsibilities with GP (who will monitor, who will treat)

Every clinic appointment
Weight (calculate BMI)
Waist and hip circumference (and the ratio)
Blood pressure and pulse

Every 3 months for first year, then annually
Glucose and lipid profile

Annually
Glycosylated haemoglobin

Management of abnormalities
Advice and information, e.g. on dieting, exercise
Switch to antipsychotic with less propensity to metabolic syndrome
Treat diabetes, hypertension, hyperlipidaemias in usual way

evidence that they increase the risk of stroke (Chapter 13). Caution should also be applied in all elderly patients.

Clozapine

Clozapine is a unique antipsychotic, being effective in 30% of patients with schizophrenia resistant to, or intolerant of, all other antipsychotics. Unlike in depression, treatment resistance in schizophrenia is clearly defined: it is a failure to respond to two 6-week treatment trials of antipsychotic medication (at least one of which is an atypical antipsychotic). Clozapine may also reduce suicide risk in schizophrenia.

- It is not clear how clozapine achieves its greater efficacy. It may block dopamine receptors in a different way, or it may be the particular combination of additional receptors that it blocks.
- Clozapine does not have clearly greater efficacy against negative or cognitive symptoms.

Unfortunately, clozapine causes agranulocytosis. Although rare (1–2%), it means that:

- Clozapine is reserved for patients with schizophrenia who have not responded to, or are intolerant of, at least two other antipsychotics.
- Regular (weekly) blood tests are mandatory to monitor the white cell count, and patients must be registered with a monitoring service. This means the drug often needs to be stopped if the white cell count falls; it also makes the drug expensive.
- Other important side effects of clozapine are weight gain, metabolic syndrome, hypersalivation and sedation. Seizures can occur at high dose. Plasma levels can be monitored.

Anticholinergics

These drugs (e.g. procyclidine, benztropine) are used to counteract EPS resulting from the use of antipsychotics. They have no therapeutic role in themselves.

- **Mode of action**. They block muscarinic receptors. Their use may seem paradoxical given that other side effects of antipsychotics are attributed to the same action (Table 7.3). The rationale is that they restore a dopaminergic–cholinergic balance in the basal ganglia.
- **Practical usage**. *Procyclidine* can also be given parenterally to reverse acute dystonias.
- **Side effects**. Can exacerbate psychosis and cause delirium, memory impairment and euphoria. The

anticholinergic side effects of the antipsychotic may be worsened.

- **Cautions and contraindications**. Prophylactic and long-term use, though widespread, should be avoided for three reasons: (1) the efficacy of antipsychotics is maximal at a dose below that at which EPS occur, so reducing the dose is the logical response to these side effects; (2) the long-term use of anticholinergics may increase the risk of tardive dyskinesia; and (3) anticholinergics may be misused because of the euphoric effect so it is important to establish the objective presence of EPS rather than rely on patient self-report.

Drugs for dementia

Several drugs are now licensed to treat Alzheimer's disease (Chapter 13). They have a small, beneficial effect on cognition in the short to medium term, but do not modify the course of the disease.

Cholinesterase inhibitors

Acetylcholinesterase inhibitors (e.g. donepezil, rivastigmine, galantamine) are used in the treatment of mild to moderate Alzheimer's disease.

- **Mode of action**. Inhibit the synaptic breakdown of acetylcholine, which is decreased in Alzheimer's disease and is necessary for memory and cognitive functioning. Galantamine also stimulates nicotinic cholinergic receptors.
- **Uses**. Modestly improve cognitive function. Do not modify the disease process.
- **Practical usage**. Limited to specialist clinics and require formal assessments before and during treatment, including tests of cognitive, global and behavioural functioning, and activities of daily living.
- **Side effects**. Anorexia, nausea, vomiting and diarrhoea can occur.

N-Methyl-d-aspartate (NMDA) receptor antagonists

Memantine is licensed for moderate and severe Alzheimer's disease.

- **Mode of action**. Memantine blocks the effects of glutamate at the NMDA receptor, decreasing the potential neurotoxic effects of increased glutamate that may occur in Alzheimer's disease.
- **Practical usage**. As for cholinesterase inhibitors.
- **Side effects**. Usually well tolerated but may cause dizziness, headache and hallucinations.

Drugs for substance dependence

Drugs are available to help withdrawal, maintain abstinence or control intake of various substances. The beneficial effect of these drugs is relatively modest.

Alcohol dependence

Disulfiram (Antabuse)

- **Mode of action**. Interferes with alcohol metabolism by blocking one of the enzymes involved. If alcohol is consumed, acetaldehyde accumulates, leading to flushing, headache, choking sensations, tachycardia and anxiety.
- **Uses**. As a deterrent to drinking alcohol in people motivated to use the drug.
- **Practical usage**. Usually employed in specialist practice in combination with non-drug treatments.
- **Side effects**. Sedation and nausea.
- **Cautions and contraindications**. Avoid in heart disease, suicide risk, psychosis or severe liver disease.

Acamprosate

- **Mode of action**. Unknown, probably acts via GABA and glutamate receptors.
- **Uses**. Used to reduce craving in abstinent patients.
- **Practical usage**. Used in specialist practice, in combination with other non-drug treatments.
- **Side effects**. Diarrhoea, nausea.

Opiate dependence

Opiate agonists

- **Mode of action**. *Methadone* is an opiate agonist with a half-life of around 24 hours. It is an effective substitute for other opiates such as heroin. *Buprenorphine* is a partial agonist, effective in patients with moderate dependence, but which may precipitate withdrawal in patients with severe dependence.
- **Uses**. To reduce craving and withdrawal symptoms.
- **Practical usage**. Used by specialists in combination with other medical and psychological treatments.
- **Side effects**. Drowsiness, nausea and vomiting, constipation, respiratory depression.
- **Cautions and contraindications**. Acute respiratory depression or raised intracranial pressure.

Opiate antagonists

- **Mode of action**. *Naltrexone* blocks the effects of opiates and precipitates withdrawal symptoms.
- **Uses**. To block the effect of opiates in patients after withdrawal.

- **Practical usage**. Used only in specialist clinics at a usual dose of 50 mg daily.
- **Side effects**. Nausea and vomiting.
- **Cautions and contraindications**. Do not use in patients currently dependent on opiates or with acute hepatitis or liver failure.

Prescribing in specific groups

Special care is needed when prescribing for patients who are pregnant or breastfeeding, and in children or the elderly. Many drugs are not approved for use in these groups, but nevertheless are widely used. As a rule:

- Choose a well-established drug, and the lowest possible dose.
- Consult the British National Formulary or other expert source first.
- Review the need for, and contraindications to, every drug.
- Ensure the patient (or carer) is aware of possible side effects.
- Monitor closely. If in doubt, stop drug and review.

Pregnancy

Strike a balance between the wish to avoid all drugs for the sake of the foetus, and the potential adverse effects on mother (and foetus) of leaving the psychiatric disorder untreated. Few drugs are established as completely safe in pregnancy (or when breastfeeding), so use all drugs cautiously and ensure that the mother is fully aware of the known risks and benefits, and also the uncertainties.

- *Antidepressants*. TCAs and SSRIs (and ECT) are not contraindicated. There is some evidence of an increase in the risk of congenital malformations and persistent pulmonary hypertension with SSRIs, and the use of TCAs near term may result in a 'twitchy' baby. The dose requirement increases in the third trimester.
- *Mood stabilizers*. As a rule, avoid lithium and valproic acid, especially around conception and first trimester, due to a small but clear teratogenicity risk. Use of lithium near term may result in neonatal hypothyroidism.
- *Anxiolytics and hypnotics*. These are best avoided.
- *Antipsychotics*. EPS may occur in the baby if these are taken near term.

Breastfeeding

Most drugs are excreted into the breast milk. Therefore, weigh up the need for medication against the mother's wish to breastfeed and the risks of doing so. As in pregnancy, always proceed with caution and seek expert advice.

- *Antidepressants*. TCAs (especially amitriptyline, imipramine) and SSRIs are probably safe. MAOIs are not recommended.
- *Mood stabilizers*. If lithium is used, the baby should be monitored. Carbamazepine, valproate and lamotrigine are probably safe.
- *Anxiolytics and hypnotics*. Avoid benzodiazepines as they can make the baby lethargic and cause failure to thrive.
- *Antipsychotics*. These can sedate the baby and are not recommended.

Children

The prescribing of psychotropic drugs for children is best left to child psychiatrists. See Chapter 16.

The elderly

In general, prescribe at lower doses or increased intervals to compensate for the slower metabolism and excretion in the elderly. Always consider medication as a cause of delirium (Chapter 13).

- *Antidepressants*. TCAs may cause delirium (due to their anticholinergic effects) and falls (due to postural hypotension). SSRIs are therefore preferable if sedation is not needed.

- *Mood stabilizers*. These are not contraindicated.

- *Antipsychotics*. Best avoided in dementia (see above).

- *Anxiolytics and hypnotics*. Notorious for causing delirium and falls. Avoid.

Other biological treatments

Electroconvulsive therapy (ECT)

ECT is an effective and safe treatment for severe depression although it can have some negative effects on cognitive function, especially memory. Its bad press reflects understandable fears, misinformation and its past misuse. Current guidelines are intended to ensure its use is limited, and made as safe, effective and acceptable as possible.

- **Mode of action**. Unknown. ECT has many effects in the brain. It may act on monoamines, producing the same result as antidepressants.

- **Clinical indications**. ECT has the best evidence of effectiveness in severe depression including depressive stupor and depressive psychosis. The response is often better than drug therapy and may be dramatic. It is also used for puerperal psychosis and treatment-resistant depression and mania.
- **Practical usage**. Obtain informed consent, or use the Mental Health Act (MHA). Always do a physical examination, and obtain an ECG and routine blood tests first in addition to testing cognitive function. During a brief general anaesthetic with muscle relaxant, an electric charge (~300 mC) is passed across the head to produce a generalized seizure of 30–60 seconds. Treatment can be bilateral, with one electrode on each temple, or unilateral into the non-dominant hemisphere. Bilateral ECT is slightly more effective but causes more short-term memory impairment. ECT is usually given twice a week for 6–12 treatments. A good response is predicted by a greater severity of depression, and a past response to ECT.
- **Side effects**. Anaesthetic effects – nausea, dry mouth and headache. Memory loss occurs for the hours surrounding the seizure. Significant long-term memory loss is sometimes reported by patients although overall memory often improves with the remission of depressive symptoms; objectively, subtle deficits in recall of personal memories may occur (but it is unclear if this is due to ECT or to the depressive disorder). Nonetheless, it should be discussed when obtaining consent. No neuropathological effects of ECT have been found, even following multiple treatments.
- **Cautions and contraindications**. Few, and mainly related to anaesthetic risk. Avoid if the patient has a suspected intracranial lesion (as intracranial pressure rises during seizure). ECT can be given in conjunction with antidepressants and antipsychotics. ECT is extremely safe, with a mortality rate of 5 per 100 000 treatments.

Psychosurgery

In the 1940s and 1950s – prior to the introduction of antidepressants and antipsychotics – thousands of patients each year were operated on to sever pathways between frontal lobes and limbic structures. Psychosurgery is still used very occasionally for intractable OCD and depressive disorder, but only after wide consultations under the MHA and never without informed consent. Modern stereotactic procedures avoid most of the earlier complications (haemorrhage, seizures and death).

- Recent case series suggest worthwhile improvement in one-third of patients – at the expense of some frontal lobe impairment, and with continuing ethical concerns about the principle.

Psychological treatments (the psychotherapies)

All medical treatments require an interaction between doctor and patient. This interaction is a major determinant both of the patient's satisfaction with the consultation and of their subsequent adherence to the recommended treatment. 'Psychotherapy' in the sense of a helpful relationship is consequently a part of all medical practice, whether the doctor realizes it or not. However, the term is normally applied to specific psychological treatments, the main ones being psychodynamic psychotherapy, behavioural therapy, cognitive therapy and cognitive behavioural therapy (CBT). We first consider non-specific factors common to all psychotherapies, and then the specific characteristics of each one.

Factors common to all psychotherapies

All psychotherapy is based on general or non-specific therapeutic factors. The therapist:

- Is credible and has a plausible rationale for what they do.
- Behaves in an empathic and interested fashion.
- Instils hope of improvement in the patient.

Similarly, to be successful, all forms of psychotherapy need attention to several practical issues:

- *Select the right therapy for the right patient.* Take account of factors predictive of good outcome to psychotherapy in general (e.g. motivation) as well as pros and cons of a specific therapy.
- *Prepare the patient for therapy.* Many people have either no idea, or the wrong idea, of what psychotherapy is and what it involves.
- *Ensure the therapy is available.* Many treatments are not widely available, or have long waiting lists.

The evidence base for psychotherapy

Psychotherapies have been less well evaluated than drugs, partly due to the practical difficulties of doing so and partly because of the absence of pharmaceutical industry funding for trials. However, there have now been many good randomized trials and systematic reviews, and there is good quality evidence for specific psychotherapies, especially cognitive and behavioural therapies, in several disorders, as outlined below.

Adverse effects of psychotherapy

Like all medical treatments, psychotherapy can have adverse as well as beneficial effects. These are more likely with poorly trained and unsupervised therapists and with therapists who are in a position to exploit the patient.

- Even well-delivered therapy can be ineffective or harmful. For example, it is harmful for patients who have suffered a trauma to be required to talk about it in great detail to a therapist (so-called *debriefing*).

Simple forms of psychotherapy

Simple psychotherapies are formalized versions of the therapeutic component of all doctor–patient relationships, as mentioned in Chapter 1 and at the start of this section.

- *Psychoeducation* is the provision of information to people to help them to understand and cope with the illness. Psychoeducation may take place individually or in groups, and will usually take the person's own strengths and coping strategies into account.
- *Counselling* is a loosely defined activity whereby people are helped to overcome or cope with life's problems. The counsellor serves as a support, a facilitator of emotional expression, a source of information and as someone off whom ideas can be bounced. Counselling is provided in many settings, mostly non-psychiatric. There is evidence for its short-term effectiveness in mild neuroses and stress-related disorders.
- *Supportive psychotherapy* is a formalized version of what a good friend might provide: listening, accepting and encouraging. All health professionals – as well as relatives and friends – provide supportive psychotherapy whether they realize it or not. It does not aim to produce change, but rather to help people cope with adversity or insoluble problems over a sustained period.
- *Problem-solving therapy* is a structured mix of counselling and CBT. It helps the patient learn to deal actively with life's problems – by specifying them, selecting an option for tackling each one,

trying out solutions and reviewing the effect. It is effective in mild neurotic and depressive disorders and can be given effectively by GPs and nurses.

The major types of specific psychotherapy

The major psychotherapies can be divided into two classes: those that are descendants of psychoanalysis (i.e. psychodynamic psychotherapy) and those that are based upon behavioural and cognitive theories. The key differences are highlighted in Table 7.7.

Psychodynamic psychotherapy

Psychodynamic therapy is usually a time-intensive and lengthy process that may go on for months or even years. With the arrival of the more evidence-based, briefer (and more widely available) psychotherapies outlined below, psychodynamic psychotherapy now has a lesser role, and its provision on the NHS is very limited. Nevertheless it remains important to know about its principles and its contemporary indications. Several psychodynamic concepts also remain useful throughout medicine (Box 7.4).

> ▣ **Box 7.4 Psychodynamic concepts of continuing value**
>
> - *Transference.* The feelings and attitudes a patient develops toward their therapist. They are considered to have been transferred onto the therapist from another relationship, usually that with a parent. It is important to consider transference during any doctor–patient relationship, especially if a patient starts to behave in an unexpected or unusual way (e.g. inappropriate signs of affection, or threatening self-harm if an extra appointment is not given).
> - *Counter-transference.* The feelings the therapist may develop toward the patient (e.g. excessive involvement, attraction or dislike). Counter-transference is a response to the patient's transference but is also influenced by the therapist's own past experiences and relationships. It is important for all doctors to be aware of the emotions invoked in them by patients, to try to understand their origins and ensure they do not affect their ability to treat the patient effectively.
> - Psychological *defence mechanisms* (see Table 6.2).

The principles of psychodynamic psychotherapy are:

- Emotional and interpersonal problems result from unconscious processes, driven by psychological mechanisms and internal representations (of people and things) developed early in life.
- The therapist is particularly interested in the patient's pattern of previous relationships, evidenced most directly by the way the patient interacts with the therapist (transference; Box 7.5).

Table 7.7 Comparison of the two major classes of psychotherapy

	Psychodynamic psychotherapy	Other psychotherapies
Examples	Psychoanalysis Psychodynamic therapy	Behaviour therapy Cognitive behavioural therapy
Focus	Unconscious phenomena	Observable phenomena and behaviour
Time focus	The past (as evidenced in the present)	The present
Aim	Insight and self-understanding, thence altered interpersonal behaviour	Direct, practice-driven change in behaviour and/or cognitions
Practical issues	Therapist listens and interprets Sessions unstructured	Therapist explains Sessions highly structured
Therapist	Extensive training (years) Key is therapist's skills and attributes	Briefer training (months) Key is adherence to treatment manual
Duration	Unspecified, can be prolonged (years)	Agreed number of sessions (e.g. 8)
Efficacy	Largely unknown	Proven in trials
Main indications	Difficulties with relationships Some personality disorders	Depressive disorders Neuroses and somatoform disorders Eating disorders

- The therapist makes interpretations about what the patient says, and draws connections between events and feelings, which he or she conveys to the patient.
- During therapy, the patient is expected to gain insight into their emotions and behaviour as a result of the interpretations.
- The therapeutic effect may emerge directly from greater self-understanding, and be promoted (reinforced) by new patterns of behaviour that arise from it.

Psychodynamic therapy is now used mainly for people with 'personality difficulties', especially recurrent problems with relationships. It also has a role in chronic neuroses and depressive disorders resistant to other drug and psychological treatments. It should be avoided in people with paranoid or antisocial personality disorder, and in those with psychosis.

- *Brief psychodynamic psychotherapy* compresses psychodynamically oriented therapy into a more feasible 10–20-session course. The therapist takes a more active role than in traditional psychoanalysis and focuses on particular issues. There is evidence for its efficacy in depression.

Behaviour therapy

Behaviour therapy arose from the behavioural theories of experimental psychology. The central idea is that adaptive behaviours can be learned and maladaptive behaviours unlearned. It is effective in anxiety disorders (especially phobias and OCD) and in behavioural problems in people with learning disability.

Exposure is a key component of behavioural treatment. Either the patient is reintroduced (re-exposed) to a situation or behaviour they have come to avoid (e.g. an agoraphobic leaving the house), or they learn to stop an inappropriate, excessive response (e.g. recurrent hand washing in OCD). Exposure is usually graded (graded exposure).

- Sudden and prolonged exposure (*flooding*) – such as shutting a claustrophobic in a lift until the panic subsides – also works, but is too unpleasant for routine use.

The elements of graded exposure are:

- The therapist assesses the problem behaviour, its antecedents and consequences. She or he explains the nature of the treatment and its rationale to the patient.

- A step-by-step programme is developed jointly with the patient. Homework tasks are set which re-expose the patient to the situation to a degree that produces a tolerable level of anxiety. The patient finds that each extra exposure increases anxiety, but that it then subsides. In this way the patient is desensitized to the stimulus.
- Subsequent sessions review progress and problems, and set the next series of tasks.

 Clinical scenario

Mr Q had not been out of his house for 2 years, fearful he might faint in the street. His therapist elicited a detailed account of the problem, how it started and its effect on Mr Q. She explained what behavioural treatment was and how it worked. She agreed a plan with Mr Q to do a task he felt he could just manage: to walk to his front gate and stand there for 20 minutes. He felt anxious doing so, but achieved this goal several times in homework sessions. He found that as he stood there the anxiety subsided. He was then encouraged to move to the next steps by walking increasing distances from his house. He was able to do the shopping again, which reinforced his feeling of success. During the agreed 12 sessions he made steady progress that was maintained thereafter.

Many other treatments and techniques are based on the premise that changing behaviour and other bodily functions, such as muscular tone and posture, helps mental well-being. They include relaxation training, assertiveness training, biofeedback and social skills training. They are available in occupational therapy and physiotherapy departments, from private therapists and by using self-help manuals.

Cognitive therapy

The aim of cognitive therapy is to correct inaccurate or unhelpful ways of thinking, with the aim of improving mood, reducing anxiety and allowing return to normal behaviour. The main components are:

- The therapist obtains a detailed description of the problem, paying particular attention to the thoughts (cognitions) the patient has when experiencing the problem.
- The therapist provides an explanation (formulation) of the role of cognitions in perpetuating the problem to the patient.
- The patient is then taught how to become aware of and to challenge the negative and inaccurate

cognitions and to practise thinking in more accurate and helpful ways.

- The therapeutic techniques include education about the role of cognitions and their consequences on emotion and behaviour; becoming more aware of the occurrence of particular thoughts and inferences using diaries; and doing 'experiments' to test cognitions against alternatives.

 Clinical scenario

Ms R had a depressive disorder. Her therapist helped her identify a number of negative cognitions that made her feel depressed (including 'nobody likes me' and 'there's no point trying to change anything, it won't help'). The therapist formulated the depression as being maintained by the effect of these cognitions on her mood and behaviour. He helped Ms R become aware of the distorted and negative slant to her cognitions. Ms R was helped to make alternative cognitions ('not everybody likes me but I have evidence that some people do' and 'some things probably will help and if I don't try I won't find out') and practised challenging the thoughts and replacing them with more positive ones. She became skilled at doing this and her mood and activity improved. At follow-up a year later she remained well, and was using the techniques she had learned whenever she felt negative cognitions or low mood creeping back.

Cognitive behavioural therapy (CBT)

In practice, cognitive and behavioural treatments are usually combined as CBT. In phobic anxiety, for example, this would involve working both on cognitions and on graded exposure. There is good evidence for the efficacy of CBT (with varying proportions of C and B) in many disorders:

- In mild to moderate depressive disorder, CBT is at least as effective as antidepressant drugs.
- In panic disorder and phobic anxiety, CBT is probably the most effective treatment; the benefits are more persistent than with anxiolytics, and avoid the problems of the latter.
- There is good evidence of efficacy in other neuroses, including somatoform disorders and OCD.
- A modified form of CBT is the most effective treatment in bulimia nervosa.
- CBT has some effect against psychotic symptoms in schizophrenia.
- There is inconsistent evidence that CBT prevents relapse in bipolar disorder.

Other psychotherapies

Hybrid therapies

The distinction between the two major types of therapy in Table 7.7 is oversimplified and there are several hybrid therapies (Figure 7.2), and other therapies that have additional components. None is widely available in the UK.

- *Cognitive analytical therapy* (CAT) combines a cognitive approach and psychoanalytic concepts. It is used in depression and other conditions.
- *Interpersonal therapy* (IPT) uses cognitive, behavioural and psychodynamic concepts and techniques to focus on the patient's relationships and the problems arising from them. Limited evidence suggests similar efficacy to CBT in depression and bulimia nervosa.
- *Dialectical behavioural therapy* (DBT) was developed specifically for people with borderline personality disorder. It combines psychoeducation with behavioural skills training, creating a strong therapeutic relationship.
- *Eye movement desensitization and reprocessing* (EMDR) is used in people with post-traumatic stress disorder. Mentalisation based therapy is used for people with borderline personality disorder. It helps people to understand that thoughts and feelings relate to mental states not just in themselves but also in others.

Group therapy

Many of the psychotherapies have been adapted to treat several people at once. Group therapy originated from the view that it is therapeutic to share experiences and feelings, and to examine the relationships that form in a group.

- Most therapies including CBT can be given effectively in a group format for the same indications as individual therapy. Some patients like groups but others don't.

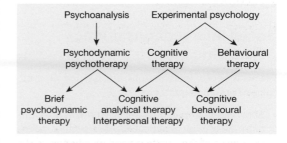

Figure 7.2 Links between the psychotherapies.

- A therapeutic community is a form of psycho-dynamic group therapy where the participants are resident for 6–12 months. It is mainly used in attempts to treat personality disorder.

Family therapy

Family therapy is based upon the theory that the problem is located in the family rather than in the (child) patient. The family 'system' is therefore the therapeutic target. Psychodynamic, behavioural and other concepts are used. There is some evidence for its efficacy in children with conduct disorder, substance misuse, eating disorders, schizophrenia and bipolar disorder.

Social treatments

Social factors have major roles in the aetiology and maintenance of many psychiatric disorders. Social factors also determine the environment in which therapy is given and affect its outcome. Equally, social treatments – intervening to change some aspect of the person's circumstances – are themselves important therapeutic interventions.

Acute social interventions

- *Psychiatric admission* is a major social intervention. In general admission is reserved for those for whom community treatment is no longer feasible because the risk to themselves or others is too great or if there is a risk of ongoing deterioration in their health. Admission can be traumatic for patients particularly if it involves detention under the Mental Health Act (see Chapter 19). In all instances the least restrictive means of providing treatment should be sought.
- *Crisis* intervention is provided by specialist teams who provide home treatment and support in order to prevent admission to hospital. They provide intensive input to patients in the community, including brief psychological interventions, medication, home visits and telephone support.

Social interventions during psychiatric care

Practical social interventions are needed at some stage in most patients' care.

- Accommodation and financial problems are common. Help with practical matters such as housing, rescheduling debts, etc. can be therapeutic by reducing the stressors that are maintaining the disorder. Increasingly this form of support is provided by voluntary organizations such as the Citizens' Advice Bureau.
- Family support and education can be an important part of care, even if specific family therapy is not being carried out.
- Social isolation is often a problem for people with psychiatric illness. This can be addressed by home visits, attendance at day centres, putting the person in touch with self-help groups, etc.
- In chronic psychiatric disorder, social and occupational skills and self-confidence are often damaged. Rehabilitation involves continuing support of the kinds outlined above, as well as more extensive interventions such as sheltered accommodation and supported employment.

The wider social environment

Preventing domestic violence, child abuse and unemployment would no doubt improve the psychological well-being of the population. Whilst such utopian ('primary prevention') goals are not relevant for the management of individual patients, there are measures that can affect their prevalence or impact:

- *Public education.* To increase awareness of psychiatric disorders, and decrease the stigma attached to them and to their treatment.
- *Social policy.* Political decisions alter the social fabric and influence behaviours associated with psychiatric disorder. For example, taxation affects alcohol consumption, and legislation determines the extent of compulsory treatment. Some events are, however, beyond control – for example, the effect of national football results on rates of self-harm.

⚷ KEYPOINTS

- Psychiatric disorders are treated with drugs (psychopharmacology) and/or psychological methods (psychotherapy). Social interventions are also important.

- The choice of treatment depends upon the diagnosis and on other contextual factors, including the patient's preference and history, and treatment availability.

- There is good evidence for the efficacy of most commonly used drugs, but all also have limitations and side effects. CBT is of proven benefit for several disorders but has limited availability.

- Involve patients fully in treatment decisions.

FURTHER READING

Anderson I, Reid IC (2006) *Fundamentals of Clinical Psychopharmacology.* Informa Healthcare.

Stahl SM (2011) *The Prescriber's Guide (Stahl's Essential Psychopharmacology),* 4th edn. Cambridge University Press.

Taylor D, Paton C, Kapur S (2011) *The Maudsley Prescribing Guidelines in Psychiatry,* 11th edn. Wiley-Blackwell.

? SELF-ASSESSMENT

1 An 18-year-old boy presents with auditory hallucinations and believes there is a conspiracy to have him murdered. He is, however, eating and drinking sufficiently and feels safe with his parents. You diagnose a first episode of psychosis (schizophrenia). What would be your first line of treatment?

a Olanzapine

b Clozapine

c ECT

d Referral for CBT

e Lithium

2 A 72-year-old lady has become severely depressed after the death of her husband. She believes her body is rotting away. She has stopped eating and drinking and is becoming very frail. What would be your preferred treatment modality?

a Olanzapine

b Clozapine

c ECT

d Referral for CBT

e an SSRI antidepressant

3 A 28-year-old office-based secretary finds herself becoming increasingly anxious about leaving home. She worries about fainting and 'making a fool' of herself in crowds. She has panic attacks when she tries to leave the house. What would be the preferred treatment?

a Benzodiazepines

b Olanzapine

c Referral for CBT

d ECT

e an SSRI antidepressant

8

Psychiatric services and specialties

Learning objectives

✓ To be able to describe the various psychiatric subspecialties and services available to patients and the roles of individuals within the patient's care team

---

This chapter covers how psychiatric services are organized in the NHS. It is via these services that the treatments discussed in this book are delivered. It then describes the main features of the various psychiatric specialties.

- Psychiatrists see only a small (and rather unrepresentative) fraction of all people suffering from psychiatric disorders, and the services provided are 'biased' accordingly. In particular, the perspective from general practice – where most patients with psychiatric needs are managed – is very different. This issue is covered in Chapter 18.
- Service organization and service delivery in psychiatry vary markedly from one healthcare system to another. As with mental health legislation, there are also some differences within the NHS between England and Wales, Scotland and Northern Ireland.

Organization of psychiatric services

Trends in service delivery and organization

Over the past 30 years, psychiatric services have progressively moved out of psychiatric hospitals (asylums) to the other settings shown in Figure 8.1. The shift of psychiatry to the community has occurred for several reasons:

- The community is where psychiatric disorders present, and provides their context.
- Public preference and social attitudes.
- In-patient care is sometimes unnecessary and may sometimes be harmful.
- Economic and political pressures.

Despite these trends, in-patient care remains an important component of psychiatry for several groups:

- Assessment of suspected severe psychiatric disorder.
- Those at significant risk of suicide.
- 'Asylum' for those in crisis.
- Those who may be dangerous to others as a result of psychiatric disorder.
- Treatment of acute schizophrenia, mania and severe depression.
- Longer term care of some patients with dementia, chronic schizophrenia and learning disability.

As the number of psychiatric hospital beds has fallen, the threshold for admission has risen and an increasing percentage of in-patients are psychotic, disturbed and detained compulsorily. This is especially true in inner cities, and has stimulated efforts

---

Psychiatry Lecture Notes, Eleventh Edition. Gautam Gulati, Mary-Ellen Lynall and Kate Saunders. © 2014 John Wiley & Sons, Ltd. Published 2014 by John Wiley & Sons, Ltd.

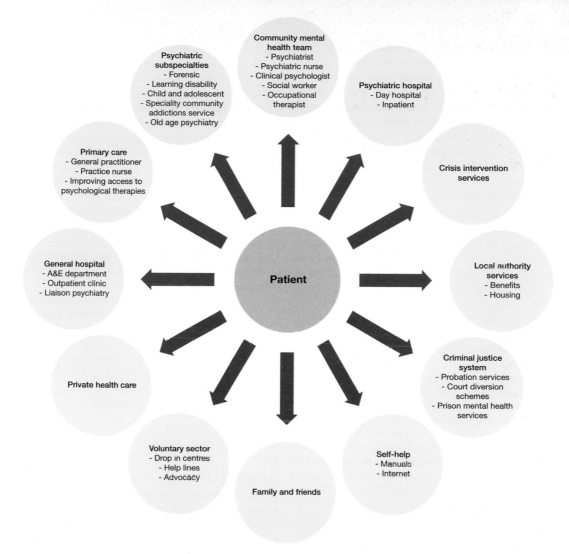

Figure 8.1 Psychiatric services.

to ease the pressure on in-patient facilities. Research suggests that admission can be avoided in approximately 40% of cases by using day hospitals or 'crisis teams'. Crisis teams are generally available 24 hours a day, 7 days a week. They comprise a variety of mental health professionals (psychiatrists, community psychiatric nurses, social workers, etc.) and provide short-term, intensive packages of care to patients in the community, avoiding the need for admission.

Making the move from hospital to community-based care has posed problems and has led to a gap between the intention and reality of community care:

- Hospital services have been removed before community services are fully in place.
- Community care is not in fact a cheap option, and has been under-resourced.
- A considerable burden is placed upon relatives and carers.
- It is difficult to provide care for some groups of people – the homeless, those with complex psychiatric and social problems, and those whose illness interferes with adherence to treatment.

Community care

Logically, this term should refer to the management of all psychiatric problems outside a hospital setting; numerically this would mainly comprise common psychiatric conditions (depression, anxiety, etc.) managed by GPs. Usually, however, community care means care *within psychiatric services* – patients who tend to be more severely and chronically ill, especially with schizophrenia, severe mood disorder and comorbid conditions.

The main features of contemporary community care in psychiatry are:

- Psychiatric problems are managed at the patient's home, in GP surgeries or in local mental health centres. To facilitate this, the psychiatrists usually divide their responsibility into geographical sectors.
- Care is usually provided by a *community mental health team* (CMHT; see below).
- Management includes social interventions as well as drug and psychological treatments.
- Admission is reserved for severe episodes of illness and crises.
- Most patients are treated with their consent. A few need some form of legal coercion, under the Mental Health Act (or similar legislation in other jurisdictions, see Chapter 19).

Multidisciplinary teams

As psychiatry has moved into the community, there is a trend towards the specialty becoming less 'medically dominated'. Some psychiatrists now work as members of multidisciplinary CMHTs, as one of many 'mental health professionals'. However, it remains the role of the psychiatrist to provide leadership to the clinical team. The psychiatrist's particular roles in the team generally centre on making diagnoses, prescribing medication, the use of the Mental Health Act (although psychiatrists are no longer necessarily the 'Responsible Clinician'), taking medico-legal responsibility and acting in a supervisory role to other members of the clinical team.

The other members of multidisciplinary teams usually comprise:

- *Community psychiatric nurses* (CPNs). CPNs perform much of the day-to-day psychiatric work of the CMHT. CPNs are often the designated *key worker* (see below); they do many of the initial and follow-up assessments and they give medication. Some have additional therapeutic skills (e.g. in CBT) and are called *nurse practitioners*.
- Social services departments have statutory responsibilities affecting psychiatric patients, which *social workers* attached to the team fulfil. For example, the social worker takes the lead role in assessing social circumstances and arranging accommodation, helping with benefits, etc. Some social workers are Approved Mental Health Professionals, with particular roles under the Mental Health Act.
- *Secretary/administrator.* Teams generate a lot of paperwork and its members are often out and about. A central person who handles the administration, takes messages and arranges meetings is therefore a key figure.
- *Clinical psychologist.* Many teams have a clinical psychologist, who helps in assessments and in providing psychological treatments.
- *Other team members* may include occupational therapists, support workers, accommodation officers, befrienders, etc.
- *Voluntary organizations* and *self-help groups*, though not formally part of the CMHT, provide important additional sources of support and help for many people – including those with needs but who are not receiving formal psychiatric care.

The key worker

Every patient under the care of more than one member of a multidisciplinary team has a *key worker* (the actual term used may vary) who:

- is usually a CPN or social worker;
- coordinates and administers treatment;
- knows about local resources and how to access them;
- liaises with the GP and other agencies;
- assists in planning and monitoring of the care package, usually as part of the *care programme approach* (CPA; see below);
- informs others of changes in the patient's mental state or needs.

The Care Programme Approach (CPA)

The way in which adult mental health services are delivered in the community varies markedly between countries, due to differences in the structure of health and social care services, and the relationship between them. It is also subject to rapid changes in policy, emphasis and terminology.

Since 1991 the specified model for community psychiatric care in the United Kingdom has been the CPA. The aim of the CPA was to improve and standardize the planning and provision of care for psychiatric patients. The key aspects of CPA are that:

- It starts with a detailed assessment. This covers psychiatric, medical and social needs, and assessment of risk to self and others.
- A key worker is assigned.
- A *care plan* records the identified needs, how they will be tackled and by whom. The care plan is drawn up in consultation with the patient and nearest relative. Both get a copy, as do all the professionals involved.
- Progress of the case is monitored by the key worker, who reports regularly back to the CMHT.
- Formal 'CPA meetings' are held to review and plan care, usually 6-monthly. The meetings involve all people/agencies involved in the case, together with the patient, and carers or significant others who the patient wishes to be present. The record of the meeting, and decisions made is then sent to all parties.
- All patients have a right to refuse CPA, unless detained under the Mental Health Act.

Until 2008, CPA applied to all patients. Now it has been restricted to those with a wide range of needs from a number of services, or who are at most risk. Ultimately this has made little difference in practice.

- Regardless of whether the CPA 'badge' is in use, the principles of good communication within the CMHT, inclusion of the patient and their significant others in care decisions, and careful assessment of the patient's medical and social needs, should always be applied.

Other services

Assertive outreach is another form of community care 'package', with smaller caseloads per staff member and more intensive support than the usual CMHT. According to research Assertive Outreach Teams have little effect on in-patient admissions but are significantly better than CMHT care in maintaining engagement with difficult-to-reach patients.

Early Intervention is a service designed for patients in the first episode of a psychotic illness, or those at high risk of developing psychosis. These services normally work with patients for a fixed period of time (e.g. 3 years) before handing care over to another agency (e.g. CMHT or GP). There is some evidence that Early Intervention Services can reduce length of admission, number of relapses and suicide.

Psychiatric specialties

Psychiatric subspecialties are delineated by the patients' age and/or the type of disorder:

- General adult psychiatry
- Psychiatry of old age (psychogeriatrics)
- Child and adolescent psychiatry
- Liaison psychiatry (psychological medicine)
- Substance abuse
- Forensic psychiatry
- Learning disability

The main elements and distinguishing features of each specialty are now described. Most of the main features of service organization noted above (e.g. move to community care, CMHTs, etc.) are common across the various specialties.

General adult psychiatry

Adults with psychiatric disorders are looked after by general adult psychiatrists unless their problems come into the domain of another subspecialty, and their care is transferred to it. The precise boundaries of general psychiatry will depend on the availability of specialist services. Schizophrenia and other psychoses have traditionally been the focus of most general psychiatry services. Although this remains the case, general adult psychiatrists increasingly work in partnership with primary care, and assist GPs in the management of patients with the more common psychiatric disorders.

 Clinical scenario

Ms D is 27 and has been admitted informally with schizophrenia. At the ward round, Rob, a CPN from the CMHT, agrees to be her key worker. Ms D has been made homeless and unemployed and remains vulnerable to abuse and neglect. Rob liaises with the social worker and sorts out financial arrangements and accommodation in a group home, and, with her consent, contacts Ms D's parents with whom she had lost touch. A pre-discharge CPA meeting is held, at which all professionals, Ms D, and her parents are present. After discharge, Rob visits weekly, giving Ms D her depot medication and monitoring her mental state. The psychiatrist sees Ms D every 3 months or whenever there is cause for concern. An exacerbation of her illness is managed at home with support and increased medication. Rob begins therapy with Ms D's family, who are supportive but have become over-involved. However, Ms D relapses and is found wandering the street in a state of neglect. She is detained under Section 3 of the Mental Health Act. When almost ready for discharge, a CPA meeting plans her future care.

Psychiatry of old age (psychogeriatrics)

Most old-age psychiatrists deal with the whole range of psychiatric disorder in the elderly and not just dementia.

- Concurrent medical problems and medications affect the presentation and management of psychiatric disorders. For example, constipation is common in the elderly and is therefore a less useful diagnostic sign for depression; it may also produce delirium and may limit the dose of antidepressant that can be given.
- Psychiatrists in old-age CMHTs have close ties with both geriatric medicine and social services. This is necessary given the prevalence and nature of dementia and the frequency of associated physical and social problems of the elderly mentally ill.

 Clinical scenario

Mr A is 75 and has become forgetful. He lives with his healthy wife. A domiciliary visit revealed cognitive impairment and depressive symptoms. A trial of antidepressants did not help, and his cognitive impairment has got worse. Routine investigations were negative and you diagnose probable Alzheimer's disease. An occupational therapist visits to assess his daily living skills. His wife can care for him with help from 'meals on wheels' and visits from a CPN. You liaise with the GP regarding Mr A's leg ulcers (which make him delirious when infected); the GP prescribes antibiotics and contacts a district nurse. Two years later Mr A has become severely demented and aggressive, seemingly in response to hallucinations. His wife is not coping. The psychologist gives advice about managing his behaviour, which settles with this. You help his wife by organizing day care and a 2-week respite admission for him. The next year she dies. Mr A is admitted to a nursing home. A social worker sorts out the finances. Six months later Mr A breaks his hip. After discussion with his son, conservative management is agreed on. Mr A is kept comfortable in the nursing home and dies the next day.

Child and adolescent psychiatry

Children's psychiatric problems differ in important respects from those of adults, and the approach to their assessment and management is also different (Chapter 16).

- A child psychiatrist requires a detailed understanding of physical and psychological development. Some are also trained in paediatrics.
- The first referral to child psychiatric services may come from the GP, paediatrician or school educational psychologist.
- A child psychiatry team includes specialized social workers, nurses and psychologists. Some of the team may concentrate upon family therapy.
- On the rare occasions when in-patient care is needed, other members of the family may be admitted too, to help in evaluation. The in-patient team includes teachers who assess the child's problems in an educational setting, as well as continuing the child's education whilst in hospital.

Clinical scenario

L is a 15-year-old girl who has previously been known to community child and adolescent mental health services. She has a 2-year history of an eating disorder, and has lost a lot of weight in the last 3 months. She has a long history of self-harm and has taken six non-lethal overdoses of paracetamol in the last few months. In addition she reports the development of depressive symptoms. She was subject to sexual abuse at the hands of a teacher at primary school. She lives with her parents and younger sister, who report that they are finding it hard to cope at home and fear for L's safety. After discussion with her family, CPN and other members of the clinical team it is agreed to admit L informally to the adolescent unit for further assessment and treatment. She attempts to abscond on the second day of her admission and is found to have made a noose from her bedding. A Mental Health Act assessment is arranged and she is subsequently detained in hospital under Section 2. She undergoes some family therapy sessions with her parents and sister and an experienced psychologist and is treated with antidepressant medication. There is also input from a dietician. Her Section 2 is converted to a Section 3 (for treatment) after 3 weeks. Her weight returns to the normal range and her depressive symptoms gradually remit, as do her self-harming and suicidal ideation. She is eventually discharged back to her family home after a 3-month admission.

Liaison psychiatry (psychological medicine)

Liaison means link, and liaison psychiatrists provide an important link between psychiatric services and medical and surgical services. Such linking services are often referred to as departments of psychological medicine. They are usually based in general hospitals and are principally concerned with three patient groups:

- People who present to A&E having self-harmed. Some hospitals have trained counsellors to carry out screening of all self-harm patients; elsewhere it is left to the medical or nursing staff to decide when to refer to a psychiatrist.
- Patients whose doctors suspect they have a psychiatric problem (such as delirium, depression or substance misuse) contributing to, arising from or complicating their medical disorder.
- Patients whose somatic symptoms are unexplained by demonstrable medical disease.

Liaison psychiatrists offer specialist opinions on these patient groups; they may then offer treatment themselves, or refer on to other local psychiatric services.

 Clinical scenario

You are asked to see Mr B in A&E. He is 49 and has taken an overdose. He is not suicidal but does have depressive and anxiety symptoms. You suspect he has an adjustment reaction after recent life events. You offer him an appointment next week, give him a number to call if he feels the urge to self-harm again, and phone his GP. On review, the severity of depression becomes clearer. He starts antidepressants. You discuss the case with the local CMHT who take over his care. Six months later you are called to see him on a surgical ward where he is awaiting a cholecystectomy. The houseman discovers his psychiatric history and wants your opinion on his mental state. Mr B is fine, but you note that his antidepressant (a monoamine oxidase inhibitor) may interact with analgesics. You alert the anaesthetist.

Substance abuse psychiatry

Abuse of alcohol and drugs leads to a wide range of psychiatric disorders and related problems (Chapter 14), which are dealt with by this subspecialty (also known as *specialist community addictions service*). Increasingly they work in conjunction with CMHTs (e.g. in patients with dual diagnoses of mental illness and substance abuse) and other organizations (e.g. charities offering psychosocial interventions). The workload comprises:

- Management of psychiatric disorder resulting from alcohol or drug abuse.
- Management of the psychological and social consequences of substance misuse. Many people have complex and multiple needs that both cause and result from their substance abuse.
- In-patient care for detoxification (in some units).
- Outpatient maintenance and detoxification prescribing (e.g. methadone) and prescription of other medications linked to substance abuse (e.g. disulfiram and acamprosate in alcohol abusers).
- Advice and support for people wanting to stop abusing drugs or alcohol.
- Advice to other doctors managing patients in whom substance abuse may be a factor.
- Public education and local health initiatives about the dangers of drug and alcohol abuse.

Counsellors and outreach workers play important roles in this specialty in addition to the CPNs and social workers. Considerable efforts are made to make contact with people with drug or alcohol problems who are unwilling to attend a medical setting. Cooperation with physicians is important because of the medical problems that often coexist.

 Clinical scenario

Mr C presented to the emergency department having suffered a seizure. While in hospital, he became agitated and confused and was diagnosed with delirium tremens (due to alcohol withdrawal). After his recovery, a liaison psychiatrist referred him to the drug and alcohol clinic. You take a history and discuss his medical condition with his GP. He is given information about alcohol and introduced to a CPN who will visit regularly to review progress and give support. A social worker investigates his benefit problems and contacts his ex-wife about access to his children. Mr C does not want medication to help him abstain. Things go well until he loses his job. He starts to drink heavily and drops out of care. He turns up later wanting admission for detoxification. Needle marks are noticed. He admits to injecting heroin and is found to be hepatitis B positive. He again cuts down his alcohol and denies taking other drugs thereafter. He gets a new job and his wife returns to him. He has had no relapse when seen a year later.

Forensic psychiatry

Forensic means 'of the courts'. All psychiatrists become involved in forensic issues for various reasons:

- Writing psychiatric court reports or attending court on behalf of a patient.
- Assessment of local offenders/prisoners with suspected psychiatric disorder. Court diversion schemes are being developed to reduce the delay such people experience before receiving psychiatric help.
- A forensic history (e.g. of assault) may affect management decisions even if not directly related to current psychiatric problems.

Forensic psychiatrists concentrate on work in three areas:

- Psychiatric assessment of persons charged with serious crimes.
- Providing treatment for convicted prisoners with a psychiatric disorder. This includes running psychiatric care in Regional Secure Units and the Special Hospitals (e.g. Broadmoor).
- Giving advice to other psychiatrists encountering forensic issues – for example, when assessing dangerousness.

In practice, the decision as to when a patient with a 'forensic history' should be transferred to the forensic psychiatric services depends on the crime, the likelihood of recidivism, the nature of mental disorder and the availability of resources.

 Clinical scenario

Mr R is a 30-year-old gentleman. He has a history of paranoid schizophrenia and substance misuse and has been under the care of local CHMT and community addictions service. He has been remanded into custody on suspicion of attempted murder having stabbed a fellow resident at his shared accommodation. You have been asked to see him by a CPN from the Prison Mental Health Inreach team, who has concerns about Mr R's mental state. Mr R reports that he stopped taking his oral antipsychotic medication 2 weeks prior to the stabbing. In prison he presents as floridly psychotic and has refused all oral medication in prison as he believes staff are trying to poison him. He is aggressive towards prison staff. You decide to transfer him urgently to his local medium secure unit under the Mental Health Act for further assessment. Given the severe nature of Mr R's mental illness he is felt suitable for a Hospital Order with Restrictions

at time of sentencing. He spends 3 years in a secure hospital and undergoes psychological intervention targeted at previous violence, substance abuse and relapse prevention alongside holistic rehabilitation. He is prescribed a depot antipsychotic and is eventually discharged to semi-supported accommodation under the care of the community forensic mental health team.

Learning (intellectual) disability psychiatry

The definition of a learning (or intellectual) disability is an IQ below 70 with difficulties in adaptive functioning. The difficulties must have occurred before the age of 18.

Learning Disability (LD) services have a range of patients with a variety of IQs from mild (IQ 55–70) to profound (IQ less than 20). There is usually a separate team that cares for those up to 18 years of age followed by 'transition' into adult services. LD services tend to be 'lifelong' services caring for those with LD into old age.

Specialist services are required due to:

- Differences in presentation of psychiatric conditions, especially in those with lower IQs.
- The high rates of sensitivities those with LD have to psychiatric medications and the high rate of polypharmacy for a variety of conditions.
- The high incidences of those with autistic spectrum disorders.
- The high incidence of epilepsy.
- Physical conditions that can occur with certain genetic syndromes as well as 'behavioural phenotypes'.
- Safeguarding issues around vulnerable patients.
- The close relationship necessary between social services and psychiatric services.

Part of the role of the LD team is to advocate and educate in the area of LD. It is often necessary to liaise with other health teams when, for example, the patient is admitted as an in-patient to a general hospital. The Mental Capacity Act is used on a daily basis, and LD psychiatrists are often asked to assist in completing assessments for everything from capacity to consent to complicated medical procedures to capacity to consent to marriage.

 Clinical scenario

Mr C is a 30-year-old man with a moderate LD (IQ of 50) who communicates using makaton. He lives in a supported living house with three other residents. He has no psychiatric history. Carers who have known him for 10 years report occasional episodes where Mr C becomes agitated and aggressive. He hits anyone who comes close to him during these episodes but does not target anyone in particular. After a period of about 30 minutes, this behaviour resolves. Mr C is seen by a psychiatrist from the Learning Disabilities team, who requests an EEG, which shows epileptic activity. He is treated with sodium valproate and the episodes do not recur.

Groups with special psychiatric needs

Because of their circumstances, several groups have particular psychiatric needs, or are more likely to have needs unmet by the services.

The homeless

Difficulties

- Multiple social and medical needs
- High prevalence of psychiatric disorder, especially schizophrenia and substance misuse
- Lack of a supportive network – family, friends, GP
- Hard to engage in treatment and follow-up

Solutions

- Flexible CMHT care packages
- Outreach workers
- Realistic goals

Ethnic minorities

Difficulties

- Psychiatric disorder harder to diagnose because of cultural differences in presentation
- Language barrier
- Concerns about racial prejudice and stigmatization
- Increased rates of some psychiatric disorders

Solutions

- Awareness of cultural differences in how psychiatric disorders present, and of their social significance in different cultural groups
- Trained interpreters
- Staff reflect the ethnic make-up of the community

People with psychiatric comorbidity (multiple psychiatric diagnoses)

Difficulties

- Worsens prognosis
- Hampers management
- Increases risk of violence (especially the combination of psychosis, substance misuse and personality disorder)

Solutions

- Recognition
- Extra resources
- Prioritize management plans – target major and solvable problems

Healthcare workers

Difficulties

- Reluctance to admit to psychiatric problems
- May knowingly mislead or conceal symptoms
- Increased risk of alcohol abuse and suicide
- Hard to maintain confidentiality
- Blurring of boundaries between being a colleague and being a patient

Solutions

- Confidential, publicized, accessible local arrangements
- For UK doctors, the National Counselling Service for Sick Doctors (0870 241 0535)

Prisoners

The prison as an alternative setting bears specific mention due to a high degree of psychiatric morbidity. There are an estimated 80–85 000 prisoners in the United Kingdom. When compared to the general population, the prison population is significantly more likely to have psychosis, major depression, and is approximately ten times more likely to have antisocial personality disorder. Despite the high incidence and prevalence of psychiatric disorders within the prison population, management of these disorders has been a cause for concern, with many cases of mental ill health going undetected and untreated. Prison Mental Health Inreach teams were established about 9 years ago with the aim of improving prisoners' health. These Inreach teams work with prisoners, prison officers and prison GPs to diagnose and treat mental disorders in the prison population. Their core functions also involve linking with agencies leading up to the prisoner's release so as to ensure continuity of care. The Mental Health Act is not applicable within the prison setting in England and Wales, and prisoners therefore need to be transferred to hospital if they are ill and in need of compulsory treatment.

 KEYPOINTS

- Most psychiatric patients are treated in the community. Care is delivered by a community mental health team (CMHT).
- In a CMHT, the psychiatrist works with psychiatric nurses, social workers and other disciplines.

- Psychiatric admission is reserved for cases where there is known or suspected severe psychiatric disorder coupled with a significant risk of harm to self or others.
- A variety of subspecialty services address specific aspects of psychiatric need.
- Most psychiatric disorders are managed not in specialist care, but in general practice.

 FURTHER READING

A useful web-based resource by for psychiatric subspecialties can be accessed at the website of the Royal College of Psychiatrists: www.rcpsych.ac.uk

? SELF-ASSESSMENT

1 Which of the following services (a–e) would be most appropriate for the three cases (i–iii) detailed below?
 a Standard Community Mental Health Team
 b Assertive Outreach Team
 c Primary Care Psychological Intervention
 d Forensic Psychiatry
 e Specialized Community Addictions Service

 i Mr D is a 19-year-old university student. He presents with a 6-month history of increasing social withdrawal and self-neglect. His tutors have become increasingly concerned with his academic performance. During the university holidays his parents have brought him to see his GP due to his odd behaviour. He reports that the television has been talking about him and believes that his bedroom may have been bugged. He describes recently beginning to hear voices. He is subjectively distressed by these experiences and wishes to seek help. He drinks a moderate amount of alcohol and has smoked cannabis once or twice in the last year, but not for the last 3 months. He denies any other drug use and does not report any suicidal thoughts or thoughts of violence.

 ii Mrs F is a 33-year-old housewife. She has presented to her GP with a 5-week history of low mood and reduced energy, and reports that she does not find anything enjoyable. She has a disturbed sleep pattern but her appetite is normal. She denies other symptoms or any thoughts of suicide. There is no history of drug misuse and she drinks alcohol rarely. Mrs F was divorced 2 years ago, and continues to work as a secretary for a local solicitors' firm. She

is otherwise fit and well and reports that she Is not keen on taking medication. She reports that she has accessed self-help resources on the internet, which she has found useful in the past.

 iii Mr G is a 45-year-old gentleman with a diagnosis of paranoid schizophrenia. He has had four admissions to psychiatric hospital in the last 2 years, all of them under the Mental Health Act. He responds to oral antipsychotic medication but has a history of poor compliance in the community and limited insight into his illness. He lives in a shared house in the city centre and has a history of not attending out-patient appointments with his psychiatrist and of limited engagement with his Community Psychiatric Nurse. When unwell he becomes floridly psychotic and has attempted to end his life on several occasions by taking overdoses during relapses. He does not have a history of interpersonal violence. He has used crack cocaine in the past, although reports that this has not been the case for the last few months. During his most recent admission to hospital he was started on a long-acting depot antipsychotic injection.

2 Which of the following CMHT professionals (a–f) would be most appropriately involved for the interventions below (i–iv)?
 a Psychiatrist
 b Clinical Psychologist
 c Community Psychiatric Nurse
 d Social Worker
 e Occupational Therapist
 f Support Worker

i Mr C is a 25-year-old gentleman who is under the care of the local Community Mental Health Team. He has been taking oral olanzapine (an antipsychotic) medication for the last 3 months after being admitted to hospital for the first time 4 months ago for a 5-week admission. He has a diagnosis of paranoid schizophrenia. He reports that he is no longer happy to continue taking his medication as he is suffering unpleasant side effects including excessive sedation and significant weight gain (15 kg in the last 3 months). He wishes to discuss alternative pharmacological therapies.

ii Mrs E is a 30-year-old lady with a history of bipolar affective disorder. She has taken lithium for several years and has responded well. She has not been admitted to hospital for the last 3 years and lives with her husband and 8-year old daughter. She has recently disclosed that she was subject to physical and emotional abuse at the hands of her father during her teenage years. Her father died the previous year. She reports that she is finding herself recalling the abuse frequently and finds the thoughts extremely distressing. She has had thoughts of harming herself by cutting her wrists superficially to relieve emotional tension but has not done so. She denies any thoughts of suicide.

iii Mr F is a 44-year-old gentleman with a history of schizoaffective disorder and infrequent substance abuse. During a recent manic phase he spent significant amounts of money on credit cards buying a new car and a motorbike. He has recently left his job in a local supermarket and has lost his tenancy on his latest accommodation having damaged some property during his recent relapse. He is currently staying with his elderly parents who are supportive, but there have been some difficulties as they live in a small, one-bedroom flat.

iv Mr P is a 20-year-old student who is recovering from a recent episode of depression. He is taking antidepressants and has completed some cognitive behavioural therapy (CBT). He has a long-standing interest in athletics but struggles to attend his local club alone due to a high level of anxiety. He would like someone to accompany him during his first few visits there.

9

Mood disorders

Learning objectives

✓ To be able to describe the presentation, aetiology, assessment and management of mood disorders with an emphasis on depressive disorder and bipolar affective disorder

Variation in mood is part of normal human experience. It is only when a disturbance of mood is sufficiently severe to cause impairment in the activities of daily living that we think of it as disordered. The two major diagnostic categories are depressive disorder and bipolar disorder; however, other diagnoses such as abnormal grief reaction and perinatal mood disorders are also covered in this chapter.

Depressive disorder

The term 'depression' is widely used to describe low mood, but in order for a diagnosis of depressive disorder to be made there are a number of key features that must be present for at least 2 weeks (see Box 9.1). Low mood may be diurnal in nature (worse in the morning).

 Box 9.1 ICD-10 criteria for depressive disorder

A

Persistent low mood; and/or

Loss of interest or pleasure (anhedonia)

Fatigue or low energy (anergia)

B

Reduced concentration and attention

Reduced self-esteem and self-confidence

Ideas of guilt and worthlessness

Hopelessness about the future

Suicidal thoughts

Disturbed sleep

Diminished appetite

The severity of the episode is determined by how many of these features are present

Mild: 2 or more from A + 2 from B

Moderate: 2 or more from A + 3 from B

Severe: All 3 from A + 4 or more from B

If there has been more than one discrete episode this is termed recurrent depressive disorder.

Depressive disorder is also associated with a number of other symptoms that relate to these core diagnostic features. These include psychomotor retardation (slowed movements and thinking) or agitation, loss of libido, constipation and amenorrhoea. This group of symptoms are sometimes referred to as *somatic syndrome*.

 Clinical scenario

Mrs J has a 6-week history of low mood, anhedonia, tearfulness and early morning waking. She is off her food and has lost weight. Every day is a struggle and she finds it hard to concentrate or motivate herself to go to work or look after her children. However, she is just about coping and has no suicidal ideation. She had a similar episode 3 years ago. There is no evidence of an organic mood disorder. Your provisional diagnosis is that she has a recurrent depressive disorder and is currently in a depressive episode of moderate severity.

Psychiatry Lecture Notes, Eleventh Edition. Gautam Gulati, Mary-Ellen Lynall and Kate Saunders. © 2014 John Wiley & Sons, Ltd. Published 2014 by John Wiley & Sons, Ltd.

Dysthymia

This term is used to describe longstanding mild depressive symptoms. Dysthymia is often associated with other psychiatric or physical illness and can also co-occur with depression – a condition sometimes termed 'double depression'.

Psychotic depression

Depression at its most severe becomes *psychotic depression* (also called *depressive psychosis*). Worries and perceived misdemeanours become delusional in intensity. The patient may believe that they, or a part of them, is dead (*Cotard's syndrome*); they may experience *auditory hallucinations,* which are often derogatory in nature. Suicide risk is high.

Psychomotor retardation can increase to the point where the person sits motionless and mute – *depressive stupor*. This often used to be fatal (from dehydration); it now calls for emergency electroconvulsive therapy (ECT).

Psychotic depression must be distinguished from other psychoses (Chapter 12). This is based on the presence of other depressive symptoms, and the *mood congruity* of the delusions and hallucinations.

Atypical depression

For some individuals depression is associated with increased sleep, increased appetite and phobic anxiety. This is often termed atypical depression and tends to respond better to monoamine oxidase inhibitors (MAOIs) rather than selective serotonin reuptake inhibitors (SSRIs).

Reactive and endogenous depression

This dated classification divided depression into 'reactive depression', brought on by a stressful life event, and 'endogenous' depression, supposedly occurring from within the patient, with no clear external cause. Endogenous depression was thought to be more heritable and more responsive to antidepressant treatment. Research into depression has shown that such a division does not exist, and these terms are rarely used now.

Mixed anxiety and depressive disorder

Anxiety symptoms are common in depressive disorder and when symptoms of both disorders are present but not individually sufficient enough to meet criteria for a diagnosis of a mood disorder or an anxiety disorder this is described as a mixed anxiety and depressive disorder.

Epidemiology of depressive disorder (Table 9.1)

Depressive disorder is common. The risk is greatest in women and in those with a positive family history. The reason for higher rates is women is unclear but may be related to:

- Genetic predisposition.
- Sex hormone influences.
- Social pressures.
- Greater willingness to acknowledge the presence of depressive symptoms.
- Comorbid conditions: for example, men are more likely to develop alcohol abuse than women.

For all other mood disorders, a mixture of genetic, biological, psychological and social factors contribute to varying degrees (as in the rolling vignette in Chapter 6). There is a moderate genetic predisposition to depression (heritability ~40%), more so in early-onset cases. The predisposition is shared between the various types of depressive disorder and overlaps with those associated with anxiety disorders, but not bipolar disorder. The number and identity of genes are unknown.

Environmental influences contribute substantially to depressive disorders (Table 9.2).

- Hypofunction of monoamine neurotransmitter systems – 5-HT (serotonin) and NA (noradrenaline) – in conjunction with altered hypothalamic-pituitary-adrenal (HPA) regulation is implicated. However, though these systems are all altered in

Table 9.1 **The epidemiology of depressive disorders**

Lifetime risk	15%
1-month prevalence	5%
Sex ratio (M:F)	1:2
Mean age of onset	Late 20s
Risk to first-degree relatives of a patient with a depressive disorder:	
of bipolar disorder	2%
of depressive disorder	15%

Table 9.2 Aetiological factors in depressive disorders

Biological
Genes
Medical conditions (organic mood disorder)
Neurochemical changes:
    Monoamine abnormalities
    Altered HPA axis function

Psychological
Childhood environment:
    Emotional deprivation
    Parental loss
Abnormal cognitions
Learned helplessness
Personality factors – neuroticism

Social
Life events
Unemployment

HPA, hypothalamic-pituitary-adrenal.

depression, their causal role and interrelationships remain unclear.

- Psychological models have centred on the role of abnormal ways of thinking, with a tendency to think negatively about the self, the future and the world (the cognitive theory of depression). The personality attributes of *'neuroticism'* (anxiety, obsessionality, poor coping with stress) and low self-esteem are also associated with depressive disorder.
- Current approaches to understanding mood disorders integrate findings from neuropsychology, psychopharmacology and neuroimaging. People who become depressed have negative biases in emotional processing, which may involve a failure in the frontoparietal regulation of processes in the amygdala. These biases can be reversed by antidepressant drugs.
- Adverse experiences in childhood, recent life events and lack of social support are major risk factors.
- Focal lesions of the subcortical white matter, visible on magnetic resonance imaging (MRI) scans, are a risk factor for late-onset depressive disorder and are associated with a poor prognosis.
- Other structural brain changes reported in depressive disorder include a reduction of glial cells in the prefrontal cortex, and hippocampal atrophy. It is not known if these changes are cause, consequence or coincidence.

Management of depressive disorders

The first requirement is an ability to recognize depression in all its guises. Depression frequently goes undiagnosed and untreated. Psychiatrists only see a small percentage of people with depressive disorder, so all doctors need to be confident about its diagnosis and first-line treatment. Treatment depends largely on severity. In the absence of previous episodes, mild depressive episodes are often self-limiting and antidepressant drug treatment may not be indicated. Information, advice and simple measures such as self-help guides to problem-solving may be adequate. There is evidence that increased physical exercise and activity helps. On the other hand, if there have been previous episodes of at least moderate severity that have responded to treatment, then treatment should be started while symptoms are still mild.

Drug treatment

The first-line treatment for a depressive episode of at least moderate severity is usually an antidepressant drug. However, before prescribing, consider several factors (Table 9.3). Over 70% of depressive episodes respond to an antidepressant, either an SSRI or a tricyclic antidepressant (TCA), although only as few as one-third of patients may respond to first-line therapy (Chapter 7). The chances of successful treatment can be increased if simple measures are taken (Table 9.4).

- In practice, SSRIs are now prescribed much more commonly than TCAs, based mainly on tolerability and safety.
- There are small differences in efficacy and tolerability between SSRIs and, while the likelihood of specific adverse events should be discussed with the patient, a good first-line choice is sertraline.
- It is important to *monitor for emergent suicidal ideation* as this may occur as the patient improves, and may actually be increased by SSRIs, especially in younger people. However, there is no evidence that SSRIs are associated with an increase in suicidal acts.

 Clinical scenario

Mr S has a moderate depressive episode. He is married and unemployed. He initially doesn't accept he's depressed and blames his problems on what he feels are his own inadequacies. You explain that he has a depressive disorder that would benefit from treatment. You summarize what depression

Table 9.3 Factors affecting management decisions in depression

Question	Implication
Is there a serious suicide risk?	May need admission. Use SSRI not TCA as less toxic in overdose
Are there psychotic symptoms?	Add an antipsychotic to the antidepressant, or use ECT
What are the main symptoms?	Affects choice of drug, e.g. use sedative antidepressant if insomnia
Is there a past history of response?	Use the treatment that worked last time
Is there a past history of mania?	Caution with antidepressants; consider mood stabilizer
Are there medical problems?	Avoid TCAs after recent myocardial infarction
What does the patient want?	May have a preference for drug or psychological therapy

ECT, electroconvulsive therapy; SSRI, selective serotonin reuptake inhibitor; TCA, tricyclic antidepressant.

is and how antidepressants work, including their possible side effects and delayed onset of action, but also emphasize that they will help him sleep and reduce his anxiety. You recommend he takes 50 mg sertraline. His wife is present and agrees to supervise his tablets. You will see him in a week to review progress. You gradually increase the dose of sertraline to 150 mg.

- After recovery, continue treatment at the same dose for at least 6 months. The dose is then tapered off over several weeks. Continuing treatment in this way reduces the high risk of relapse in the months after a depressive episode, and tapering off reduces the risk of 'withdrawal' symptoms.
- There is no good evidence that long-term use of antidepressants is harmful.

 Clinical scenario *(continued)*

Mr S took his tablets as prescribed. His sleep and agitation improved rapidly. The depressive symptoms responded over the next few weeks, though it was necessary to increase the sertraline to 200 mg/day for a full response. He subsequently accepted that he had been ill, and conceptualized

the sertraline as correcting a chemical imbalance, which helped him solve life's problems more effectively. He no longer blamed himself for his redundancy and found a new job. His wife confirmed the improvement. On your advice, he remained on medication for a further 9 months.

Psychological treatment

Cognitive behavioural therapy (CBT), interpersonal therapy (IPT) and probably other psychological treatments, such as problem-solving therapy (Chapter 7) or brief psychodynamic therapy, are effective alternatives to antidepressants in mild and moderate depressive disorder, especially for patients who prefer psychological therapies to drug treatment.

- CBT is much the most widely available psychological treatment, but is nevertheless of restricted availability due to a shortage of trained therapists. New NHS initiatives using internet- and phone-based CBT appear promising and mean that the treatments can be provided to more patients.
- Combining an antidepressant with CBT is a bit more effective than either alone and should be considered when CBT is available.

Table 9.4 Prescribing antidepressants effectively

Principle	Examples
Educate patient	About efficacy, onset of effects and side effects, and non-addictiveness
Attend to the psychosocial aspects	Restore hope; education about depression; give practical advice
Give an adequate dose	Know dose ranges for specific SSRIs and TCAs
Check drug being taken	Non-adherence is common reason for non-response
Give the drug for long enough	Therapeutic trial should be 6–8 weeks, at adequate dose

SSRI, selective serotonin reuptake inhibitor; TCA, tricyclic antidepressant.

There are no established predictors of who will benefit from psychological rather than pharmacological treatment of depression. A few pointers suggesting good psychotherapeutic response are:

- Depression not severe (as defined in Table 9.1).
- 'Psychological mindedness' (the ability and willingness to think about psychological matters).
- Willingness to engage in therapy and carry out homework tasks.
- Preference for psychological treatment or reluctance to take medication.

Non-response to first-line treatment

In up to two-thirds of cases, a depressive episode does not respond to a first-line antidepressant (or to a psychological treatment). If so:

- Check the antidepressant has been taken as prescribed.
- Increase to the maximum tolerated and recommended dose.
- Review the case. Is the diagnosis right? Could there be powerful perpetuating factors, such as an endocrine disorder, marital strife or alcohol misuse? Can their impact be reduced?

If the patient has still not improved, there are various options to consider. The most common option is to switch from one class of antidepressant to another – e.g. SSRI to SNRI (selective serotonin and noradrenaline reuptake inhibitor) – or to try a second drug from the same class (SSRI to SSRI). There is limited evidence in favour of either strategy. Alternative options, with at least some evidence of efficacy, are:

- Add lithium, if depression is severe. This has a good evidence base but the risks and drawbacks of lithium limit its popularity.
- Add mirtazapine to an SSRI; the sedative effect of mirtazapine is useful if insomnia or agitation is a problem.
- Add a second-generation antipsychotic, such as olanzapine or quetiapine, especially if there are psychotic symptoms, or agitation and insomnia.
- Add CBT or other psychological treatment.
- Switch to an MAOI, especially in atypical depression. Remember MAOI cautions (Chapter 7).
- Psychiatric referral, if this has not already occurred (see below).
- Consider ECT for severe and drug-resistant depression.

Psychiatric referral for depression

Referral for psychiatric assessment or ongoing care of depressive disorder is appropriate when:

- The patient has not responded to treatment.
- There is a substantial risk of harm to self or others.
- A second opinion on diagnosis or treatment is required.
- Combinations of drugs or rarely used agents are being considered.
- To access specialized psychological treatments, occupational therapy, etc.
- The patient is severely unwell and hospital admission or ECT may be required.

Prevention of relapse

Following an initial depressive episode patients should be advised to continue antidepressant treatment at the same dose for at least 9 months from when they recovered. Continuation of an antidepressant after recovery cuts relapse rates by at least 50% in patients with recurrent depressive disorder and should be recommended to all appropriate patients. Psychological treatments such as CBT may also be effective, by reducing negative cognitions or by teaching strategies for recognizing and treating re-emergent symptoms.

- In people who do relapse, reinstitute the treatment that worked the first time but continue it for longer. Some patients appear to benefit from prolonged antidepressant treatment.

Prognosis

Over 50% of people who have had one depressive episode will have another. The more severe the depression, the worse the prognosis; most people with psychotic depression suffer multiple episodes, and 10% never recover fully.

- The proportion with severe, recurrent and chronic illness is higher in psychiatric care than in general practice.
- The risk of suicide is increased at least 10-fold in people with depressive disorder. About 4% of patients who have had depression will die by suicide, rising to 15% in those ill enough to have required psychiatric admission at some stage.
- Mortality is also increased from natural causes, notably cardiovascular disease, accidents and substance misuse.

Bipolar disorder

Bipolar disorder is a relapsing and remitting condition that is characterized by the presence of periods of elated mood (mania/hypomania) and depressed mood, although the presence of elated mood alone is sufficient for the diagnosis to be made.

 Box 9.2 Symptoms of mania

A. Mood that is predominantly elevated, expansive or irritable and definitely abnormal for the individual concerned.

B. At least three of the following must be present (four if the mood is merely irritable):

  1 Increased activity or physical restlessness.

  2 Increased talkativeness ('pressure of speech').

  3 Flight of ideas or the subjective experience of thoughts racing.

  4 Loss of normal social inhibitions resulting in behaviour inappropriate to the circumstances.

  5 Decreased need for sleep.

  6 Inflated self-esteem or grandiosity.

  7 Distractibility or constant changes in activity or plans.

  8 Behaviour that is ill advised or reckless and whose risks the subject does not recognize, e.g. spending sprees, foolish enterprises, reckless driving.

  9 Marked sexual energy or sexual indiscretions.

Hypomania

Hypomania is a happiness and zest for life in excess of that which is normal. The degree of functional impairment is variable. A daily routine may be just about maintained, though with less need for sleep and more nocturnal activities (e.g. spring cleaning, writing a novel). Though subjectively productivity may be increased, tasks are rarely done well or completed. *Concentration* is impaired and *distractibility* is usual. The infectious gaiety easily switches to irritability.

- Hypomania may progress to a full manic episode, especially in those with a past history of mania.
- Note that there is no satisfactory category or term for manic symptoms lasting less than 4 days (Table 9.5).
- People whose elated mood never goes beyond hypomania are described as having bipolar-2 disorder (see Table 9.5).

Table 9.5 Distinguishing hypomania and mania

Features of hypomania	Features of mania
Present for at least 4 days	Present for at least 7 days or needing hospital admission
Core features mild or moderate	Core features marked
Mild or moderate dysfunction	Substantial dysfunction
Partial insight preserved	Minimal or absent insight
No psychotic features	Psychotic symptoms may occur

Mania

In moderate and severe mania the symptoms cause substantial impairment of occupational and social functioning (Box 9.2). Thought processes become disordered and jumpy (*flight of ideas*), accompanied by *pressure of speech* (p. 28). Psychotic symptoms may emerge. These are mood congruent and *grandiose*: a patient may believe themselves blessed with special powers (e.g. that they can fly or have been sent to save the world). They may hear voices supporting these beliefs. Unfortunately, reality or gravity supervene, and people with mania do things they later regret. For example, they may suffer consequences of promiscuity or generate huge debts.

Mixed affective states

In *mixed affective states*, manic and depressive symptoms coexist within the course of a day. The disorder is not rare, but it is difficult to diagnose. It may be triggered by antidepressant treatment in a patient with a tendency to bipolar disorder. The treatment of mixed states usually focuses initially on the manic symptoms.

Cyclothymia

Cyclothymia is a mild, chronic bipolar variation of mood. Like dysthymia, it is sometimes viewed as a personality trait. Psychiatric help is rarely sought since the mild mood elevations are pleasant and associated with a sense of productivity and creativity.

- A history of cyclothymia or a family history of bipolar disorder are significant in someone presenting with a depressive episode; they increase the chances that the patient will actually turn out to have bipolar disorder. They may also increase the risk that antidepressants induce a manic episode.

 Clinical scenario

Mrs J presents with depressive symptoms, but informs you that she recalls two periods several years ago when she felt elated, slept little, became unusually gregarious and spent money uncharacteristically. After each episode she was embarrassed and distressed by her actions, but she had not sought treatment. You diagnose bipolar (II) disorder, currently in a moderate depressive episode.

Bipolar disorder is strongly heritable (80%). The monozygotic (MZ):dizygotic (DZ) twin concordance is 75:25%. Relatives of someone with bipolar disorder have an increased incidence of both bipolar and unipolar depressive disorder (Table 9.6).

- Many chromosomal loci and genes are implicated, and overlap with those for schizophrenia (Chapter 13). Current leading bipolar disorder candidate genes include the HLA (human leucocyte antigen) complex, *ANK3* and *CACN1C*. There is some evidence for inheritance down the maternal line.
- No childhood risk factors are known. Life events can precipitate the initial episodes; once the disorder is established, its course is increasingly immune to environmental circumstances.

Table 9.7 Causes of organic mood disorder

Usually depression	Usually mania
Cushing's disease	Hyperthyroidism
Addison's disease	Steroids
Hypothyroidism	Amphetamine (acute)
Hypercalcaemia	L-DOPA
Diabetes mellitus	Antidepressants
Carcinomas	Bromocriptine
β-Blockers	Isoniazid
Digoxin	
Amphetamine (chronic)	

Either depression or mania
Multiple sclerosis
Cerebrovascular disease
Systemic lupus erythematosus
Epilepsy
Brain tumours

- Most of the neurobiological abnormalities described for depressive disorder are also implicated in bipolar disorder, although there may be differences in the abnormalities in emotional processing.
- Always consider drug-induced mania (an example of organic mood disorder) in young people with no family history of bipolar disorder. In someone first presenting in middle age, exclude cerebrovascular disease, tumours and medication side effects (Table 9.7).

Table 9.6 The epidemiology of bipolar disorder

Lifetime risk	1%
1-month prevalence	0.4%
Sex ratio (M:F)	1:1
Mean age of onset	Early 20s
Risk to first-degree relatives of a patient with bipolar disorder:	
of bipolar disorder	10%
of depressive disorder	15%

Management of bipolar disorder

Treatment of mania and mixed episodes

Patients with mild manic symptoms can be successfully treated as out-patients, if the patient has insight that they need treatment. More severe mania, especially if psychotic, usually requires admission, often compulsorily.

- Antipsychotics (e.g. risperidone, olanzapine) or valproate and lithium are effective antimanics. Antipsychotics are probably slightly more effective, but cause more sedation and weight gain. Benzodiazepines are used, as required, for sedation.

- The choice of drug is influenced by the patient's existing medication – they may already be on a mood stabilizer. If they are on an antidepressant, stop it. If the patient is on lithium, check the blood level to assess recent adherence.
- Some patients learn to recognize prodromal symptoms of mania (e.g. initial insomnia, increased energy). If so, a short course of antipsychotic or valproate may successfully treat the episode.
- ECT can be highly effective in patients with severe mania that does not respond to drug treatment.

Mania can last for months if untreated. Death from 'manic exhaustion' was well recognized before treatments became available.

Treatment of depressive episodes

Depressive episodes and symptoms in bipolar disorder ('*bipolar depression*') can cause severe dysfunction and can be difficult to treat. There is increasing evidence that optimal drug treatment of bipolar depression is quite different from that described for unipolar depression.

- Quetiapine, an atypical antipsychotic, is the treatment with the best evidence and can be highly effective, with a rapid onset of action. Sedation and weight gain may limit longer term acceptability.
- Antidepressants may be less effective than in unipolar depression and they should be used in combination with an effective antimanic drug (see above) because antidepressants used alone can precipitate mood destabilization or mania.
- Lamotrigine, an antiepileptic drug, is probably also effective, although it needs to be started slowly.
- For severe depression, antipsychotics, ECT and psychiatric admission may all be necessary.

Prevention of relapse

- The guiding principle should be that the patient needs to understand their own illness and learn to recognize signs of mood instability.
- Long-term mood monitoring by the patient can be extremely helpful.
- Relapses in bipolar disorder are often heralded by non-specific symptoms (e.g. deteriorating sleep), as mentioned above. Some patients become adept at recognizing and responding to these warning signs.
- Conventionally, long-term drug treatment is not offered until a patient has had at least two manic episodes, or one manic and one depressive episode. However, the effective early treatment of bipolar disorder may improve its long-term outcome, and increasingly the trend is to start long-term treatment after one serious episode, especially when there is a family history of bipolar disorder. The decision is an important one and the patient should be given sufficient information and time to make a properly informed choice.
- Long-term lithium treatment is the standard prophylaxis for bipolar disorder and is supported by the most robust evidence. Lithium reduces the risk of both manic and depressive relapse by 40–50%. Long-term lithium treatment should not be initiated unless both patient and doctor intend to continue it for at least 2 years. Valproate and olanzapine also reduce the risk of manic relapse. Lamotrigine reduces the risk of depressive relapse. Other drugs such as carbamazepine may also be used, although the evidence is limited.
- Psychological approaches such as CBT or family therapy may also help in preventing relapses.

Organic mood disorders

Mood disorders that have a known physical cause are termed organic mood disorders. Recognized causes of organic mood disorder are summarized in Table 9.7. See also Chapter 13.

- Even when an organic diagnosis is made, psychological and social factors may still be relevant to course and treatment.

 Clinical scenario

A 65-year-old man presented with insomnia, anorexia, back pain and weight loss. He also felt fed up and irritable. The provisional diagnosis was depression with somatic symptoms. However, physical examination revealed bony tenderness over his lumbar spine and a hard nodular prostate. Blood tests showed hypercalcaemia and anaemia. He had metastatic carcinoma of the prostate. His depressive symptoms resolved as the hypercalcaemia was treated, along with an antidepressant.

Other aspects of mood disorders

Puerperal (postpartum) disorders

The postnatal period (puerperium) is a hormonally, and often psychologically, turbulent time. It is traditional to group psychiatric disorders that occur at this time together as puerperal disorders, partly because their clinical picture and management differ somewhat from similar disorders occurring at other times.

Maternity blues

The 'blues' refer to a tearful, irritable, labile mood that affects over 50% of mothers on the third or fourth postnatal day. Symptoms resolve within days without treatment, though explanation and reassurance are appropriate. There is no association of the blues with mood disorder.

- Maternity blues may be due to the precipitous fall in sex steroids after delivery, as well as to the impact of childbirth and concerns about mothering.

Postnatal depression

Postnatal depression tends to start within a month of delivery; one in seven mothers are affected. The symptoms are unremarkable, with the negative thoughts tending to focus on the woman's perceived failings as a mother or on her baby's well-being. Physical exhaustion exacerbates matters.

- As well as the standard mood and risk assessments, remember to consider the mother–baby relationship. Postnatal depression may put the baby at short-term risk and, if untreated, may lead to problems with bonding and child development.
- Most cases are managed at home. Use supportive measures, including explanation and reassurance. Mobilize resources (e.g. the local mothers' group), and liaise with the GP, midwife and health visitor. Many cases resolve within a few weeks, but antidepressants or psychological treatment should be considered if the disorder is moderate or severe. If admission is necessary, it should ideally be to a mother-and-baby unit, to maintain and observe their relationship.
- Before prescribing antidepressants, check whether the mother is breastfeeding (Chapter 7).

- Postnatal depression is more common in women with a history of psychiatric disorder and in those lacking support. A postnatal change in sensitivity of the dopaminergic system is implicated.

Puerperal psychosis

Puerperal psychosis is a rare condition, which occurs in 1–2 per 1000 births. The disorder can be severe. Perplexity and a delirium-like state are characteristic. Onset is usually in the second postnatal week.

- Risk factors include a past or family history of puerperal psychosis, a diagnosis of bipolar disorder and being a primigravida.
- The baby is at potential risk because of the mother's delusions, or because she is so preoccupied by her symptoms that baby is neglected. The assessment should specifically address these issues.
- Admission to hospital is usually necessary. Treatment is with antipsychotics and antidepressants, and with a low threshold for ECT – which often produces a dramatic response. Full recovery is usual, but there is a 25% relapse rate after the next delivery and a 50% lifetime risk.

Premenstrual syndrome

Up to 80% of women suffer from symptoms in the days before their period: irritability, depression, abdominal bloating and breast tenderness. However, a specific premenstrual syndrome has proved difficult to validate (and is not included in ICD-10). The term *premenstrual dysphoric disorder* is sometimes used for women with prominent psychological premenstrual symptoms.

- If a woman complains of premenstrual syndrome, establish the symptoms and their relationship with the menstrual cycle. Ask her to keep a diary – it may transpire that the symptoms are present at other times too.
- There is limited evidence that drug treatments are successful and the placebo response is very high. However, the effectiveness of SSRI treatment during the premenstrual period is gaining an evidence base.

Other psychiatric issues specific to women

Abortion, sterilization, hysterectomy and the menopause have all been said to cause psychiatric distress, especially mood and anxiety disorders. There is no good evidence for any of these claims. Each of these events may, however, act as stressors that are relevant to the understanding, presentation or treatment of a disorder occurring soon afterwards.

Grief

Many of the features of grief overlap with those of depression. Psychiatrists and other doctors are asked to assess or support people during these times, so it is necessary to know:

- The characteristic psychological reactions to impending death and to bereavement.
- The features that distinguish these from depressive disorder.

Normal grief

People may grieve a death (*bereavement*) or other major loss, or may grieve an impending event (*anticipatory grief*). The responses are forms of adjustment reaction (Chapter 10). Three stages have been described:

- *Shock and disbelief.* On being informed of the event there is an initial numbness that usually lasts a day or two. Behaviour may be acutely disturbed.
- *Preoccupation.* This central phase involves a preoccupation with the deceased. In the early stages anger is common, and may be directed at doctors, God or other targets of blame. Uncontrollable crying, low mood, social withdrawal and somatic symptoms akin to those of depression may be pronounced. The voice or image of the deceased may be vividly perceived, though usually with an 'as if' quality rather than being truly hallucinatory.
- *Acceptance and resolution.* With time, the person comes to terms with the event, symptoms subside

and life begins to return to normal. This phase may take several months to start, and several more to be completed. Recurrence of grief is common around anniversaries.

In uncomplicated grief, *bereavement counselling and support* (e.g. from Cruse) may be useful. Such grief should not be labelled as a disorder but viewed as a natural, if painful, process. The therapist should, however, be vigilant for signs of abnormal grief or depressive disorder.

Abnormal (pathological) grief

Grief can be abnormal in three ways:

- *Absent or delayed grief.* There may appear to be no outward signs of grief despite an event of grief-inducing proportions (absent grief). Grief usually begins a few weeks later (delayed grief).
- *Prolonged grief.* A term used if there are prominent symptoms more than 6–12 months later. At this time, actively consider a developing depressive disorder and the need for treatment.
- *Excessive grief.* The intensity of grief is unusually great – this may reflect the person's closeness to the deceased, their personality or a depressive disorder.

Grief and depression

A depressive disorder occurs in one in three grieving people, and is severe in one in five. It is not always easy to decide when the threshold from grief to depression is crossed. The distinction is made largely on the basis of excessive intensity or duration of symptoms, but other features may also help (Table 9.8). The person may need persuading that their suffering is no longer just the pain of normal grief but is now a depressive disorder meriting treatment.

Table 9.8 A comparison of depression and grief

	Depression	Grief
Suicidal thoughts	Common, driven by low mood	Transient, driven by wish to be with the deceased
Blame for situation	Self	Other people or fate
Psychomotor retardation	Yes	No
Psychotic features	If severe; mood congruent	No, but may 'see' or 'hear' the deceased
Symptom course	Pervasive	Fluctuating

KEYPOINTS

* Mood disorders involve excessive deviations or fluctuations of mood. They affect 1 in 6 people at some stage in their lives. Unipolar depressive disorders are much more common than bipolar disorder.

* The core features of depression are low mood, lack of energy, and anhedonia. Many other psychological and somatic symptoms also occur.

* Depression may present with somatic symptoms such as fatigue and weight loss, and should always be considered in the differential diagnosis of these symptoms.

* Suicidal risk needs detailed and regular assessment in everyone with mood disorder.

* Antidepressants are the usual first-line treatment for depressive disorder. Give an adequate dose and continue for at least 9 months after recovery. CBT is as effective as antidepressants for mild and moderate depression: availability is increasing but there can still be long waits. ECT is reserved for severe cases.

* Mania is treated with antipsychotics and/or mood stabilizers. Long-term treatment with the latter reduces the risk of relapse.

 FURTHER READING

Anderson I, Ferrier IN, Baldwin RC, *et al.* (2008) Evidence-based guidelines for treating depressive disorders with antidepressants: A revision of the 2000 British Association for Psychopharmacology guidelines. *Journal of Psychopharmacology* 22(4): 343–396.

National Institute for Health and Care Excellence (NICE) (2006) Clinical guideline 38. Bipolar disorder: The management of bipolar disorder in adults, children and adolescents, in primary and secondary care. NICE.

National Institute for Health and Care Excellence (NICE) (2009) Clinical guideline 90. Depression in adults (CG90). NICE.

Saunders KEA, Goodwin GM (2010) The course of bipolar disorder. *Advances in Psychiatric Treatment* 16: 318–328.

 SELF-ASSESSMENT

1 Marion complains of a low mood and low energy which have been present for the past 6 weeks. She has lost approximately a stone in weight. She says she had a similar episode 4 years ago following the birth of her first child. What is the most likely diagnosis?
   a Postnatal depression
   b Bipolar 2 disorder
   c Dysthymia
   d Depressive episode
   e Recurrent depressive disorder

2 Brian is described by his wife as someone who is 'glass half empty'. He rarely gets enjoyment out of activities and expresses a generally negative outlook on life. However, up until the last 3 weeks he has functioned well both at work and home. At present he is preoccupied with the fact that his bowels are rotting away and that he is undeserving of food. He says very little in the assessment and appears psychomotor retarded. Which is the most likely diagnosis?
   a Schizophrenia
   b Psychotic depression and dysthymia
   c Bipolar depression
   d Drug-induced psychosis
   e Bowel cancer

3 Which of the following statements is true about bipolar disorder?
   a Antidepressants are the mainstay of treatment.
   b Bipolar 2 disorder is associated with the need for hospital admission when mood is elated.
   c Bipolar disorder can be limited to episodes of mania.
   d Bipolar disorder is more common in women.
   e Puerperal psychosis is less common in women who have a history of bipolar disorder.

Neurotic, stress-related and somatoform disorders

Learning objectives

✓ To be able to describe the presentation, aetiology and assessment of common neuroses

✓ To be able to describe the general principles relating to the management of common neuroses

---

General characteristics of neurosis

Neurotic symptoms and syndromes

We all experience anxiety and worries. Sometimes these become so persistent and inappropriate that they can be regarded as an illness. *Neurosis* ('to do with the nerves') or *neurotic disorders* are the traditional terms for those symptoms when they are not due to an organic brain disease, psychosis or personality disorder. The symptoms of neurosis are emotional, cognitive, behavioural and somatic. Neuroses are often but not always associated with an external stressor.

- Anxiety is the primary emotion in all these disorders, although depressed mood is often present.
- The cognitions are worries, fears and concerns that are inappropriate or excessive but (by definition) not delusional.

- Behaviours include avoidance and other strategies intended to reduce anxiety, such as repeated checking.
- Somatic ('physical') symptoms, not explained by a medical disease but associated with tension, autonomic arousal and hyperventilation (such as aches and pains, bowel disturbance and breathlessness), are common.

Neurotic disorders may present with the emotion of anxiety (e.g. attacks of panic) but may also present with one of the other symptoms such as cognitions (e.g. recurrent worries about having a serious medical condition), behaviour (e.g. the agoraphobic unable to leave her house) or somatic symptoms (e.g. palpitations).

- Neuroses are common in primary care and also in medical clinics where the diagnosis is easily missed
- Neuroses are not necessarily 'minor' illnesses; they can be chronic and disabling.

The individual *neurotic disorders* are listed in Table 10.1. Mild cases sometimes cannot be placed into any one of these specific categories and are best

---

Psychiatry Lecture Notes, Eleventh Edition. Gautam Gulati, Mary-Ellen Lynall and Kate Saunders. © 2014 John Wiley & Sons, Ltd. Published 2014 by John Wiley & Sons, Ltd.

Table 10.1 Classification of neurotic, stress-related and somatoform disorders

Neurotic disorders (neuroses)
Anxiety disorders:
  Phobic anxiety
  Panic disorder
  Generalized anxiety
Obsessive-compulsive disorder (OCD)
Dissociative disorders
Neurasthenia (chronic fatigue syndrome)
Depersonalization-derealization syndrome

Stress-related disorders
Acute stress reaction
Adjustment disorders
Post-traumatic stress disorder

Somatoform disorders
Hypochondriasis
Dysmorphophobia
Somatization disorder
Other somatoform disorders

described as *undifferentiated neurosis* or *minor emotional disorder*.

- Depressive symptoms are common in patients with neurosis, and neurotic symptoms are very common in patients with depressive disorders. Indeed, in many patients seen in primary care, anxiety and depressive symptoms coexist in similar proportions. A diagnosis of *mixed anxiety-depression* is appropriate for such cases.
- Culture specific variants of neurosis occur. These include *amok* (dissociative disorder in Indonesia), *koro* (severe anxiety about penis shrinkage in Chinese men) and *dhat* (semen-loss anxiety in Asian men).

Stress-related and somatoform disorders

The term 'neurosis' has been used to describe patients with predominantly somatic symptoms and also for symptoms clearly caused by stress. In the current classification (Table 10.1) these types of neurosis have each been given their own category: somatoform and stress-related disorders, respectively.

- If somatic symptoms (e.g. palpitations, pain) are unexplained by a medical disease or other psychiatric diagnosis the diagnosis is *somatoform disorder*. This diagnosis is controversial because of its assumption that such medically unexplained symptoms are better regarded as a psychiatric than as a medical condition.
- If there is a major external stressor that appears to explain the symptoms, a *stress-related disorder* may be diagnosed.

Diagnosing neuroses

If a patient presents with symptoms suggestive of a neurotic disorder, ask two questions:

1 *Do the patient's symptoms warrant any diagnosis?*
- Gauge whether the symptoms are diagnostically significant from their intensity, number and pervasiveness, and from the resulting *dysfunction* – are they interfering with the person's life? – and do they need treatment (e.g. see social phobia)?
2 *Is an alternative diagnosis more appropriate?*
- Neurotic symptoms can occur as part of another psychiatric or medical condition, especially depression, but also substance misuse, psychosis, eating disorders and certain organic conditions (e.g. anxiety due to thyrotoxicosis). Life-long symptoms could be indicative of an underlying personality disorder.

Epidemiology of neurosis

Neurosis is very common indeed, afflicting about 15% of the population at any one time. Most neurotic disorders are significantly more prevalent in women, save for OCD and panic disorder. The onset is generally between early adulthood and middle age, though children may have neuroses. Prevalence increases with low household income. Comorbidity with depression is common.

Management of neurosis

Management should consider biological, psychological and social factors. Neuroses all respond to certain drugs and psychological treatments. However, some neurotic disorders respond better to certain types of treatment than others:

- Antidepressants and anxiolytic drugs are both effective, though anxiolytics are less commonly used because of concerns about dependence. Antidepressants are effective even when there are few, if any, depressive symptoms.
- Simple psychological interventions such as reassurance and explanation are important. Specific psychological therapies, especially cognitive behavioural therapy (CBT), are at least as effective as medication for most neuroses and especially effective for some (e.g. panic disorder). The specific type of CBT used differs between neurotic disorders.

- Social interventions such as removal of stressors and improvement of social support where possible can also be helpful.

Prognosis of neurosis

The majority of cases of neuroses in primary care are acute and transient. Psychiatrists tend to see the small proportion of cases that are severe, chronic or disabling. The prognosis is better when there is no personality disorder, the patient is strongly motivated to get better and the duration of the illness is short.

Aetiology of neurosis

Neuroses have a multifactorial aetiology that is best considered from a combination of biological, psychological and social perspectives:

- Biologically, neuroses are moderately heritable, are associated with alterations in the 5-HT, noradrenergic and associated brain systems. Neuroimaging studies have demonstrated altered brain function and even altered brain structure (e.g. hippocampal atrophy in post-traumatic stress disorder).
- Psychologically, cognitive factors and behavioural conditioning are important, especially in phobias and panic disorder.
- Socially, relevant factors include life stressors, unhelpful responses by the medical system and lack of social support.

The precise combination of these factors in an individual patient in predisposing, precipitating and perpetuating a neurosis can be described in an aetiological formulation.

The specific disorders

So far, this chapter has considered the factors common to neurotic syndromes. The rest of the chapter considers factors specific to the individual disorders listed in Table 10.1.

Anxiety disorders

These disorders are dominated by the emotion of anxiety together with the anxious thoughts, avoidance behaviour and the somatic symptoms of sympathetic arousal that accompany it (Table 10.2). Anxiety disorders are divided into three main subtypes: *phobic, paroxysmal* (*panic*) and *generalized* (Table 10.3).

Table 10.2 Common symptoms of anxiety

Component	Prominent features
Emotion/mood	Anxiety, irritability
Cognitions	Exaggerated worries and fears
Behaviour	Avoidance of feared situations Checking Seeking reassurance
Somatic symptoms	Chest tightness Shortness of breath Palpitations 'Butterflies' Tremor Tingling of fingers (due to hyperventilation) Aches and pains Poor sleep Frequent desire to pass urine and defecate

- Somatic symptoms of anxiety (e.g. chest pain) may cause the patient to present initially to general medical services.

Phobic anxiety

Phobic anxiety is said to be *situational*, and is largely restricted to the experience or anticipation of a particular situation. This situation may be a specific concern (e.g. heights, spiders) or a more general one (e.g. agoraphobia). As a result of this anxiety the person tends to *avoid* these situations (e.g. a severe mouse phobic may avoid old houses or nature programmes). Although avoidance produces immediate relief from anxiety, it is ultimately counter-productive because it reinforces the fear. Overcoming avoidance is therefore a key part of psychological treatment for phobias.

- The main differential diagnosis is from the other anxiety disorders. Occasionally, phobic anxiety may arise secondary to delusions (e.g. fear of others because they are believed to be aliens). A phobia of having a serious disease is classified separately, as hypochondriasis (see below).
- Behavioural therapy for phobia is based on graded exposure to the situation (either in reality or in imagination). In CBT, a cognitive component is added to help the patient more accurately evaluate the dangerousness of the stimulus (e.g. a flight phobic may be encouraged to find out the actual statistical risk of dying in a plane crash).
- Antidepressants and anxiolytic drugs have a role.

Table 10.3 Features distinguishing the three types of anxiety disorder

	Phobic anxiety	Panic disorder	Generalized anxiety
Occurrence of anxiety	Situational	Paroxysmal	Persistent
Associated behaviour	Avoidance	Escape	Agitation
Associated cognitions	Fear of situation	Fear of symptoms	Worry
Somatic symptoms	With exposure	Episodic	Persistent

Agoraphobia

One of the most common phobias is *agoraphobia* (literally 'fear of the market place') (Table 10.4). Intense anxiety is provoked either by open, or large, spaces that are crowded and difficult to escape from (e.g. supermarket queues). Panic attacks are commonly associated, and having a panic attack may itself become the feared situation. The appropriate diagnosis is then *panic disorder with agoraphobia*.

- The associated cognitions commonly concern fainting, dying or another catastrophe, rather than a fear of shops or spaces per se.
- The condition can be severe, and the avoidance can lead the person to become housebound.
- On average, symptoms have been present for over 2 years before help is sought. It is most common in young women.

Social phobia

Social phobia is a fear of other people associated with anticipation of negative evaluation by them (Table 10.5). It must be distinguished from normal shyness, and from social withdrawal due to depression. In social phobia there is often a history of low self-esteem and a triggering incident when the person feels they made a fool of themselves. The anxiety may lead to shaking or blushing, which becomes a focus for further anxiety.

- Treatment is with CBT and antidepressant drugs, particularly SSRIs.
- Alcohol misuse may develop as a result of self-medication.

 Clinical scenario

Paul is a 30-year-old man who recently presented to his GP complaining of anxiety symptoms. Of note, Paul is due to be married in 6 months' time. He described how he wanted to marry his fiancée, but that he feared being humiliated on the day as he walked down the aisle in front of a large congregation of people. He stated that he usually avoided large family gatherings or work parties, and described how he usually consumes alcohol to help him cope with these situations. Paul's doctor diagnoses him with social phobia. He refers Paul for a course of cognitive behavioural therapy. The option of adding an antidepressant such as paroxetine was discussed but Paul is not keen on medication.

Panic disorder

Panic attacks are episodes of severe paroxysmal anxiety. They are associated with somatic symptoms and

Table 10.4 Symptoms of agoraphobia

Component	Prominent features
Emotion	Situational anxiety – in shops, crowded large places
Cognition	Thoughts of collapsing and being left helpless in public
Behaviour	Avoidance of panic-provoking situations
Somatic symptoms	Physical sensations of panic
Associations	Strong association with panic disorder

Table 10.5 Symptoms of social phobia

Component	Prominent features
Emotion	Situational anxiety in social gatherings
Cognition	Being judged negatively by others
Behaviour	Avoidance of social occasions
Somatic symptoms	Blushing, trembling
Associations	Secondary alcohol misuse

Table 10.6 **Symptoms of a panic attack**	
Component	**Prominent features**
Emotion	Severe, incapacitating anxiety
Cognition	Of dying, going mad or otherwise losing control
Behaviour	Escape
Somatic symptoms	Prominent symptoms of sympathetic arousal (Table 10.2)
Associations	Agoraphobia, depression

Table 10.7 **Symptoms of generalized anxiety disorder**	
Component	**Prominent features**
Emotion	Anxiety
Cognition	Excessive, disproportionate, uncontrollable worry
Behaviour	Easily startled, on edge
Somatic symptoms	Multiple chronic aches, headache, tension, sweating
Associations	Depression

unpleasant feelings of depersonalization or derealization (Table 10.6). In *panic disorder*, the attacks are recurrent over a period of at least 1 month. The somatic symptoms may be severe and lead to a misdiagnosis of angina, epilepsy or other medical disorders.

- The differential diagnosis is from panic attacks occurring only as part of a phobia or occasional panic occurring as part of other neuroses and depressive disorder. Also certain medical conditions can occasionally be a cause of paroxysmal anxiety.
- CBT is very effective for panic. It is aimed at helping the patient to see their symptoms as the result of anxiety and not as indicators of an impending catastrophe (such as a heart attack). Antidepressants are also effective, although patients with panic disorder may find them hard to tolerate as they may exacerbate panic before reducing it.
- Aetiologically, patients with panic disorder appear to have a low biological threshold for anxiety. Cognitive factors such as a tendency to catastrophically misinterpret somatic symptoms (e.g. *'the chest pain means that I am having a heart attack'*) are also important. Panic attacks may start during a period of stress.

Generalized anxiety disorder

Generalized anxiety is persistent anxiety associated with chronic uncontrollable and excessive worry (Table 10.7). It may fluctuate in severity but is not paroxysmal (as with panic), situational (as with phobia), life-long (as with a personality disorder) or clearly stress related (as with a stress-related disorder).

- Chronic somatic symptoms such as aches and pains and bowel symptoms may lead to medical presentations.
- Treatment is based on the same pharmacological, psychological and stress-reducing methods used in other anxiety disorders, but their efficacy may be lower.

Obsessive-compulsive disorder (OCD)

In OCD, obsessions and compulsions are the most prominent and persistent symptoms (Table 10.8), but one does not require both symptoms for a diagnosis. The main differential diagnoses are depressive disorder (in which obsessional symptoms are common), psychotic disorder (obsessions are usually regarded as untrue and are uncomfortable for the sufferer, unlike delusions where beliefs are seen as a reality) and obsessional (anankastic) personality disorder.

- 5-HT-predominant antidepressants (SSRIs, clomipramine) are effective, as is behavioural therapy. A higher dose of antidepressant than in depression is often required.
- If untreated, the prognosis is poor. The disorder is prone to chronicity.
- Aetiological factors include genetic vulnerability, an anankastic personality and social stressors. The condition is perpetuated by the avoidance of

Table 10.8 **Symptoms of obsessive-compulsive disorder (OCD)**	
Component	**Predominant features**
Emotion	Anxiety about the topic of the obsessional thought
Cognition	Preoccupation with obsession(s)
Behaviour	Compulsions
Somatic symptoms	Tension, especially if prevented from doing compulsive act
Associations	Depression, anankastic personality disorder, Tourette's syndrome

situations that trigger the obsessions, and by the performance of the compulsions; both of which stop the anxiety habituating.

- OCD is unusual amongst neuroses in being equally common in men and women.

🔍 Clinical scenario

June is a 25-year-old woman who recently presented to her GP with a history of compulsions. She has fears of contamination, and washes her hands excessively, to the extent where the skin on her hand has been sore and damaged. She recognizes that her fear of contamination is excessive and unreasonable, and has attempted to resist carrying out her compulsive behavior, but to no avail. June has a history of hoarding, and often doubts that she has carried out routine actions, like turning off the cooker or locking her door, and this has resulted in checking behaviour, which has become excessive in recent years. She is diagnosed with obsessive-compulsive disorder, and offered a prescription of fluoxetine as, although June is willing to participate in cognitive behavioural therapy, she is keen to get on with treatment whilst awaiting a place with a CBT practitioner.

Dissociative and conversion disorders

In dissociative disorders, also called *conversion disorder*, there is a loss of function, either psychological or physical, that is not explained by organic disease (Table 10.9).

- These disorders were called *dissociative* because they were thought to represent a loss of the normal association between different mental processes

Table 10.9 Symptoms of dissociative disorder

Component	Prominent features
Emotion	May be suppressed, with denial of anxiety
Cognition	Denial of psychological impact of stressors
Behaviour	Loss of function
Somatic symptoms	Loss of function, e.g. paralysis
Associations	Acute stressors, depression

such as personal identity and memories, sensory and motor function.

- The term *conversion* was used for loss of physical function because of the unsubstantiated theory that psychological conflicts got converted into physical symptoms, thereby resolving the mental conflict (so-called *primary gain*) and often providing practical benefits such as the attention of others (so-called *secondary gain*).
- Dissociative disorders were previously known as *hysterical*; this archaic term (suggesting causation by a wandering uterus) has now been abandoned.

Presentations include loss of psychological function such as memory (psychogenic amnesia), wandering in a trance (fugue), loss of motor function (paralysis, pseudoseizures) or loss of sensory function (glove and stocking anaesthesia).

- When the possibility of a dissociative disorder is raised, organic causes for the loss of function must be excluded. This may require extensive medical investigation.
- Dissociative disorders (which are regarded as originating in unconscious processes) must be distinguished from consciously motivated symptoms. The latter in turn are divided into *factitious disorder*, in which symptoms are produced deliberately to obtain medical care, and *malingering*, which is behaviour that is designed to achieve personal gain (see towards the end of this chapter). Deciding if someone is feigning illness is difficult and requires evidence of marked inconsistency (e.g. limping into the consulting room and then running for a bus).
- The current diagnostic criteria require that there should be a plausible 'psychogenic' explanation for the symptoms, in terms of severe internal conflicts or a traumatic life event; this is, however, often difficult to establish in practice.
- There have been very few randomized treatment trials. Clinical experience suggests that important components of management are: (a) to accept the reality of the patient's symptoms but to explain that they are potentially reversible; (b) to encourage a gradual return to normal function; (c) to treat coexisting depression; (d) to refer for psychotherapy in some cases; and (e) to refer for physical rehabilitation for chronic disorders that impair motor function.

Neurasthenia (chronic fatigue syndrome, or CFS)

The term neurasthenia is now rarely used in the United Kingdom or the United States but remains in common usage in China and some other countries.

There is substantial overlap with the functional syndrome of *chronic fatigue syndrome* (CFS). Although classified separately, neurasthenia has much in common with somatoform disorders, in that physical complaints predominate, no definite medical disease has been identified and the presentation is usually to non-psychiatric services. The main feature is persistent, disabling mental and physical fatigue, often accompanied by pain and other symptoms (Table 10.10).

The differential diagnosis is from fatigue associated with medical conditions and from depressive and anxiety disorders. A simple explanation that the symptoms are real and not imagined but reversible rather than fixed can be helpful.

- There is good evidence for the efficacy of CBT and graded increases in activity, but less for antidepressants.
- The prognosis is often poor, with a tendency to chronicity. Avoidance of physical activity and belief in a physical cause are associated with a worse outcome.
- The aetiology is very controversial. Biological, psychological and social factors are involved. Biologically, there is evidence for disturbed cerebral 5-HT function and reduced cortisol. Although many patients report onset after a viral infection, and patients with documented Epstein–Barr virus (EBV) infection can develop a fatigue syndrome, the aetiological role of retroviruses overall remains uncertain. Psychologically, depression, anxiety and excessive concern with symptoms leading to inactivity is common. Socially, a fear of a stigmatizing psychiatric diagnosis and widely available misinformation may shape patients' illness beliefs and help-seeking behaviour.

Table 10.10 Symptoms of neurasthenia (chronic fatigue syndrome)

Component	Prominent features
Emotion	Exhaustion, tiredness, irritability
Cognitions	Concern about fatigue and its causes, poor concentration
Behaviour	Avoids physical exertion
Bodily symptoms	Physical and/or mental fatigue after minor exertion, muscular pain (myalgia), headache, patchy sleep
Associations	Depression

- A similar constellation of symptoms is also referred to as *myalgic encephalomyelitis* (ME). This condition is thought by some to be better regarded as a neurological disorder and distinct from CFS, although this is also controversial.

Depersonalization-derealization syndrome

Depersonalization and derealization are symptoms that can occur in all neuroses. Occasionally they are the predominant feature, in which case this rarely used diagnostic category applies. The differential diagnoses include a depressive or anxiety disorder, psychosis, or organic causes, especially complex partial epilepsy. The usual guidelines for managing neurosis apply. Antidepressants may help, but the prognosis for established cases is poor.

Stress-related disorders

In some cases presenting with neurotic symptoms, the stressor appears to be of such overwhelming importance in causing the symptoms that they are classified as 'reactions to stress'. The whole range of neurotic symptoms may occur, commonly in a diffuse picture of distress, anxiety and depression. The subtypes of stress-related disorders are:

- *Acute stress reaction* – beginning and ending within hours or days of the stressor.
- *Adjustment disorder* – beginning less acutely and lasting several months.
- *Post-traumatic stress disorder (PTSD)* – a delayed response to an extreme stress associated with particular symptoms and especially the re-experiencing of the trauma in dreams or imagination.

Acute stress reactions

These are transient, but severe, emotional reactions immediately following an exceptional stressor (e.g. rape) and are colloquially referred to as 'nervous shock' (Table 10.11). The differential diagnosis includes the initial stages of other neuroses, acute psychosis (behaviour can be very odd and out of character) and delirium. Management is by removal of the stressor (if possible), reassurance and the provision of support. A short course of benzodiazepines may sometimes be used to reduce arousal.

- Trials show that early 'debriefing' (requiring that the patient tells a therapist about the stressful incident in detail soon after it has occurred) is

Table 10.11 **Symptoms of acute stress reaction**

Component	Predominant features
Emotion	'Dazed'
Cognition	Amnesia or denial of event
Behaviour	Overactivity or withdrawal
Somatic symptoms	Many autonomic symptoms
Association	Acute stressor

unhelpful and may even worsen outcome for some patients.

Adjustment disorders

Also called *adjustment reactions*, these are reactions to stress that are more prolonged than acute stress reactions. The symptoms typically begin within a month of the stress and do not last longer than 6 months (Table 10.12).

- Grief reactions and psychological reactions to medical conditions are types of adjustment reaction.

Management includes helping the patient to address a continuing stressor more effectively (perhaps by problem-solving therapy), discouraging unhelpful coping strategies such as substance misuse, and treating depressive or anxiety symptoms as necessary.

Post-traumatic stress disorder (PTSD)

PTSD is a delayed response to an exceptionally severe traumatic event (e.g. serious road accident, major disaster, severe assault). It was initially described in

Table 10.12 **Symptoms of adjustment disorders**

Component	Prominent features
Emotion	Depression, anxiety, poor concentration, irritability
Cognition	Preoccupation with event
Behaviour	Angry outbursts
Somatic symptoms	Moderate autonomic symptoms
Associations	Chronic stressor

Vietnam War veterans and, more recently, it has been recognized in UK law as a basis for personal compensation claims.

The onset may be months or years after the original trauma. A central feature is an involuntary re-experiencing of the traumatic event in nocturnal dreams or as intrusive 'flashbacks' often triggered by reminders of the trauma (Table 10.13).

Management includes treating any comorbid psychiatric disorder or substance misuse, and encouraging a return to normal activities. Antidepressant drugs are modestly effective. There is also an evidence base for the effectiveness of trauma-focused CBT.

- A treatment called *eye movement desensitization and reprocessing* (EMDR), in which the patient is asked to think about an image of the traumatic event whilst moving their eyes from side to side, is also effective, although controversy remains about how it works.
- The prognosis for PTSD is generally good, with a gradual resolution in most cases. However, a minority of cases become chronic. Associated alcohol misuse and depression are common.

Somatoform disorders

The somatoform disorders category was created to accommodate those patients who present with predominantly somatic complaints where neither depression and anxiety nor a medical condition provides a better explanation (Table 10.14). It includes many subcategories. There are two main groups:

- Conditions in which the main feature is concern about having disease (*hypochondriasis*) or deformity (*dysmorphophobia*).

Table 10.13 **Symptoms of post-traumatic stress disorder (PTSD)**

Component	Prominent features
Emotion	Anxiety and irritability, numbness and detachment
Cognition	Repeated reliving of the event in images ('flashbacks') and nightmares
Behaviour	Avoidance of situations associated with the trauma
Somatic symptoms	Exaggerated startle response
Associations	Substance misuse, depression, severe previous stressor

Table 10.14 Symptoms of somatoform disorders

Component	Prominent features
Emotion	Anxiety and depression usually present (but not predominant)
Cognition	Concern with physical symptoms, disease or deformity
Behaviour	Medical help seeking
Bodily symptoms	Prominent, defining
Associations	Depressive and anxiety disorders, iatrogenic harm from inappropriate medical care (e.g. surgery)

- Conditions in which the main feature is concern about somatic symptoms (*somatization disorder, persistent autonomic dysfunction, persistent somatoform pain disorder* and *undifferentiated somatoform disorder*).

To make the diagnosis of a somatoform disorder:

- The concerns and/or symptoms must be unexplained by or disproportionate to any organic disease, severe enough to cause distress and have persisted for at least 6 months.
- Depressive and anxiety symptoms are insufficient to justify a diagnosis of depressive or anxiety disorder.
- The symptoms are not delusional (e.g. distinguish from a psychotic disorder with somatic hallucinations).
- The symptoms are not deliberately manufactured (cf. factitious disorder, malingering), nor is there prominent loss of a specific function (cf. dissociative and conversion disorder).
- Aetiologically, childhood deprivation and abuse are risk factors. A predisposition to health anxiety and serious (and perhaps mismanaged) illness in a relative are also common.

Assessment and management of somatoform disorders

The principles of managing neuroses also apply to somatoform disorders. However, since such patients (and sometimes their doctors) often believe these somatic symptoms indicate medical disease rather than a psychiatric condition, the patients may seek and receive medical rather than psychiatric care. Patients are often hostile to the idea that their symptoms are 'psychogenic' or that they will benefit from psychiatric

treatment. The effective management of somato[...] disorder therefore requires a close liaison between G[...] physician and psychiatrist. The principles are:

- Take the patient's somatic concerns seriously. Neither dismiss them as 'just psychological', nor collude with unfounded beliefs about unproven medical causes.
- Medical investigations should be determined by the doctor's interpretation of the symptoms, not by the patient's demands. People with somatoform disorder are no more likely to die of undiagnosed organic disease than the general population, although they are at risk of harm from unnecessary medical tests and treatments. It is worth remembering that (perhaps counterintuitively) the more somatic symptoms a patient has, the less likely they are to have a medical disease.
- Ensure a clear and consistent explanation for the symptoms is given that, if possible, is agreed on by all doctors involved.
- Treat coexisting depression and anxiety in the usual way.
- Antidepressants are beneficial in most somatoform disorders, even when there is no good evidence of depression. However, their use needs careful explanation if they are not to be rejected as inappropriately 'psychiatric'.
- CBT is of proven value but must be adapted to be consistent with the patient's predominantly somatic concerns.
- Encourage a return to normal functioning and a decrease in illness behaviour.

Hypochondriasis and dysmorphophobia

The characteristic feature of these somatoform disorders is a preoccupation with the possibility of having a serious physical disease or deformity.

- The main differential diagnoses are depressive disorder (in which hypochondriacal worries and concerns about appearance are common) and psychotic disorders (with hypochondriacal delusions or somatic hallucinations).

Hypochondriasis

Patients with hypochondriasis are preoccupied with the idea that they have a serious medical condition when they do not. Patients repeatedly seek medical reassurance and investigation, but are not reassured by either.

- Repeated requests for investigation to exclude a serious disease may be the presenting feature.

nts and CBT can be effective. It ___ to help the patients to restrict ___ eek reassurance or check their ___ behaviours tend to perpetuate the condition.

- The prognosis is variable: transient hypochondriasis is common (e.g. in medical students), but once established the condition can last many years and lead to extensive medical investigations.

Dysmorphophobia

This disorder, also called *body dysmorphic disorder*, is characterized by a preoccupation with a subjectively abnormal physical appearance (e.g. perceived ugliness or deformity) that is not objectively present and often associated with avoidance of social interaction.

- Management follows the principles described for somatoform disorders in general. Patients often request cosmetic surgery, which may sometimes be helpful but which can also lead to further dissatisfaction. Specialist assessment is advisable before surgery is performed.

Somatic symptom disorders (somatization disorder and associated diagnoses)

Somatic symptoms, such as fatigue and pain, that are not adequately explained by medical disease are very common. When these are persistent and associated with disability and or distress they may appropriately be regarded as illnesses and consequently require a diagnosis. Such patients comprise about one-third of all attenders in medical out-patient clinics, and so are clinically important.

- Confusingly, medicine and psychiatry have developed parallel diagnostic systems for these problems. Medicine uses diagnoses of so-called 'functional disorders' describing the symptoms in terms of the bodily system they relate to (see Table 10.15). Psychiatry uses somatoform diagnoses based mainly on the number of symptoms and their duration. The current psychiatric classification is as given below.

Somatization disorder (Briquet's syndrome)

These patients, almost always women, present with multiple different medically unexplained symptoms that have occurred over many years. They have often had normal abdominal organs surgically removed, an observation that highlights the risk of iatrogenic harm. They have been described as adopting 'illness as a way of life'. Recurrent major depression and personality disorder are common associations – indeed, some regard the condition as a personality disorder.

- Management is based on 'damage limitation' and containment by long-term follow-up. There is no specific treatment, but active treatment of associated recurrent depression and anxiety may be helpful.
- The prognosis is very poor. Iatrogenic problems, such as drug reactions and abdominal adhesions, may result from unnecessary medical and surgical interventions.

Undifferentiated somatoform disorder

This is the diagnosis used instead of somatization disorder when the patient has few symptoms.

Persistent somatoform pain disorder

This diagnosis is used when the main symptom is pain that is inadequately explained by a medical disease. Antidepressants are useful; tricyclic antidepressants (TCAs) and selective serotonin and noradrenaline reuptake inhibitors (SNRIs) are more effective than selective serotonin reuptake inhibitors (SSRIs). CBT may be helpful.

Somatoform autonomic dysfunction

This is a rarely used diagnosis for cases where the symptoms are thought to be clearly explicable in terms of autonomic arousal and associated overbreathing (e.g. breathlessness, chest pain, flushing, diarrhoea and tremor).

Functional somatic syndromes and their relationship to somatoform disorders

The medical classification of functional somatic symptoms (Table 10.15) is a parallel one to the psychiatric classification of somatoform disorders. Functional somatic syndrome diagnoses are commonly made in most medical specialties and account for a very substantial number of the patients seen. For example, irritable bowel syndrome is the most common diagnosis made in many gastroenterological clinics; the majority of cases of acute chest pain are 'non-cardiac', and often associated with panic disorder. Similarly, numbness, weakness and

Table 10.15 **Common functional somatic syndrome diagnoses**
Medically unexplained pain syndromes Non-cardiac chest pain Facial pain Pelvic pain Back pain Irritable bowel syndrome Muscular pain and fibromyalgia
Medically unexplained chronic fatigue Chronic fatigue syndrome

tingling are frequent symptoms in neurology clinics, yet are often 'functional'. It should also be noted that more than one-half of patients with a functional somatic syndrome satisfy criteria for depressive or anxiety disorder rather than a somatoform disorder. This is important for treatment. Because the diagnostic systems overlap, but emphasize different aspects of the presentation, a combined medical and psychiatric diagnosis may be preferred – for example, irritable bowel syndrome and generalized anxiety disorder or chronic fatigue syndrome and somatization disorder.

Factitious disorders and malingering

The relationship between bodily symptoms and psychiatric disorder is complicated further by patients who consciously elaborate or even deliberately make up symptoms. These are not neuroses but are included here because of their importance in the differential diagnosis of patients presenting with somatic symptoms.

- If the behaviour appears to be aimed at receiving medical treatment it is called *factitious disorder*. People with persistent, severe factitious disorder who travel from one hospital to another have been described as having *Munchausen's syndrome* (after Baron von Munchausen, who told stories of fantastic exploits). The degree of conscious manipulation is often unclear.
- If the behaviour is for fraudulent purposes (e.g. to avoid legal proceedings or military conscription) it is referred to as *malingering*. Factitious disorder is a psychiatric disorder; malingering is not.

If there is suspicion that symptoms are being manufactured, discrete but determined efforts to verify the person's details and history should be made. Once a factitious disorder has been confirmed, the patient should be gently confronted with the evidence. However sympathetically handled, self-discharge commonly results. People with factitious disorder can sometimes make doctors feel angry and manipulated. It is important to take care not to generalize these negative feelings to the larger group of patients who have medical problems you cannot explain by a disease diagnosis.

 KEYPOINTS

- Neuroses are syndromes of emotional, cognitive, behavioural and somatic symptoms that are not secondary to another disorder. Neurotic symptoms occur commonly in other psychiatric disorders.
- Neuroses afflict 15% of the population, women more than men. They may become chronic and disabling. The main subtypes are anxiety disorders and somatoform disorders.
- Stress-related disorders are neuroses in which there is a clear relationship to a major psychological stressor.
- Somatoform disorders encompass medically unexplained symptoms (somatization) and fears about having physical disease (hypochondriasis), and are closely related to other neuroses. They are usually seen in non-psychiatric medical settings.
- Neuroses, stress-related disorders, and somatoform disorders can all be treated psychologically (especially with CBT) or with antidepressants. Anxiolytics can also be useful in the short term.

 FURTHER READING

National Institute for Health and Care Excellence (NICE) (2005) CG31 Obsessive-compulsive disorder: Core Interventions in the treatment of obsessive compulsive disorder and body dysmorphic disorder. NICE.

National Institute for Health and Care Excellence (NICE) (2006) CG26 The management of PTSD in adults and children in primary and secondary care. NICE.

National Institute for Health and Care Excellence (NICE) (2011) CG113 Generalised anxiety disorder and panic disorder in adults. NICE.

? SELF-ASSESSMENT

1 Charles is a 24-year-old man who presents with thoughts of shouting obscenities in a church setting. His psychiatrist thinks that these are 'obsessional' in nature. Which of the following is true about obsessional thoughts?
   a They are egosyntonic.
   b They are necessary to make a diagnosis of OCD.
   c They can take the form of vivid imagery.
   d They do not respond to pharmacotherapy with SSRIs.
   e They are commonly associated with antisocial personality disorder.

2 A 32-year-old sergeant returned from an advanced military post in a conflict zone 6 months ago and is being assessed for the development of post-traumatic stress disorder. Which of the following would you consider *not* to be a recognized feature of PTSD?
   a Flashbacks
   b Nightmares
   c Disinhibited behaviour
   d Exaggerated startle response
   e Anxiety

3 Which of the following statements about anxiety disorders is true?
   a Agoraphobia is more common in men.
   b Primary and secondary gain are associated with somatoform disorders.
   c Glove and stocking anaesthesia is a recognized feature of dissociative disorders.
   d Malingering is a psychiatric disorder.
   e Somatization disorder only occurs in females.

Eating, sleep and sexual disorders

Learning objectives

✓ To understand the diagnostic differences between different eating disorders

✓ To be able to describe key aspects in the management of eating disorders

✓ To develop an understanding of common sleep disorders

✓ To develop a framework for the assessment of sexual dysfunction

Disorders of eating, sleeping and sex are grouped together in the diagnostic manual ICD-10 because they are syndromes associated with a disturbance in 'basic' desires and behaviours. Here, we describe the features, assessment and management of these disorders, although the assessment of eating disorders is covered in Chapter 3.

Eating disorders

Eating disorders can present in many different ways to in all branches of medicine. To a great extent they are culturally bound, predominating in industrialized countries where thinness is valued and where easy access to food means obesity is a real possibility. Most eating disorders begin between the ages of 7 and 13 and are characterized by a preoccupation with weight and the development of anxieties about weight gain, changing body shape and unrealistic goals of an idealized clothing size. Around 40% of children in this age group are worried about becoming fat. Dieting behaviours often emerge at puberty when body shape changes considerably.

Eating disorders are conventionally separated into *anorexia nervosa* and *bulimia nervosa*, as described below. Anorexia has been recognized for a number of centuries but bulimia was only first described in 1979. However, bear two clinical realities in mind:

- Many patients – around 50% – do not meet all the criteria for either disorder, or have some features of both. They are labelled *atypical eating disorder* – or *eating disorder not otherwise specified (EDNOS)*. This does not mean their disorder is any less severe.
- Many patients move from one category to another over time.

 Box 11.1 Eating disorders in men

- Males represent around 1 in 6 cases of eating disorder in community settings.
- Dieting is often for specific goals, e.g. athletic performance, to avoid teasing.
- Males are more sensitive about shape from the waist up (women are the opposite).
- Males start dieting from a higher weight and feel fat at relatively higher weights compared to women.
- Men are less likely to seek diagnostic evaluation perhaps because of perceived stigma.

Psychiatry Lecture Notes, Eleventh Edition. Gautam Gulati, Mary-Ellen Lynall and Kate Saunders. © 2014 John Wiley & Sons, Ltd. Published 2014 by John Wiley & Sons, Ltd.

Anorexia nervosa

Clinical features

As well as the core features above, the key elements of anorexia nervosa are:

- *Self-induced weight loss*, induced primarily by restriction of food intake.
- *Weight ≥15% below normal* (BMI <17.5).
- Irrational fear of fatness/intense drive for thinness.
- Body image distortion and excessive reliance on weight or shape for self-esteem.
- *Amenorrhoea* (if post-menarche and not using hormonal contraceptive). Part of a wider endocrine disturbance that includes elevated cortisol and growth hormone levels.
- Two subtypes are defined: (i) *restrictive* (ANR), and (ii) *binge-purge* (ANBP).

Additional features include:

- A range of bodily symptoms and signs, which become more pronounced as weight loss progresses (Table 11.1). The medical complications can be serious and life-threatening, especially if the effects of starvation are exacerbated by the metabolic consequences of vomiting, or diuretic or laxative abuse.
- The core psychological features (e.g. 'fear of fatness') become paradoxically worse as weight is lost (maybe because it increases the 5-HT dysfunction, which is thought to contribute to the disturbance). The disorder thus tends to be self-perpetuating – reinforced by the fact that achieving a lower weight has certain rewards: it may enhance feelings of self-control, result in perceived approval from peers, avoid sexual development or gain parental attention.
- Depressive and obsessional symptoms.
- If the onset is before puberty, secondary sexual development is delayed.
- Depression, fatigue and irritability, especially as weight loss becomes pronounced.
- Social withdrawal and narrowing of interests.
- Use of diuretics, laxatives, excess exercise or self-induced vomiting to enhance weight loss.

 Clinical scenario

Miss T, 14, was noticed to be losing weight although this was partially disguised by baggy clothing. She enjoyed cooking for the family and took up regular aerobics. She became vegetarian and avoided all fattening foods. When the issue of her weight was raised, Miss T became upset, insisting that she was fat. She had a history of obesity. The GP found she was underweight (BMI = 15) and suspected anorexia nervosa.

Table 11.1 Physical features and medical complications of anorexia nervosa

Physical symptoms
Sensitivity to cold
Gastrointestinal symptoms – constipation, bloating
Dizziness
Amenorrhoea
Poor sleep

Physical signs
Emaciation
Cold extremities
Dry skin, sometimes orange (hypercarotinaemia)
Downy hair ('*lanugo*') on back, forearms and cheeks
Poorly developed or atrophic secondary sexual characteristics
Bradycardia, postural hypotension, arrhythmias
Peripheral oedema
Proximal myopathy

Abnormalities on investigation
Low LH, FSH, oestradiol, T_3
Increased cortisol, growth hormone
Hypoglycaemia
Hypokalaemia, hyponatraemia, metabolic alkalosis
ECG: prolonged QT interval (serious)
Hypercholesterolaemia
Osteopenia and osteoporosis
Low WBC and platelets
Delayed gastric emptying
Acute gastric dilatation (due to over-rapid refeeding)

ECG, electrocardiogram; FSH, follicle-stimulating hormone; LH, luteinizing hormone; T_3, triiodothyronine; WBC, white blood cells.

Epidemiology and aetiology

Anorexia mainly affects females (sex ratio 10:1) although it is an increasing and overlooked problem in men (see Box 11.1). The average age of onset is 15–16 years. The prevalence in Western societies, including the United Kingdom, is about 1% in females aged 12–18. Social pressure to be thin has been blamed. The other risk factors are summarized in Table 11.2.

- Note that most risk factors are shared with bulimia nervosa.
- The familial risk of anorexia nervosa does not seem to be genetic in origin (in contrast to most other psychiatric disorders).

Differential diagnosis

The classic picture of anorexia nervosa is unmistakable. In the early stages it must be distinguished from other causes of weight loss. The psychiatric

Table 11.2 **Risk factors for eating disorders**
General factors
Female (sex ratio ~10:1 in clinical sample, 6:1 in community)
Adolescence and early adulthood
Living in a Western society
Family history
Eating disorder
Depression
Substance misuse (bulimia nervosa)
Obesity (bulimia nervosa)
Premorbid experiences
Adverse parenting – low contact, high expectations, arguments
Sexual abuse
Family dieting
Critical comments about eating, weight or shape
Pressure to be slim
Premorbid characteristics
Low self-esteem
Perfectionism (anorexia nervosa)
Impulsivity (bulimia nervosa)
Anxiety
Obesity (bulimia nervosa)
Early menarche (bulimia nervosa)
Specific groups
Ballet dancers
Models
Jockeys
Gymnasts

differential diagnosis includes depressive disorder, substance misuse, obsessive-compulsive disorder (OCD) and body dysmorphic disorder. The medical disorders include diabetes, inflammatory bowel disease, malabsorption syndromes, hypopituitarism and cancer. The distinction is made by:

- Detecting the core psychological symptoms of anorexia nervosa.
- Excluding physical and other psychiatric causes of weight loss.

Management

The objectives of treatment of anorexia nervosa are:

- Altering the person's attitude to weight and body shape via psychological treatments.
- Helping them increase weight.
- Detecting and treating medical complications.

The second and third components can be achieved reasonably successfully, at least in the short term;

the first component is difficult as the core beliefs are often resistant to treatment. Some principles of management are:

- Establish a good therapeutic relationship – many patients are reluctant to accept treatment. Help them to see they need help, and maintain motivation thereafter. Agree some goals: what weight is the person prepared to work towards? At what rate? How much exercise is appropriate?
- Encourage early weight gain to break the cycle and to overcome the problem that starvation interferes with psychological treatments. Weight gain is promoted by behavioural strategies – for example, contingent rewards.
- The key element of therapy is to change attitudes towards weight and shape, and the person's preoccupation with them. A modified type of cognitive behavioural therapy (CBT) ('transdiagnostic CBT') is commonly used while most adolescent patients respond well to a specific form of family therapy.
- Drugs (antidepressants or antipsychotics) do not have an established role in management, though they are sometimes used to treat comorbid disorders such as depression.
- Monitor physical condition. Serum potassium should be checked regularly. Multivitamins and supplements may be used.

In-patient treatment

In-patient care is indicated if weight loss is intractable and severe (e.g. BMI <14), or if there is a serious risk of death from suicide or medical complications. Admission is preferably to a specialist unit. It usually lasts 8–12 weeks. The purposes are to:

- Manage medical complications.
- Actively encourage refeeding but avoid refeeding syndrome (see Box 11.2).
- Allow intensive psychological treatments.
- Compulsory admission is rarely used, and considered only if life is in immediate danger. Forced refeeding is also used occasionally and controversially.

 Clinical scenario *(continued)*

Miss T is now 15 and has collapsed. For the past year, despite denials to her parents, she had dieted and exercised excessively. She weighed 29 kg (BMI = 12.5), was hypothermic and had a low blood potassium. After medical stabilization she passively accepted admission to an eating disorder unit. She began a behavioural programme with a target to gain 0.5 kg/week for 2 months. A psychiatrist and nurse therapist explored eating and weight issues in individual and family sessions. Her potassium was monitored regularly. Ten weeks later her BMI was 15 and she became an out-patient.

 Box 11.2 Refeeding syndrome

This is a potentially catastrophic syndrome that arises as the result of the depletion of cardiac muscle secondary to starvation. This may be amplified by changes in serum phosphorus, magnesium and potassium that occur with insulin release when food intake increases. The resulting low phosphate may further amplify cardiac problems leading to heart failure.

Refeeding can be avoided if the following principles are followed:

- Measure all serum electrolytes prior to refeeding and monitor every 5–7 days.
- Start at 1200 kcal/day and gradually increase every 5 days.
- Monitor for tachycardia and oedema.

Prognosis

The outcome of anorexia nervosa is variable. About 20% have a good outcome, with a short-lived disorder and full recovery. Another 10–20% develop a chronic and intractable disorder. The rest progress to another eating disorder, have a relapsing illness or have residual features.

- The mortality rate is increased 10-fold in the first 10 years of illness, with a 10–20% death rate in long-term follow-up studies. Compared to the general population the mortality rate in anorexia is 12 times higher and more than twice that of psychiatric in-patients. Death is usually from complications of starvation (approximately 60% as a direct effect of the illness), sometimes from suicide (27%).
- Poor outcome is associated with: long duration prior to presentation; onset in adulthood; severe weight loss; vomiting.

 Clinical scenario *(continued)*

Miss T is now 27 and a beautician. She has a BMI of 16 and has occasional scanty menstrual periods. She continues to be preoccupied with her appearance, and gains self-esteem from her control over eating and weight. She diets continually and works out twice a day. Now and then she has a large binge followed by self-induced vomiting and extra gym sessions. She avoids doctors.

Bulimia nervosa

Bulimia refers to uncontrolled eating binges. Many people binge and feel bad about it, but in bulimia nervosa it is excessive, repetitive and associated with self-induced vomiting and other means to negate the calorific effect of the binges. It punctuates an otherwise anorexia nervosa-like pattern of dietary restriction.

Clinical features

In addition to the core features of eating disorders, bulimia nervosa is characterized by:

- Recurrent binge eating (more than twice a week); 1000–4000 kcal (4–8 MJ) are typically consumed in a binge.
- 'Loss of control' during binges.
- Compensation after bingeing by purging (vomiting, diuretics or laxatives), excessive exercise or restriction.
- Regret or shame after bingeing.
- Irrational fear of fatness/distortion of body image.
- Does not meet diagnostic criteria for anorexia nervosa.
- Two subtypes: (i) purging (80%); and (ii) compensation, e.g. exercising or restricting (20%).

The combination of dieting and bingeing means body weight is usually unremarkable – the most obvious difference from anorexia nervosa. The first binge is often triggered by diet-induced hunger and followed by compensatory purging. However, this behaviour often generalizes over time to become a means with which to deal with difficult emotional states. A small proportion of bulimia nervosa cases occur in women with borderline personality disorder who self-harm (often by cutting) and misuse alcohol or drugs. This is a much rarer combination than sometimes believed.

If body weight is decreased, some of the physical features and complications of anorexia nervosa may be present (Table 11.1). Otherwise, fewer abnormalities are seen in bulimia nervosa. Those that are present reflect the self-induced vomiting, or abuse of laxatives or diuretics:

- Repeated vomiting may produce pitted teeth (eroded by gastric acid), calluses on the knuckles ('Russell's sign', from putting fingers down throat), hoarse voice, salivary gland enlargement, and metabolic disturbances (Table 11.1).
- Diuretic use: electrolyte disturbances and renal dysfunction.
- Laxatives: electrolyte disturbances and colonic motility problems.

Epidemiology and aetiology

Bulimia nervosa occurs in 2% of women aged 16–35 years. Based on community surveys, only 10% of cases ever present for help. Many of the risk factors are shared with anorexia nervosa (Table 11.2). There is a genetic predisposition, which overlaps with that for anxiety disorders.

- The genetic contribution to bulimia nervosa is controversial. Some studies suggest a surprisingly large heritability – over 80%.

 Clinical scenario

Miss V is 23. She has several episodes of bingeing and vomiting each week. In an hour she can eat 10 packets of crisps, 10 chocolate bars and a couple of loaves of bread washed down with a bottle of wine. She then makes herself sick. She is preoccupied with her weight and shape and feels fat (though her BMI is normal). She has a history of taking overdoses when particularly distressed. She was obese as a child, and sexually abused by an uncle. There is a family history of obesity and depression.

Differential diagnosis

- Anorexia nervosa with bulimic features (anorexia trumps bulimia, diagnostically, although in reality a better term would be 'eating disorder NOS', as explained above).
- Sporadic bingeing in other psychiatric disorders (e.g. atypical depression)
- Medical causes of vomiting.
- Binge eating disorder – recurrent binges occur but without extreme weight control behaviour. This is a recent entity but one that contributes to 25% of medical obesity. Unlike bulimia nervosa it is characterized by bingeing only and often relentless grazing. Its presentation is often gradual and it most commonly affects people in their 30s and 40s.

Management

Treatments are markedly more effective (and better evaluated) than in anorexia nervosa. Take a 'stepped care' approach, depending on the severity of the problem and the patient's wishes.

Self-help manuals are a cost-effective and increasingly used first-line treatment.

- A modified form of CBT is effective in 60–70% of patients, with the majority remaining well 5 years later. CBT aims to help the patient: (a) understand the links between bingeing, vomiting and dieting; (b) regulate their diet and break the vicious cycle

between the three behaviours; and (c) decrease their preoccupation with body shape.
- Interpersonal therapy (IPT) also works, but takes longer. IPT emphasizes the role of relationship problems in the disorder.
- Antidepressants reduce the frequency of bingeing and vomiting. The best evidence is for fluoxetine. High doses (60–80 mg/day) may be required, and the disorder often relapses on stopping.

Prognosis

The prognosis of bulimia nervosa is probably better than that of anorexia nervosa (the mortality rate is certainly lower), though there are few good data.

- People have had bulimia nervosa for an average of 5 years at presentation; 30–50% still have an eating disorder (bulimia nervosa or atypical eating disorder) 5–10 years later.
- Poor prognostic factors include: premorbid childhood obesity, low self-esteem and personality disturbance.

Sleep disorders

Sleep problems are usually secondary to a psychiatric or medical disorder, but sometimes a sleep disorder is the primary diagnosis. ICD-10 records over 80 sleep disorders, but essentially, there are three types of problem:

1 Too little sleep (insomnias).
2 Too much sleep (hypersomnias).
3 Unusual sleep behaviours (parasomnias), e.g. sleep-walking, sleep-talking.

The assessment of sleep disorders is covered in Chapter 3.

Insomnia

Insomnia is a disturbance of normal sleep patterns, commonly difficulty in initiating sleep. One-third of adults complain of it but it is highly subjective and although a typical adult sleeps 7–9 hours per night this varies widely from night to night as well as varying greatly between different people. It causes much distress and is a risk factor for premature death; 80% of cases of insomnia are related to anxiety and depressive disorders. Most of the rest are secondary to medical disease (e.g. it is common in Parkinson's disease), chronic pain and substance misuse. The remaining fraction (<10%) is *primary insomnia*. To distinguish these cases, exclude the presence of an underlying psychiatric or medical disorder (e.g. restless legs syndrome, lymphoma). Ask about other factors that affect sleep such as shift working, medication, alcohol, caffeine, etc. A sleep diary and corroboration from the sleeping partner are helpful. Whilst 30–48% of people report insomnia symptoms, only 6% meet criteria for a diagnosis of insomnia.

Treatment of insomnia

Treat any associated disorder (e.g. use a sedative antidepressant if insomnia is due to depression). Interventions for insomnia include:

- *Stimulus control.* An effective method to restore a good sleep routine. The person should go to bed only when sleepy, put the light out straight away, get up if awake for more than 20 minutes, get up at a regular time and avoid daytime naps.
- *Sleep hygiene* – this approach pays attention to health practices (e.g. use of caffeine and alcohol) and stimuli (e.g. noise, light) that affect sleep.
- *Relaxation therapy* – behavioural, cognitive and biofeedback routines to reduce arousal. The person should wind down 90 minutes before bedtime and practise relaxation when in bed.
- *Hypnotics* – short-acting benzodiazepines and related drugs. Effective in the short term and widely used, but may cause daytime drowsiness, and long-term use should be avoided because of dependence.
- *Melatonin* – a naturally occurring hormone that regulates circadian rhythm. At present it is licensed only for short-term treatment of insomnia in those over the age of 55. It should not be taken for more than 3 weeks.

Excessive daytime sleepiness

Excessive daytime sleepiness can be caused by:

1 insufficient sleep;
2 fragmented sleep;
3 primary disorder of excessive daytime sleepiness – the *hypersomnias* (see Table 11.3).

The diagnosis of *hypersomnia* can only be made if the excessive daytime sleepiness is not due to other sleep disorders.

In *narcolepsy* there are repeated attacks of daytime somnolence usually leading irresistibly to sleep. It usually begins in the second decade and is associated with *cataplexy* (abrupt loss of muscle tone), *hypnagogic hallucinations* (on falling asleep) and *sleep paralysis* (the patient wakes but is unable to move). An autoimmune origin is suspected as 98% have the DR15

Table 11.3 Causes of hypersomnia

Psychiatric disorders
Depressive disorder
Neurasthenia (chronic fatigue syndrome)

Medical disorders
Narcolepsy
Klein–Levin syndrome
Sleep apnoea syndrome
Chronic physical disease

Other
Side effects of drugs (prescribed or illicit)

variant of HLA-DR2. Pathologically, there is a loss of hypothalamic hypocretin-producing neurons. Stimulants (amphetamines or modafinil) are the main treatment; clomipramine is also used for the cataplexy.

Parasomnias

Parasomnias are abnormal episodic events during sleep – sleepwalking, nightmares, etc. They are part of normal development in children; in adults they usually reflect emotional stress.

- Distinguish parasomnias from other causes of odd nocturnal behaviour, such as epilepsy.

Sexual problems

Psychiatrists are sometimes portrayed as being obsessed with sex – a relic of Freudian theories, not helped by media portrayals of psychiatrists. The reality is rather different and more mundane. Nevertheless, an understanding of sexual problems and how to assess them is important in psychiatry because:

- Sexual dysfunction is a common consequence of psychiatric disorders or their treatment. For example, loss of libido in depression and ejaculatory failure due to antipsychotics.
- Sexual dysfunction may contribute to psychiatric disorder. For example, an anxiety disorder may be exacerbated by a man worrying about his impotence.
- Disorders of sexual function, preference and identity are specific mental disorders.

Sexual dysfunction

Each of the components of sex – desire, physiological arousal and orgasm – can go awry (Table 11.4). Each

Table 11.4 **Types of sexual dysfunction**
Sexual desire disorders Lack of Excess
Failure of genital response Erectile dysfunction (impotence) Vaginal dryness
Orgasmic dysfunction Premature ejaculation Anorgasmia
Other Vaginismus (involuntary spasm of vaginal musculature) Dyspareunia

type of dysfunction may be due to psychological or medical causes, or both.

- Painful intercourse, loss of sexual desire and impaired orgasm are more common in women; the main problems for men are impotence and premature ejaculation.
- Sexual dysfunction is associated with sexual inexperience, anxiety and relationship problems.

Assessment of sexual dysfunction

Asking about sex is the topic, along with suicide, that most health professionals feel least confident and most embarrassed about. This is unnecessary. Many patients are glad to be asked, since sexual problems are common and it may be their first opportunity to seek reassurance or treatment.

- Know when to introduce the subject – try to respond to cues. For example, if a depressed patient tells you he gets no pleasure from life, it is a good moment to ask whether this has also affected his interest in sex. If no cue presents itself, preface the assessment with a comment such as: 'I need to ask you some questions about your sex life, to help me understand your problem. Is this alright?'.
- Use terminology appropriate to the person's age and culture.

Assessment of sexual function covers several areas (Table 11.5). Some of the questions will be used regularly, others rarely. Below are further details of two common sexual disorders to illustrate the general approaches to assessment and treatment of sexual dysfunction.

Erectile dysfunction

Erectile dysfunction is the inability to reach erection or to sustain an erection long enough for intercourse.

Most erectile dysfunction is secondary – that is, full erection was possible at one time, but is now difficult to achieve. Primary erectile dysfunction is rare and usually has a neurological or circulatory basis.

Common causes of impotence include:

- Anxiety about sexual performance.
- Alcohol.
- Unwanted effects of prescription medicines.
- Diabetes.
- Vascular disease.

Treatment is usually with combined psychological and physical approaches. Underlying disorders should be treated. Psychological treatment is outlined below. Drug treatment with phosphodiesterase type V inhibitors (e.g. sildenafil) is now widespread and has largely replaced injections and devices.

- Prescribing of sildenafil for 'psychological' impotence is possible on the NHS, but restricted to specialist centres and for those 'suffering severe distress as a result of impotence'.

Dyspareunia

Dyspareunia is pain on intercourse. It may result from impaired lubrication with vaginal secretions (due to anxiety or inadequate arousal) or from physical scarring (e.g. after childbirth). Pain on penetration may be due to pelvic pathology.

- When dyspareunia is secondary to psychological factors, sexual therapy techniques can be used (see below).

Psychological treatment of sexual dysfunction

Sexual problems may respond to reassurance or use of self-help manuals. Others require sex therapy, which is provided by some psychiatrists and by private therapists. Sex therapy uses behavioural methods, and is effective (assuming no underlying medical cause for the dysfunction). The principles are:

- Treat the couple together.
- Educate about sex and the factors affecting it.
- Encourage open discussion of feelings and decrease anxiety and embarrassment.
- Use graded exposure (Chapter 7). The couple gradually rebuild their sexual relationship, setting aside time and commitment to follow a series of steps – starting with non-genital 'sensate focus', then moving on via genital focus before finally returning to full intercourse. Additional methods are used for

Table 11.5 **Assessment of sexual function**

Questions	Comments
Current sexual functioning	
What is the nature and frequency of sex?	
Is there a particular problem?	Get a history of each difficulty
How much interest do you have in sex? Has this changed recently?	Increased libido is rarely complained of. A feature of mania
In men	
Erectile function:	
Any problems getting or keeping an erection?	
Do you get erections in the morning?	Loss of morning erections or when masturbating suggests organic cause
Do you worry about your sexual performance?	Impotence related to performance anxiety
Ejaculatory function:	
Do you come too quickly?	Common in inexperienced, anxious men
How long after penetration?	
Do you feel anxious about this?	
In women	
Do you have pain on intercourse? When? Where?	Dyspareunia and vaginal dryness have psychological and gynaecological causes
Do you feel anxious or tense about sex?	Extreme anxiety can lead to vaginismus
Sexual development	
Estimate age of puberty	
When did your voice break? Periods start?	Problems or delays in sexual development may lead to psychological effects or indicate an abnormality (e.g. Turner's syndrome)
When did you first masturbate? First intercourse?	Affected by cultural and individual differences
Sexual orientation and preferences	
What is their sexual orientation?	
Any particular sexual preferences or fetishes?	Detailed questioning indicates if the patient views it as a problem, or in a forensic context
If so, what?	
Have they ever got you into trouble?	
Other issues	
Current psychiatric disorder?	Most psychiatric disorders, especially depression, are associated with sexual dysfunction
General health?	Medical disorders (e.g. diabetes, vascular disease) affect sexual functioning; do a physical examination
Current medication?	Many drugs have sexual side effects (e.g. thiazide diuretics, H_2 antagonists, antihypertensives–as well as antidepressants and antipsychotics)

specific forms of dysfunction. For example, dilators for vaginismus or the squeeze technique for premature ejaculation.

- Lack of sexual desire has the worst prognosis.

Other sexual disorders

In these disorders the problem is not sex itself but the object of sexual desire or sexual identity. The person may or may not agree with this view. In ICD-10, these disorders are grouped with personality disorders.

- Forensic psychiatrists may be asked to report on the psychiatric status of sex offenders.
- Homosexuality used to be classified as a psychiatric disorder.

Gender identity disorders

- In *gender dysphoric disorder* (commonly known as *transexualism*) the person, usually male, wishes to live as a member of the opposite sex. They seek hormonal or surgical treatment to match their body to their subjective gender. Sexual orientation is variable and sexual desire often low. Transsexuals may suffer great distress, and depression is common.

- *Transvestism* is the urge to dress in clothes of the opposite sex. If accompanied by sexual arousal it is called *fetishistic* transvestism. There is no desire to change sex. Transvestites are often married and cross-dress secretly. There is no specific treatment.

Disorders of sexual preference (paraphilias)

Sexual desire can centre on a wide range of animate and inanimate objects. Such pleasures only constitute a disorder if the activity is illegal (e.g. paedophilia) or if sex becomes dysfunctional and over-dependent on an object such as shoes (e.g. fetishism). Paraphilia is usually but not always a male disorder.

- In *paedophilia*, sexual interest or activity centres on prepubescent children. Psychological treatments have been used to reduce reoffending rates. Antiandrogens such as cyproterone acetate and goserelin have been used to suppress libido. There is some evidence of efficacy but the evidence base is limited. Those who are found offending are managed primarily by the criminal justice system with the use of specific legislation.
- *Exhibitionism* is the exposing of the genitals to strangers. Two groups are recognized: (1) inhibited men who struggle against the urge, feel guilty and expose a flaccid penis (type 1); (2) aggressive men who expose an erect penis and masturbate then or later (type 2). The latter shows an association with actual sexual assaults. Behavioural treatments may be beneficial. SSRIs have a limited evidence base.

🔑 KEYPOINTS

- The core psychopathology of all eating disorders is a preoccupation with body shape and weight, with extreme methods to control weight – notably dietary restriction. They occur mainly but not exclusively in young women.

- Anorexia nervosa is characterized additionally by a low body weight (BMI < 17.5), extreme dietary restriction, and amenorrhoea in women.
- Bulimia nervosa is distinguished by recurrent binge eating and self-induced vomiting.
- Half of patients with an eating disorder do not meet criteria for anorexia or bulimia nervosa.
- Bulimia nervosa responds well to CBT. No effective treatments are proven for anorexia nervosa.
- Sleep disorders comprise insomnia, hypersomnia and parasomnias (disturbances during sleep). Many are secondary to other psychiatric or medical disorders. They may be treated psychologically or pharmacologically.
- Sexual dysfunction is common and can affect the desire, the mechanics or the orgasm. Assessment of sexual function is important. Sex therapy is effective for many of the problems.

FURTHER READING

Treasure J, Claudino AM, Zucker N (2010) Eating disorders. *Lancet* 375, 583–593. doi: 10.1016/S0140-6736(09)61748-7. Access at http://www.thelancet.com/journals/lancet/article/PIIS0140-6736(09)61748-7

SELF-ASSESSMENT

1 Preoccupation with weight:
  a Is absent in bulimia nervosa.
  b Emerges in girls from the age of 7 onwards.
  c Is never seen in males.
  d Is unusual in EDNOS.

2 Which of the following should be monitored during refeeding?
  a Weight
  b Phosphate
  c Ankle swelling
  d Potasssium
  e Heart rate

12

Schizophrenia

Learning objectives

✓ To be able to describe the presentation, aetiology, assessment and management of schizophrenia

Schizophrenia is at the heart of psychiatry and is closest to the public conception of madness. Although not the most common disorder, it accounts for a significant proportion of psychiatric morbidity and the workload of psychiatric services.

- In 2008/09 patients with schizophrenia occupied 2.85 million NHS bed days; higher than for any other condition in any medical specialty.
- The economic burden of the disorder in England runs into several billions of pounds annually.

Clinical features

Schizophrenia is a psychosis, typically presenting in young adults. It is distinguished from other psychoses by:

- the presence of specific types of delusions, hallucinations and thought disorder;
- the primary disorder is not one of affective (mood) or organic aetiology;
- the clinical course.

The clinical picture of schizophrenia is complex. Here, the acute and the chronic stages of the disorders are described in turn – though in practice there is a continuum of features.

- Before proceeding, review the basic assessment (Chapter 2) and the diagnosis-focused assessment for psychosis (p. 22). These earlier sections include definitions of the cardinal symptoms of schizophrenia.

Clinical features of acute schizophrenia

The diagnostic features are shown in Table 12.1. Particular weight is placed on the presence of the 'first-rank symptoms'. A clinical diagnosis does not require a certain number of features being present, but the more there are, the more likely schizophrenia becomes.

- The predominant features vary from case to case. At one extreme, a person may present with bizarre behaviour, a full set of first-rank symptoms and florid thought disorder. At the other, the most notable symptoms may be insidious social withdrawal and academic decline, with psychotic symptoms only becoming apparent after direct questioning or observation.
- The duration criterion is to exclude transient schizophrenia-like syndromes, which have a better prognosis, and maybe a different aetiology. If the features of schizophrenia are present but for less than a month, the (temporary) label is *schizophreniform disorder*.
- Schizophrenia beginning after age 45 used to be considered a separate disorder, *paraphrenia*.
- Delusions, hallucinations and thought disorder in schizophrenia are grouped together as *positive symptoms* (in contrast to *negative symptoms*, described below).
- Many patients have non-localizing ('soft') signs on neurological examination.

Psychiatry Lecture Notes, Eleventh Edition. Gautam Gulati, Mary-Ellen Lynall and Kate Saunders. © 2014 John Wiley & Sons, Ltd. Published 2014 by John Wiley & Sons, Ltd.

Table 12.1 Clinical features of acute schizophrenia

Characteristic symptoms
First-rank symptoms:
  Thought insertion, echo, withdrawal or broadcasting
  Third person auditory hallucinations
  Running commentary
  Passivity of thought, feelings or action
  Delusional perception
Bizarre delusions
Odd behaviour
Thought disorder
Lack of insight (reality distortion)
Prodromal period of decline in performance and social
  withdrawal

Duration criterion
Symptoms present for at least 1 month

Major exclusion criteria
Not secondary to mood disorder
No demonstrable organic cause (e.g. amphetamines,
  temporal lobe epilepsy)

 Clinical scenario

Jules is a 20-year-old student who was observed by housemates having a conversation with imaginary demons. His room was covered in black paper to stop them interfering with his thoughts. His work had deteriorated markedly in the past term, and he had isolated himself. He was convinced he was part of a sinister plot and was being told what to do by unknown people whom he could hear talking about him. There was no evidence of substance misuse or mood disorder. A provisional diagnosis of paranoid schizophrenia was made.

Clinical features of chronic schizophrenia

In patients who progress to chronic schizophrenia, the acute symptoms have often largely resolved (with or without treatment). The characteristic picture becomes one of a 'burnt out' disease (Table 12.3). These features are called *negative symptoms*.

- The positive–acute/negative–chronic distinction is not absolute. Positive symptoms regularly persist or re-emerge in chronic cases, and some patients have negative symptoms in their first episode.
- Prominent, enduring negative symptoms are sometimes called *deficit syndrome*.
- *Residual schizophrenia* is a transitional state between acute and chronic schizophrenia. It describes patients with positive symptoms within the past year who have also developed negative symptoms.
- Research has shown that the symptoms of chronic schizophrenia fall more clearly into three clusters, rather than the two implied by the positive-negative distinction. The three are *reality distortion* (delusions and hallucinations), *disorganization* (thought disorder) and *psychomotor poverty* (similar to negative symptoms).

Clinical subtypes of schizophrenia

Because of the clinical heterogeneity, schizophrenia has classically been divided into several subsyndromes, based upon the pattern of symptoms (Table 12.2).

- The catatonic subtype is much rarer than it used to be. This could reflect a change in the nature or treatment of the disease, or the past occurrence of organic disorders mistaken for schizophrenia (particularly a postviral condition called encephalitis lethargica).
- The disorganized subtype is also called *hebephrenic schizophrenia*.

Table 12.2 Subtypes of acute schizophrenia

Subtype	Predominant symptoms	Other features
Paranoid	Persecutory, systematized delusions Hallucinations, usually auditory	Most common form Personality relatively preserved
Disorganized	Thought disorder Odd behaviour Fleeting, bizarre delusions Labile or inappropriate mood	Early onset Poor prognosis Premorbid schizoid or schizotypal personality
Catatonic	Motor signs	Now rare
Undifferentiated	A mixture of the above	

Table 12.3 Features of chronic schizophrenia

Negative symptoms
Flattened (blunted) mood
Apathy and loss of drive (avolition)
Social isolation
Poverty of speech
Poor self-care

Other features
Positive symptoms persist or recur at times of stress
Mild cognitive impairment is common

 Clinical scenario *(continued)*

Jules is now 45. He has had multiple admissions. Between episodes, he never regained his previous level of functioning; by 35 he was living in a group home. He spends most of his time in his room or walking the streets, often mumbling to himself. He has no specific complaints or desires. His last admission was a year ago when hallucinations worsened following a fellow resident's suicide.

Cognitive impairment in schizophrenia

Problems with memory and attention are a neglected aspect of schizophrenia. Their profile is complex.

- The most affected domains are attention, working memory and semantic memory. These deficits are superimposed on some degree of generalized intellectual deficit – though there is a wide range, and many patients score above normal.
- The impairments are, like the negative symptoms, stable and independent of the positive symptoms. Some decline probably occurs well before the onset of illness, with a further decline around the first episode. There is then a long period of stability, before deterioration in later life such that a significant minority of elderly patients with schizophrenia have moderate to severe dementia (which is not explained by any known neuropathological process).

The neuropsychological deficits of schizophrenia are thought to be central to the syndrome, and important for three reasons:

- They are the major determinant of poor functional outcome, along with negative symptoms.
- They may underlie the psychotic symptoms. By this view, psychosis is the 'fever' of schizophrenia – a problem that requires treatment, but that is non-specific and downstream of the disease process.
- They are potential targets for treatment, separate from the psychotic symptoms.

Differential diagnosis

Acute schizophrenia

Acute schizophrenia must be distinguished from other psychotic disorders (Table 12.4).

Table 12.4 Differential diagnosis of acute schizophrenia

Category of disorder	Distinguishing features/examples
Other non-organic disorders	
Delusional disorders	Absence of specific features of schizophrenia; preserved personality
Psychotic depression	Prominent depressive symptoms
Manic episode	Prominent manic symptoms
Schizoaffective disorder	Mood and schizophrenia symptoms both prominent
Schizotypal disorder	Nature of symptoms; chronic history
Puerperal psychosis	Acute onset after childbirth
Organic disorders	
Drug-induced psychosis	History of drug or alcohol misuse
Iatrogenic	Levodopa, methyldopa, steroids, antimalarials
Complex partial epilepsy	Other evidence of seizures
Delirium	Acute onset; clouding of consciousness
Dementia	Age; established cognitive impairment
Huntington's disease	Family history; choreiform movements; dementia
Systemic lupus erythematosus	Skin and renal involvement
Syphilis	Other evidence of infection

- Drug-induced psychoses (Chapter 14) pose a particular problem. At least one-third of people with schizophrenia misuse alcohol or drugs, and it can be difficult, and sometimes arbitrary, deciding whether these constitute the 'cause' of their symptoms. Judgement is based on the timing, quantity and type of substances taken.
- The organic disorders that can produce an acute schizophrenic picture (sometimes called *symptomatic schizophrenia*) are collectively common enough – about 1 in 20 cases – to require a high index of suspicion, especially if aspects of the case are atypical.

Chronic schizophrenia

In chronic schizophrenia the diagnosis itself is rarely in doubt, though occasionally neurological syndromes (e.g. a leukodystrophy) can mimic the clinical picture.

- A more common problem is to distinguish negative symptoms from depression or from the sedative and parkinsonian effects of antipsychotics.

Investigations

Schizophrenia is a clinical diagnosis. Physical investigations are mainly used to rule out the organic disorders in Table 12.4, and are chosen according to the features elicited in the history and examination.

- Brain imaging is not part of the routine assessment. It should be considered if there are neurological symptoms or signs.

Management

The management of schizophrenia is considered according to the stage of the illness (acute vs chronic) and then by the intervention (physical, psychological, social).

Management of acute schizophrenia

The key elements are summarized in Table 12.5.

- Admission for assessment is usual but not invariable. Compulsory admission may be needed, since patients are at risk from neglect or dangerous acts. Ideally, there should be several days of drug-free observation; this is rarely feasible due to shortage of beds or because the behaviour is too disturbed.

Table 12.5 Components in the management of acute schizophrenia

Intervention	Rationale
Admission	For diagnosis, investigation and starting treatment
Antipsychotic drugs	Treatment of positive symptoms
Benzodiazepines	For sedation
Establish context of disorder	
Evaluate current personal circumstances	To guide management – accommodation, work, etc.
Assessment of needs and of risk	
Education of patient and family	Improve understanding and treatment adherence

- Antipsychotics are effective against positive symptoms in a majority of patients over 2–3 weeks. Their onset is gradual; in the early stages, if behaviour is difficult to manage or the patient is very distressed, add a benzodiazepine.
- Investigate the context of the disorder, as it may give clues as to its development and prognosis. For example, comorbid substance misuse worsens outcome and may require intervention.
- Involve the family. Relatives need support and explanation, and they may be directly involved in therapy.
- First admissions can last many weeks depending on progress and external factors (e.g. finding accommodation). Future management is planned at pre-discharge Care Programme Approach meetings.
- Following an acute episode, *post-schizophrenic depression* is common, and may require treatment with antidepressants.

Early intervention

There is a trend to try to intervene earlier in schizophrenia – before symptoms become established, and even during the prodrome before unequivocal psychotic symptoms have emerged. Early intervention services have been set up to identify, engage and treat these individuals.

- The rationale is that longer duration of untreated psychosis predicts poor outcome, and thus earlier intervention may improve it.

- Though preliminary, there is some evidence that early intervention, with either cognitive therapy, antipsychotics or antidepressants, may delay, if not prevent, the transition to 'full' psychosis.
- Early intervention has its risks. Some prodromes recover spontaneously, whereas labelling and treating it may produce side effects and stigma.

Management of chronic schizophrenia

After a first episode of schizophrenia, the aims are to prevent relapse, and to optimize the level of functioning. To do this, a combination of pharmacological, psychological and social methods is used (Table 12.6).

- The amount of support and treatments needed varies markedly depending on the course and severity of the disorder – and, in practice, whether the intervention is available. The emphasis here is on cases where full recovery has not occurred after the first episode.

Table 12.6 Components in the management of chronic schizophrenia

Intervention	Rationale
Coordinated community care	Ensure medical and social needs are met
Continue antipsychotic drug	Prevent relapse
Readmission during relapse	Stabilize mental state and review management
Family therapy	Lower expressed emotion and prevent relapse
Social skills training	Improve social functioning
Cognitive behavioural therapy (CBT)	Reduce residual symptoms
Compliance therapy	Improve medication adherence
Cognitive remediation	Improve cognitive functioning
Supported employment	Financial, social and self-esteem benefits
Deal with drug or alcohol use	Improve outcome
Illness management skills training	Help coping with chronic illness
General medical care	High risk of poor physical health

- The most important specific intervention is antipsychotic medication, which significantly reduces the rate of relapse in the 2 years after an episode. Even the benefits of psychological and family interventions operate partly by improving treatment adherence. Equally, however, a sustained relationship must be established with the patient and due attention paid to their 'problems of living'. Without this commitment, the patient is unlikely to adhere to the management plan – bear in mind that over 50% of patients do not take their antipsychotics regularly.
- The value of a multidisciplinary approach is apparent from the range of patients' needs – benefits, accommodation, employment, physical health, etc. The nature of the disorder, especially the effect of negative symptoms, makes people with chronic schizophrenia vulnerable in all these areas.
- Some patients with schizophrenia remain under the Mental Health Act (in hospital or in the community) for many years.
- Patients with schizophrenia have high risks of type 2 diabetes and cardiovascular disease, contributing to their excess mortality. Some of this is attributable to side effects of antipsychotic medication. The other reasons are unclear, but probably include genetic predisposition, poor diet and lack of exercise. Regular medical review and investigations (e.g. for diabetes, lipids, blood pressure) should be an integral part of management.

Modes of treatment

Antipsychotic drugs

After a single episode of schizophrenia, antipsychotic medication is continued for 12–24 months. If the person remains well it should then be tailed off because there is little evidence that further medication is beneficial and because of the risk of tardive dyskinesia and other long-term side effects. Patients who have had multiple episodes or persistent symptoms usually remain on medication for many years, though the need for it (and the effect of cautious reductions in dose) should remain under regular review. Medication is often given in depot form if there are concerns around poor adherence.

- Antipsychotics have been described earlier in this book. Some antipsychotics, such as risperidone, olanzapine, clozapine and amisulpride, have shown greater efficacy than others in meta-analytic studies. The choice of antipsychotic is informed by the presentation of the patient, the patient's choice, the drug's side-effect profile and the patient's treatment history amongst other factors. A trial of 6 weeks at an adequate dosage is considered necessary when assessing treatment response, although some response is often seen earlier.

- Clozapine has an important role in patients who are poorly responsive to, or intolerant of, other antipsychotics. It also decreases the risk of suicide and can reduce aggression. It is the treatment of choice where there has been insufficient or no response after two 6-week antipsychotic trials including at least one with an atypical antipsychotic.
- Avoid routine co-administration of anticholinergic agents, or of combinations of antipsychotics.
- Persistent negative symptoms are not improved by antipsychotics, even clozapine. Conversely, it is a myth that the drugs cause them. Similarly, medication has little overall effect, for better or worse, on the cognitive symptoms, although atypical antipsychotics may produce small improvements.

Other physical treatments

- Benzodiazepines are useful for short-term sedation.
- Antidepressants should be used in the normal fashion for depression occurring in schizophrenia.
- Electroconvulsive therapy (ECT) is not effective, except for catatonic stupor.

Psychological treatments

Table 12.6 includes a range of psychological treatments. The two most widely used specific interventions are a form of family therapy, and CBT for residual symptoms. In addition to these specific interventions, remember that a supportive psychotherapeutic relationship is an integral part of management (as with every chronic illness).

The family approach arose from the finding that patients living with families who have *high expressed emotion* (EE) had a much higher chance of relapse than those exposed to low EE. EE is the intensity and amount of emotional involvement by the family with the patient. It was then found that high EE families could be taught to lower EE, and relapse rates fell. Family therapy focuses on education about the illness and changing the behaviour of the family. A recent systematic review confirms its (modest) effectiveness, but it has been difficult to implement widely because of practical and financial constraints (e.g. relatives are often out at work).

- The converse of high EE – a lack of stimulation – is also harmful as it exacerbates the apathy and withdrawal of chronic schizophrenia. This was first documented in institutionalized patients (and contributed to the drive to close the asylums).

CBT has some efficacy against auditory hallucinations and delusions, and is being adopted as an integral component of schizophrenia management, especially for the treatment of residual symptoms. However, its effect is rather small, the proven benefits are only short-term, and not all patients are able or willing to engage in treatment.

- Hallucinations can also benefit from simple practical manoeuvres – for example, use of ear plugs or personal stereos.

In a further recent development, *cognitive remediation therapy* and related psychological treatments, are showing some promise to improve the memory deficits of schizophrenia.

Social interventions

The nature of chronic schizophrenia means that many patients have problems with daily living. These needs should be identified and met by the multidisciplinary team working through the care programme approach (Table 12.6). Assertive outreach teams may be helpful in maintaining close contact with some patients who may have very chaotic lifestyles. Most patients are supported in the community by CMHTs (Community Mental Health Teams).

- Some patients cannot live alone or with their family. *Group homes* are houses where several patients live together, supported by their key worker and the group homes organization.

 Clinical scenario

Charlene is a 28-year-old factory worker who has had one episode of schizophrenia. She was discharged home under the care of her CMHT on a depot antipsychotic. A Community Psychiatric Nurse visited to monitor progress, give medication and advise the parents about how best to interact with the patient. After discussion with her employers, the patient returned to work part-time but 3 months later she refused medication and began smoking cannabis. She was readmitted briefly to recommence medication. This, however, became a pattern where she relapsed frequently, and eventually she lost her job. Her behaviour at home was becoming increasingly unmanageable.

She was readmitted and once her condition had settled, a meeting was held between the patient, her parents and the CMHT. She was offered a place in a group home. She agreed to take medication regularly. She was found sheltered employment in a charity shop. The CMHT social worker helped with financial issues and ensured that the patient received social benefits that she was entitled to. The patient remained relatively stable thereafter.

Prognosis

Accurate estimates for the long-term outcome of schizophrenia are surprisingly hard to obtain, because the diagnostic criteria have changed over time and because they depend on how recovery is defined. For example, some patients have persistent symptoms but live a reasonably normal life; others are functionally impaired despite minimal symptoms. Taking both symptoms and functioning into account, only about one-third of cases have the stereotyped chronic, deteriorating course; one-quarter have a very good outcome; and the remainder have a relapsing, remitting illness (Figure 12.1).

- At least 1 in 20 commit suicide. Previous estimates were higher. The risk is higher after an acute episode, when the patient may have realized the nature of their disorder and its implications, and may have developed a depressive disorder.

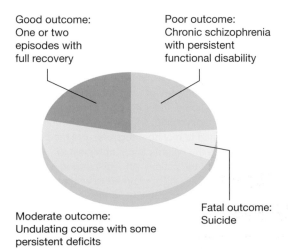

Good outcome:
One or two episodes with full recovery

Poor outcome:
Chronic schizophrenia with persistent functional disability

Moderate outcome:
Undulating course with some persistent deficits

Fatal outcome:
Suicide

Figure 12.1 Outcomes of schizophrenia.

Table 12.7 Factors associated with poor outcome in schizophrenia

Demographic characteristics
Young age at onset (e.g. under 25)
Male
Isolated, unmarried
Poor work record
Premorbid personality disorder
Substance misuse

Illness characteristics
Insidious onset
Prolonged untreated psychosis
Disorganized subtype
No mood disturbance
Early negative symptoms
Non-compliance with medication

- There is an increased mortality from natural causes too, especially cardiovascular disease, though rates of some cancers are lower than expected.
- There is an increased risk of violence (odds ratio for violence in schizophrenia and psychoses is around 4 for males and 8 for females) but recent studies show that a large proportion of increased risk to others is attributable to comorbid substance misuse rather than the disorder itself. The proportion of violence in society attributable to schizophrenia is around 5%.

Poor outcome factors are shown in Table 12.7. However, they are only weak predictors and it is impossible to foresee which category in Figure 12.1 someone presenting with schizophrenia will end up in.

- First-rank symptoms have no prognostic significance.
- The outcome of schizophrenia is better in developing than developed countries. The explanation is unknown, but probably reflects the importance of the social environment.

Epidemiology

The lifetime risk for schizophrenia is about 0.8%, with an annual incidence of 0.3 per 1000 and a point prevalence of about 5–7 per 1000 (for all psychotic disorders, the prevalence in adults is about 0.4%). The onset peaks in early adulthood,

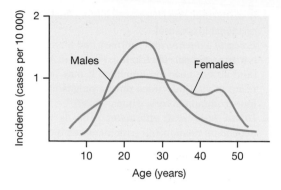

Figure 12.2 Schizophrenia: age at onset.

though the prodromal symptoms are often in adolescence.

- Men have a slightly higher incidence, and women also have a later and different age-of-onset profile, with a second peak around the menopause (Figure 12.2). Men tend to have a more severe illness and worse prognosis. Oestrogen's regulation of dopamine receptor sensitivity may explain these gender differences.
- Suggestions of a fall in incidence of schizophrenia over the past 30 years are probably the result of changing diagnostic practice and service provision, not a true decline.

- Some cases of schizophrenia begin later in life. *Late-onset schizophrenia* refers to subjects with onset over age 60. Very little is known about this subtype.

Aetiology

There have been many and diverse views of schizophrenia: as a brain disease, as a psychological disorder with no organic basis, and as a myth. Over the past 20 years, its original conception as a genetically influenced neurodevelopmental disorder again prevails.

Genetic factors

There is an increased risk of schizophrenia in people with a family history of the condition (Figure 12.3). Twin studies show that this is due almost entirely to genetic factors and that the heritability is about 80%. Adoption studies support this conclusion, in that children of a schizophrenic parent who are adopted by parents without schizophrenia retain their increased (10–12%) risk of illness.

- These studies also show that the genetic predisposition to schizophrenia overlaps with schizotypal disorder and perhaps delusional disorder. These

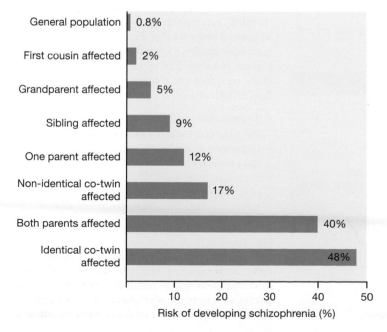

Figure 12.3 Familial risk of schizophrenia.

conditions are therefore sometimes grouped together as *schizophrenia spectrum disorders*. There are also genetic overlaps with bipolar disorder, and with autism.

- Several schizophrenia susceptibility genes have now been identified such as neuregulin and dysbindin. One common mode of action may be an influence on neurodevelopment and synaptic functioning. The mode of inheritance is not clear, but probably involves these and many other susceptibility genes, each of small effect. The genes probably interact with each other (*epistasis*) and affect a person's vulnerability to the environmental risk factors mentioned below.

- About one-quarter of people with velo-cardio-facial syndrome (VCFS), caused by a deletion of one copy of chromosome 22q11, develop schizophrenia.

Environmental factors

Although quantitatively the most important factor, genes are not the sole cause of schizophrenia. There are many known and suspected environmental risk factors, both biological and social (risk factors for schizophrenia are listed in Table 12.8). However, the interpretation of many of the factors is unclear. Taken together this information supports the view that schizophrenia has its roots in early development.

- *Obstetric complications.* The risk of developing schizophrenia in people with a history of obstetric complications is increased about four-fold. Complications associated with foetal hypoxia are par-

ticularly implicated. However, it is not known if the relationship is causal.

- *Excess of winter births* (February and March). This is a true seasonal effect, being reversed in Australia (and absent near the Equator). It may be a correlate of viral infections during pregnancy being more common in early winter.

- *Urban birth and upbringing.* This is a dose-dependent relationship (risk increased more than three-fold for a large town compared with a rural area). Its cause is unknown.

- *Migration.* There is an increased frequency (relative risk about 4) of schizophrenia in the children of Afro-Caribbeans who came to Britain in the 1950s, and in many other migrant groups in other populations. The risk is particularly high in those immigrants living in areas where they are a 'rare' ethnic group. Its explanation is controversial, with biological (genetic, viral) and sociological (racial prejudice, social deprivation) theories.

- *Early cannabis use* (pre-teens) is a risk factor, but studies have not fully controlled for use of other drugs.

- *Advancing paternal age* is thought to be a risk factor due to accumulating germ cell mutations. The risk increases with increasing paternal age.

The brain in schizophrenia

The dopamine hypothesis

The dopamine hypothesis has been the leading biochemical explanation for schizophrenia for over 30 years. It proposes that there is an excess of dopamine transmission ('hyperdopaminergia') in schizophrenia (whether due to too much dopamine, too many receptors, etc.). It was based on three main lines of evidence:

- Antipsychotic drugs are, without exception, dopamine D_2 receptor antagonists.
- Dopamine agonists (e.g. amphetamines, l-DOPA) can produce a paranoid psychosis.
- Some cerebrospinal fluid (CSF) and brain studies of schizophrenia indicate abnormal levels of dopamine, its metabolites, enzymes or receptors.

Advancing or refuting the dopamine hypothesis has proved difficult. However, the past few years have seen considerable progress, mostly through positron emission tomography (PET) and single-photon emission computed tomography (SPECT) brain imaging studies with dopamine radioligands. Dopamine does indeed appear to be closely linked to the symptoms

---

Table 12.8 Risk factors for schizophrenia

Biological
Family history
Obstetric complication
Season of birth
Advancing paternal age
Early cannabis use may be precipitating but
    psychoactive substance use is a strong maintaining
    factor

Psychological
Life stressors (precipitating and/or maintaining))
High expressed emotion in the family (maintaining)
Social
Poverty
Urban birth and upbringing
Migration (first- and second-generation migrants)

of schizophrenia, but in a much more subtle way than originally proposed:

- There is good evidence that hyperdopaminergia occurs during acute schizophrenia, in the basal ganglia (striatum).
- As well as the hyperdopaminergia during acute schizophrenia in the striatum, there is probably insufficient dopaminergic activity in the prefrontal cortex in patients with chronic schizophrenia, which contributes to the cognitive and negative symptoms.
- The dopamine system is unlikely to be the primary abnormality. Much evidence suggests that the dopamine changes are downstream of alterations in glutamate transmission. Notably, signalling via the NMDA (*N*-methyl D-aspartate) subtype of glutamate receptor is implicated both by the genetic discoveries and the fact that NMDA receptor antagonists (ketamine, phencyclidine) produce a schizophrenia-like syndrome.

Functional imaging studies

Abnormalities in regional cerebral blood flow and metabolism occur in schizophrenia, related to particular situations and neuropsychological tests. Such differences support the idea that particular neuronal circuits are impaired in schizophrenia, especially those involving the frontal cortex, hippocampus, thalamus and cerebellum.

Structural brain changes

The most robust finding is enlargement of the lateral ventricles and a slight decrease in size of the brain. There may be a preferential involvement of the temporal lobe and a loss of normal cerebral asymmetries.

- The structural brain changes are statistically robust, but not diagnostically useful since there is much overlap with controls, and the same findings can also occur in other disorders.
- Some of the abnormalities are present in people before they get ill; the other changes develop when the person develops psychosis. Thereafter, the progression of brain alterations with the course of the illness remains unclear (and is confounded by medication effects).
- The histological basis of schizophrenia is unknown, though the cytoarchitecture of the cerebral cortex – its neuronal and synaptic organization – appears altered. The white matter and its myelination may also be affected. There is no gliosis (proliferation and activation of glial cells), suggesting the absence of a neurodegenerative processes.

Psychological and social theories

The earlier psychological and social theories of the causation of schizophrenia lack convincing supporting evidence. However, psychological and social factors are clearly important in its outcome, exemplified by the effect on the patient of the emotion expressed by family members. These factors may also precipitate schizophrenia, since there is an excess of life events in the months preceding the first episode.

- Psychological interest is now directed mainly at the neuropsychological mechanisms. For example, one theory views schizophrenia as affecting the ability to distinguish actions generated by internal events (thoughts, feelings) and external stimuli (sensations).
- Schizophrenia is also being viewed as a *salience syndrome* – that is, an inability to decide which stimuli are important (salient) and to respond accordingly. This theory fits in well with the hyperdopaminergia mentioned earlier, since dopamine is a key determinant of how we decide what to respond to and what to ignore.

The neurodevelopmental model

Putting the various findings together, most researchers now view schizophrenia as a neurodevelopmental disorder. That is, it is caused by abnormalities of brain development, largely driven by genetic predisposition and early environmental factors (Figure 12.4).

- Different versions of the model emphasize the prenatal environment ('doomed from the womb'), adolescence or a combination of both.
- Ongoing factors throughout life may well contribute as well, since a pure developmental model does not explain well the age of onset, the fluctuating clinical course or cases beginning later in life. One notion is that the developmental abnormalities render the brain less able to undergo 'plasticity' – its normal adaptive response to changing environmental demands and stressors.
- Though psychosocial and family factors are neglected in the model, their influence should not be ignored, as mentioned above. These are likely to be mediated via stress and its effects upon the brain.

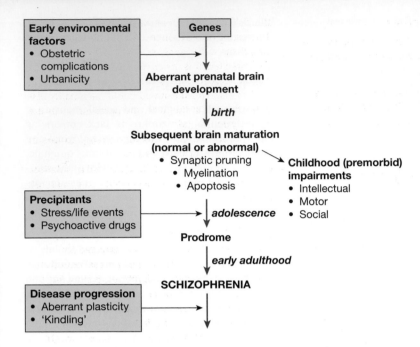

Figure 12.4 The neurodevelopmental model of schizophrenia.

The evidence in favour of the neurodevelopmental model includes:

- The fact that the neuropathological findings (e.g. ventricular enlargement) are present before the onset of symptoms.
- The histological abnormalities suggest a prenatal origin.
- Most of the robust environmental risk factors act *in utero* or early childhood.
- Children destined as adults to get schizophrenia have impaired behavioural, intellectual and motor development, demonstrable from infancy onwards.
- People with schizophrenia have increased rates of minor physical anomalies and abnormal dermatoglyphics, both of which point to prenatal developmental disturbance.

Disorders related to schizophrenia

Several other disorders are grouped together with schizophrenia, because:

- they are also psychoses that are not secondary to a mood disorder or organic disorder (in the case of schizoaffective disorder and delusional disorders); or
- they are thought to be causally related (in the case of schizotypal disorder); and
- they do not meet the criteria for diagnosis of schizophrenia (Table 12.1).

Schizoaffective disorder

Clinical features

The distinction of schizophrenia from bipolar disorder originated in the belief that these were two discrete disorders. It is reflected in the classification of bipolar disorder as a mood disorder separate from schizophrenia. However, this view is almost certainly wrong (based on epidemiological and genetic considerations). Certainly, many patients have features of both conditions, hence *schizoaffective disorder*.

- Use the diagnosis only for patients who satisfy criteria for schizophrenia *and* mood disorder *during the same episode*. Otherwise, diagnose the predominant syndrome (or neither). For example, one first-rank symptom in mania does not warrant a label of schizoaffective disorder (let alone schizophrenia). Similarly, labile mood is common in acute schizophrenia.

Management and prognosis

Mood symptoms and schizophrenic symptoms are treated on their merits. Mood stabilizers and antipsychotics are often used in combination.

- The prognosis is intermediate between schizophrenia and mood disorder. It is better in those whose predominant mood disturbance is manic rather than depressive.

Delusional disorders (paranoid psychoses)

Many patients have a psychosis without an underlying mood disturbance or organic disorder but do not satisfy the criteria for schizophrenia. Persecutory delusions are the main feature. Hallucinations are rare. Personality remains intact. These disorders are divided into acute and chronic types.

- The disorders in this 'residual' category of psychosis have had a variety of names. The preferred collective term is now *delusional disorder*, though *paranoid psychosis* is still commonly used.

Acute delusional disorder

These conditions are characterized by their acute onset, clinical features and rapid resolution.

- There are multiple, transient persecutory delusions, a sense of perplexity or suspicion, and a labile mood.
- They may be caused by drugs (in which case they are diagnosed as such) or follow extreme stresses, hence the older terms *psychogenic psychosis* and *brief reactive psychosis*. There is also an evocative French term, *bouffée délirante* (a 'puff of madness').
- Some cases will, of course, turn out to be more persistent psychotic disorders.

Persistent delusional disorder

A persistent delusional disorder is one lasting more than 3 months. *Chronic paranoid psychosis* and *paranoia* describe similar disorders.

- The delusions are usually *systematized* (i.e. stable and combined into a complex system). They often centre upon alleged (and plausible) injustices. The person may embark on litigation, or occasionally retribution, so it is important to ask about thoughts of aggression and hostility.

- The delusions are often *encapsulated*. The rest of the mental state can be unremarkable to the point that, if the delusional system is not detected, no abnormal features are elicited. Because of this, the disorder can go unrecognized for years, becoming hard to distinguish from paranoid personality disorder; though in the latter the paranoid ideas are not truly delusional.
- The appropriate diagnosis may change to one of mood disorder or schizophrenia.
- Onset is usually in middle age. Social isolation, deafness and paranoid personality traits are risk factors.

 Clinical scenario

A 50-year-old librarian, Mr Y, was arrested for threatening his boss, having been made redundant after 30 years. He had no psychiatric history. Mr Y was convinced that the boss had plotted against him. His diary revealed an increasing preoccupation with these ideas and included allegations and events known to be false. Hallucinations, thought disorder, mood disorder and substance misuse were excluded. Mr Y was single, without close friends, and had a lifelong interest in spying. He reluctantly agreed to take haloperidol, which gradually resolved the delusions and he stopped pestering his ex-boss. However, the beliefs remained in attenuated form, and he continued to suspect various conspiracies were going on.

Specific variants of persistent delusional disorders

The following variants of persistent delusional disorder are mentioned either because of their clinical importance or because they have a memorable eponym and are beloved by examiners.

- *Morbid (pathological) jealousy* is not uncommon, and is potentially dangerous. The patient, usually male, has the delusional belief that his partner is unfaithful. He may go to elaborate lengths to prove this and remains unconvinced by evidence to the contrary. He may threaten and finally attack his partner or the alleged third party. Usually morbid jealousy is a symptom of psychotic depression, schizophrenia, alcoholic psychosis or dementia, but it can be seen in isolation. The risks posed by morbid jealousy (and other psychoses with persecutory delusions with potential for violent acts) sometimes overrule patient confidentiality so the intended victim can be warned. A full risk assessment is mandatory.

- *Monosymptomatic hypochondriacal psychosis (somatic delusional disorder)* is the delusional belief that the person has an illness or deformity. It can lead to a prolonged search for inappropriate medical or surgical treatments. It must be distinguished from hypochondriasis and dysmorphophobia.
- In *de Clérambault's syndrome (erotomania)*, the patient, usually female, has a delusion that a man of high standing (a pop star, even a psychiatrist) is in love with her. Some stalkers have this disorder.
- In *folie à deux*, two people, often isolated sisters, share the same delusions. One is genuinely psychotic, the other is 'induced' to become so and is said to recover spontaneously when they are separated.
- *Capgras' delusion (illusion des soisies)* is the belief that someone close by has been replaced by an impostor or double. *Fregoli's delusion* is the belief that someone close to them is impersonating other people. Both have been called syndromes, but they are really symptoms (delusional misinterpretations). Both are very rare. They occur in schizophrenia, dementia and after right hemisphere damage.

Management and prognosis of delusional disorders

Delusional disorders, like all psychoses, can respond to antipsychotic drugs.

- Acute delusional disorders often resolve within days, especially if the triggering stressor is removed. Full recovery is the rule, although relapses may occur. Continue medication for a few months.
- Persistent delusional disorders can be resistant to treatment (or go untreated) and continue for years. Unlike schizophrenia, negative symptoms rarely occur. It has been claimed that pimozide is more effective than other antipsychotics, but without good evidence. SSRIs can also be useful.

Schizotypal disorder

Schizotypal disorder is like a chronic, attenuated form of schizophrenia, in which the beliefs stop short of being delusional, and the sensory experiences are not quite hallucinatory. The key features are:

- An aloof and suspicious manner.
- Eccentric behaviour.
- Avoidance of social contact.
- Odd beliefs and magical thinking.
- Vague, rambling or metaphorical speech.

- Tendency to odd ideas and sensory experiences.
- At least three of the above present for more than 2 years.

Schizotypal disorder is diagnosed infrequently, partly because people rarely come into psychiatric contact, and partly because it overlaps with paranoid and schizoid personality disorders.

- Schizotypal disorder appears to have a similar genetic background to schizophrenia.
- There are no specific treatments.

 KEYPOINTS

- Schizophrenia is a psychosis characterized by specific types of delusions, hallucinations and thought disorder, called first-rank symptoms. By definition, schizophrenia is not secondary to a mood or organic disorder, and the symptoms must have lasted more than a month.
- Some patients progress to a chronic state where social isolation, apathy and poverty of speech predominate. These are called negative symptoms, in contrast to the positive symptoms that characterize the acute episodes. Cognitive deficits also occur and contribute to poor functional outcome.
- Antipsychotic drugs are effective for positive symptoms but they do not prevent or treat negative symptoms. Clozapine is an atypical antipsychotic effective in some otherwise treatment-resistant cases.
- Most patients with schizophrenia need long-term, multidisciplinary support. Psychological and social interventions are an integral part of management.
- Schizophrenia is a neurodevelopmental disorder that has high heritability but is best conceptualized as arising from a gene–environment interaction.

 FURTHER READING

National Institute for Health and Care Excellence (NICE) (2009) CG82 Core interventions in the treatment and management of schizophrenia in primary and secondary care. Access at http://www.nice.org.uk/CG82

The Schizophrenia Commission (2012) The abandoned illness. Access at http://www.schizophreniacommission.org.uk/the-report/

? SELF-ASSESSMENT

1 A 22-year-old man presents with his mother. She has noted that over the last few days, he has been keeping to himself, appears perplexed and frightened, believing that a secret spy agency has conspired to murder him. He has slept with a large kitchen knife under his pillow so as to tackle any assailants. Prior to this he was attending university but his academic performance has been falling for the last few months. She is worried he may run away from home fearing for his own safety.

   Which line of management would you follow?
   a 'Wait and watch' – advise coming back in 2 weeks to see if this resolves spontaneously.
   b Refer for psychological assessment to clarify and challenge beliefs.
   c Admit for assessment and treatment.
   d Prescribe an antipsychotic and suggest taking time off university.
   e Prescribe a benzodiazepine and refer as an out-patient to the Early Intervention Service.

2 An 82-year-old nursing home resident with no previous psychiatric contact has been increasingly agitated over the last few days. She is brought to hospital where she describes seeing ghosts at the end of her bed and is frightened by them. She remains awake at night but sleeps during the day. The nursing team on the medical assessment unit feel that she is psychiatrically unwell in light of her reports and ask for a psychiatric opinion. What would you do next?

   a Suggest commencing a benzodiazepine to reduce agitation and help sleep.
   b Suggest commencing an antipsychotic drug to help hallucinations.
   c Ask for an ophthalmology opinion.
   d Ask for a urine dipstick, blood tests and a Temperature, Pulse and Respiration (TPR) chart.
   e Suggest urgent transfer to a psychiatric in-patient unit.

3 You are approached by a local citizens' group who are considering whether they should support or oppose the development of a new psychiatric unit in the neighbourhood. They have facts and statistics about schizophrenia, which they put to you. You advise them that one of the facts they have is incorrect (and talk to them about the others). Which one of their facts is incorrect and needs to be challenged?
   a The vast majority of individuals with schizophrenia are extremely dangerous.
   b People with schizophrenia are more likely to get into trouble with the law than someone without the illness.
   c People with schizophrenia are more likely to use illicit drugs than someone without the illness.
   d Some people with schizophrenia may need help and support for several years.
   e People with schizophrenia can make active contributions to society and their local neighbourhood.

13

Dementia, delirium and neuropsychiatry

Learning objectives

✓ To recognize dementia and delirium, and how to distinguish them clinically

✓ To describe the causes of dementia, the features that distinguish the different types, and an approach to the management of dementia

✓ To learn about the assessment and management of delirium

✓ To understand key aspects of other 'organic' psychiatric disorders including head injury and amnesic syndrome

✓ To think about the psychiatric manifestations of epilepsy and other disorders often considered 'medical'

Box 13.1 What does 'organic' mean?

Psychiatric disorders labelled 'organic' are those with demonstrable pathology or aetiology, or that arise directly from a medical disorder. They are contrasted with all other psychiatric disorders, which are traditionally called 'functional'. This distinction is conceptually flawed as all disorders have biological, psychological and social contributions. The term causes both practical and semantic problems, but remains in widespread use, and so is used here.

The major organic disorders are dementia and delirium. Like other psychiatric syndromes they are defined by their clinical features. However, unlike other syndromes, they are known to arise from different diseases with various aetiologies and pathologies. A complete diagnosis requires the disease as well as the syndrome to be identified. In the case of dementia, diagnosis can often be made based on clinical history, examination and neuroimaging, but the gold standard

for diagnosis remains neuropathological examination. Other organic disorders are simply psychiatric disorders that appear, in a particular case, to be caused by an identifiable medical condition. Sometimes it is the psychiatric symptoms that first bring the person to medical attention. Substance misuse disorders are organic, in that there is a specific pharmacological cause, but by convention they are classified separately. Where the psychiatric disorder is considered a *psychological reaction* to medical illness, such as becoming depressed after being told you have cancer, this is not classified as an organic disorder (see Box 13.1).

Dementia

Clinical features of dementia

Dementia is *an acquired, progressive impairment of cognition that interferes with social functioning, but without clouding of consciousness.* The cardinal

---

Psychiatry Lecture Notes, Eleventh Edition. Gautam Gulati, Mary-Ellen Lynall and Kate Saunders. © 2014 John Wiley & Sons, Ltd. Published 2014 by John Wiley & Sons, Ltd.

feature is memory impairment (short-term worse than long-term), but the clinical profile differs depending on the specific type of dementia. Common features of dementia are:

- Symptoms present for 6 months, of sufficient severity to impair functioning.
- Personality and behavioural change, for example, wandering, aggression or disinhibition.
- Dysphasias, dyspraxias and focal neurological signs may be present.
- Psychotic symptoms in half of cases at some stage.
- Lack of insight into deficits (except early on).
- Nearly always progressive (though this is not a diagnostic criterion).

The prevalence of dementia rises rapidly with age (see Figure 13.1). While specific risk factors for different dementias have been identified, and are discussed later in this chapter, none is as potent as age.

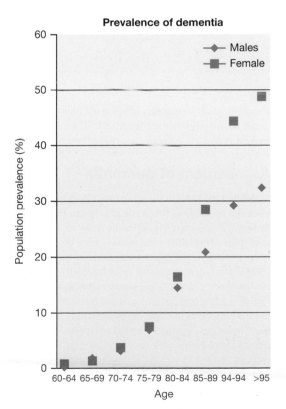

Figure 13.1 The prevalence of dementia with ageing. Data from Reynish E, Bickel H, Fratiglioni L, Kiejna A, Prince M, Georges J. (2009) Systematic review and collaborative analysis of the prevalence of dementia in Europe. *Alzheimer's and Dementia* 5(4) (Suppl.), P393.

Mild cognitive impairment (MCI) describes people who do not meet the criteria for dementia but who have evidence of a decline in cognitive function. It progresses to dementia within a year in about 30% of cases. There is much interest in this group with a view to early intervention.

Differential diagnosis of dementia

When diagnosing dementia, there are several conditions that should be considered as differentials, and which may complicate the presentation of someone with an established diagnosis of dementia (Box 13.2). For example, the symptoms of poor concentration and impaired memory may be due to depression, rather than a degenerative brain disorder. This presentation of depression is called pseudodementia (see Clinical scenario). Two factors that help distinguish depression from dementia are:

- Did low mood or poor memory come first?
- Is the failure to answer questions due to lack of ability or lack of motivation?

In older adults with depression, apathy, anxiety, irritability and forgetfulness are often more prominent than low mood. Depression is common and treatable, making it an important differential diagnosis.

 Box 13.2 The differential diagnosis of confusion or memory loss

- *Deafness* or *dysphasia* can be misinterpreted as confusion – check that the person can hear; that any hearing aids used are working correctly; that they can understand; and that they can speak.
- *Dementia* – Alzheimer's disease, vascular dementia and Lewy body dementia are the most common forms.
- *Depression*, including pseudodementia.
- *Delirium* – this is a clinical picture rather than a diagnosis and has multiple causes including CNS infection, sepsis, hypoxia, brain injury, drug toxicity, drug withdrawal syndromes and metabolic disturbance, to name a few.
- *Other psychiatric disorder*, especially late-onset schizophrenia (paraphrenia), psychosis, mania, functional disorder.
- *Transient global amnesia*.
- *Epilepsy* – post-ictal state or ongoing temporal lobe epilepsy (i.e. complex partial seizure).
- *Drugs*, especially those with anticholinergic effects, can exacerbate any cognitive impairment.

Clinical scenario: poor memory

Mrs Jones is a retired librarian, age 68, who lives alone in a village. She does not drive and finds it difficult to get out and meet people. She presented to the GP with complaints of poor memory, headache and lack of energy. She had a physical examination, bloods (FBC, UE, TFT, LFT, B12, folate, CRP) to exclude treatable organic causes for her symptoms, e.g. hypothyroidism or B12 deficiency. Due to her age and subjective memory problems, she was referred to the memory clinic. At assessment she showed some evidence of cognitive impairment, scoring 24/30 on the MMSE. This assessment allowed a more detailed conversation with her and revealed that she had low mood, poor sleep, reduced appetite and a sense of isolation and loneliness. She was started on mirtazapine and over 2–3 months showed an improvement in her mood, energy levels and cognition. She was encouraged to engage with community activities and this social rehabilitation was an important part of her recovery. Late-life depression can present with a pseudodementia and it is important to exclude this differential, particularly in someone with an atypical presentation.

Table 13.1 Causes of dementia

Common causes
Alzheimer's disease (50–60% of cases)
Vascular dementia (20–25%)
Dementia with Lewy bodies (10–15%)
Other causes account for ~10% of dementias

Degenerative disorders
Frontotemporal lobar degeneration
Huntington's disease
Prion disease
Parkinson's plus syndromes

Metabolic disorders
Alcohol-associated dementia
Vitamin B12 deficiency
Hypercalcaemia
Hypothyroidism
Hyperparathyroidism

Infections
HIV-associated dementia
Syphilis

Other causes
Normal pressure hydrocephalus
Intracranial tumours
Subdural haematoma
Head injury

The causes of dementia

The common dementias are listed in Table 13.1. Alzheimer's disease accounts for over half of all cases, with most of the rest explained by vascular dementia and dementia with Lewy bodies (DLB). The syndromes are not mutually exclusive, and the common ones often coexist. Dementia in the under 65s is termed *early-onset* (or *presenile) dementia*. In early-onset dementia, a much higher percentage of cases are due to rare genetic disorders, or are the consequence of severe head injury.

Careful clinical evaluation identifies the specific dementia (as determined by diagnostic neuropathological examination) in more than 80% of cases. Clinical features that can help to distinguish between the dementias are outlined in Tables 13.2 and 13.3. These diagnostic pointers are often more specific in early dementia, as most late-stage dementias can produce a wide variety of symptoms.

A distinction is sometimes made clinically between *cortical dementias* (e.g. Alzheimer's disease, Creutzfeldt–Jakob disease (CJD)), which predominantly affect the cortex, and *subcortical dementias* (e.g. Huntington's disease), which mainly affect the basal ganglia, thalamus and deep white matter (see Table 13.4 for the associated clinical features of each).

However, most dementias affect both regions of the brain, so the terms are misleading. It is better to try to make a specific diagnosis.

Assessment of dementia

In the history and examination (see Chapter 3), close attention to medical history is important, in order to distinguish between the different types of dementia, and their differential diagnoses. Clues could come from a history of a fall (?subdural haematoma), repeated falls (?dementia with Lewy bodies), new-onset incontinence (?normal pressure hydrocephalus, infection leading to delirium) or rapid fluctuations (?dementia with Lewy bodies). On examination you might find hypertension and a carotid bruit (?vascular dementia) or primitive reflexes (?frontotemporal degeneration). Table 13.5 shows the baseline and specialized tests that are used in the investigation of dementia.

Cognitive testing is an essential part of the routine assessment of suspected dementia, with the Mini-Mental State Examination (MMSE) most widely used as a screening tool. Used in conjunction with other measures (e.g. Hopkins verbal learning test and CLOX – a clock drawing task to test executive function), the MMSE can lead to a more informed

Table 13.2 **Diagnostic pointers in dementia (modified from Kester & Scheltens, 2009 – see 'Further reading')**

Feature	Suggestive of …
Prominent behavioural change or profound apathy early in the illness	Vascular dementia or frontotemporal degeneration
Prominent aphasia	Vascular dementia or frontotemporal degeneration (semantic dementia or progressive non-fluent aphasia)
Progressive gait disorder	Parkinson's disease (PD)-associated dementia, normal pressure hydrocephalus or vascular dementia
Frequent falls	Progressive supranuclear palsy or dementia with Lewy bodies (DLB)
Prominent fluctuations	Delirium, medication side effects, DLB, temporal lobe epilepsy, obstructive sleep apnoea syndrome or metabolic disturbance
Hallucinations or delusions	Delirium, medication side effects, late paraphrenia or DLB
Eye movement abnormalities	PD-associated dementia or Wernicke's encephalopathy

Table 13.3 **Clinical features distinguishing the dementias**

	Prominent symptoms and signs	Other clinical features
Alzheimer's disease	Memory loss, especially short term Dysphasia and dyspraxia Behavioural changes, e.g. wandering Psychotic symptoms at some stage Apathy	Progressive Survival 5–8 years
Vascular dementia	Early gait disturbance (small-step gait or parkinsonian gait) Personality change, labile mood Early urinary symptoms (frequency, urgency) Preserved insight	Stepwise progression History or signs of vascular disease elsewhere (peripheral vascular disease, ischaemic heart disease, renovascular disease, hypertension, retinopathy) Presence of risk factors for vascular disease
Dementia with Lewy bodies and Parkinson's disease dementia	Fluctuating dementia Delirium-like phases Parkinsonism Visual hallucinations REM sleep behaviour disorder	Antipsychotics worsen condition
Frontotemporal degeneration	Stereotyped behaviours Personality change Early loss of insight Expressive dysphasia Memory relatively preserved Early primitive reflexes	Slowly progressive Family history common More common in women Onset usually before age 70 Imaging shows selective atrophy of frontal and/or temporal lobes Features depend on the subtype
Huntington's disease	Schizophrenia-like psychosis Choreiform movements Depression and irritability Dementia occurs later	Presents in the 20s–40s Affected parent and other relatives
Normal pressure hydrocephalus	Mental slowing, apathy, inattention Urinary incontinence Problems walking (gait apraxia)	Most common in 50–70-year-olds Most common reversible dementia
Prion disease	Myoclonic jerks Seizures Cerebellar ataxia	Often starts at age <50 Rapid onset and progression Death within a year

Table 13.4 Typical clinical features of subcortical versus cortical dementias

	Subcortical dementia	Cortical dementia
Memory loss	Moderate	Severe, early
Language	Normal	Affected (dysphasia)
Personality	Apathetic, inert	Indifferent
Mood	Flat, depressed	Normal
Coordination	Impaired	Normal
Motor speed	Slowed	Normal

diagnosis, or it can suggest a need for more in-depth testing, for example using the Addenbrooke's Cognitive Examination.

Baseline blood tests are routinely performed in primary care, to investigate any treatable causes of cognitive impairment. All patients referred to secondary care memory clinics should also have a structural brain scan (usually a CT scan) to identify any other treatable causes, e.g. subdural haematoma or normal pressure hydrocephalus. Unless there are indications of a more unusual cause of dementia, further tests (e.g. MRI brain, lumbar puncture) rarely change the diagnosis, let alone reveal a reversible cause, beyond that provided by a careful history and examination.

In those presenting with cognitive impairment under the age of 65, further investigations may be necessary (e.g. MRI brain, lumbar puncture) in order to accurately diagnose the aetiology, to inform prognosis, and to allow appropriate genetic counselling for the individual and their family if necessary. Such patients may benefit from a neurology referral.

There is much interest in *biomarkers* to diagnose early dementia, or predict its onset, especially Alzheimer's disease. Levels of various proteins in the cerebrospinal fluid (CSF) show promise, as do some MRI measures, and some genetic tests. As yet none has the necessary sensitivity or specificity for routine use.

Table 13.5 Investigations that may be informative in the assessment of dementia. All patients should have those tests shown in bold

Test	What the test may show
Blood tests	
Full blood count	Macrocytosis (B12 deficiency), anaemia, intercurrent infection
Electrolytes including calcium	Hypercalcaemia, hyponatraemia, renal disease
Liver function tests	Alcoholic liver disease
Thyroid function	Hypothyroidism
Vitamin B12 and folate levels	Deficiencies can produce cognitive changes
ESR, ANA	Test if suspicion of vasculitis
Syphilis serology	Now rare, but overlooked
HIV test	Dementia is common in AIDS
Radiography	
Chest X-ray	Bronchial carcinoma with ?cerebral metastases
Brain imaging (CT or MRI)	Tumour; infarcts; haematoma; temporal lobe atrophy suggests Alzheimer's; pulvinar hyperintensity on MRI (new variant CJD); cortical ribbon on diffusion-weighted MRI (sporadic CJD)
EEG	Characteristic periodic bi- or tri-phasic sharp wave complexes at 1–2 Hz in prion disease
Other tests	
Lumbar puncture	Normal pressure hydrocephalus; herpes encephalitis
Cerebral blood flow studies	Parietal hypometabolism suggests Alzheimer's
Neuropsychological testing	Assess severity; profile of deficits may point to brain region most affected
Genetic testing	Available for some familial dementias
Brain biopsy	Very rarely done; mainly for suspected prion disease

ANA, anti-nuclear antibodies; CJD, Creutzfeldt–Jakob disease; CT, computed tomography; EEG, electroencephalogram; ESR, erythrocyte sedimentation rate; MRI, magnetic resonance imaging.

Management of dementia

It is important to identify and treat reversible causes of dementia (e.g. space-occupying lesion, vitamin B12 deficiency); however, the majority of presentations are irreversible, and treatment is aimed at reducing the speed of progression, and treating symptoms to optimize quality of life for patients and carers. Specific pharmacological treatments are now available, particularly for Alzheimer's disease, and these are discussed below.

Regardless of the cause of dementia, the following principles and strategies are important:

- Non-pharmacological methods should always be employed first.
- Simple interventions are effective in improving problems such as wandering (e.g. by regular exercise, or raising the door handle) and incontinence (e.g. by a toileting routine).
- Avoid antipsychotic medication due to the increased risk of stroke and association with more rapid cognitive decline and with sudden death (this is particularly important in dementia with Lewy bodies). Antipsychotics should *not* be used long term, nor for sedation, nor for behavioural problems without evidence of a psychotic basis. For psychotic symptoms that have not responded to other pharmacological and non-pharmacological measures, use antipsychotics sparingly and for brief periods only (reviewed at least every 6 weeks).

Components of treatment

1 *Treat any reversible cause.*
2 *A multidisciplinary approach and formal care plan.*
3 *Social support services:*
   a Discuss available support services and benefits, for both patients and carers.
   b Social interventions such as meals-on-wheels, day care and respite admissions help carers cope.
4 *Environment:* familiar, calm, adequately lit, visible clocks, minimize environmental change, follow routines, familiar carers.
5 *Psychological treatments* include aromatherapy, massage, reality orientation, reminiscence therapy, music therapy, art therapy, memory training.
6 *Prevent deterioration:* pay particular attention to management of cardiovascular risk factors.
7 *Treat any exacerbating factors:*
   a Pain, constipation, infection and dehydration all worsen cognitive function. Patients may be unable to express these symptoms, so you should examine for them.
   b Investigate any sudden deterioration. It may be due to a treatable cause, e.g. superimposed delirium due to a urinary tract infection.
8 *Pharmacological treatments* for dementia.
9 *Identify and treat any complications:*
   a Depression: SSRIs are better tolerated than tricyclics.
   b Disturbed sleep.
   c Aggression.
10 *Medico-legal considerations:*
   a Patients with dementia should be cautioned about the risks of driving. The Driver and Vehicle Licensing Agency (DVLA) or other relevant authority should be informed when the diagnosis is made.
   b Capacity to make specific decisions may vary depending on the severity of illness, and the nature of the decision. The 2005 Mental Capacity Act should always be taken into account – for example, regarding advance directives and deprivation of liberty safeguards.
   c In advanced dementia, palliative rather than active treatment may be indicated. Next of kin should be fully involved in these decisions.

Prognosis of dementia

Most dementias are progressive and average life expectancy is 5–8 years after diagnosis of onset, with some dementias, notably prion disease, progressing much more rapidly. Younger cases and those with focal neurological signs or psychotic symptoms have a worse prognosis. Severe dementia has a mean survival of 18 months, with death often associated with pneumonia and other febrile episodes. People with dementia should not be blood or tissue donors in view of the risk of transmission of prion disease.

Alzheimer's disease

Alzheimer's disease is the most common dementia, and there have been substantial advancements in understanding the pathology, and developing treatments.

The cardinal features of Alzheimer's dementia are neurofibrillary tangles and amyloid plaques in the hippocampus and cerebral cortex, with loss of synapses. Neuropathological diagnosis is therefore the most accurate. Neurochemically, the main abnormality is a loss of acetylcholine due to degeneration of the cholinergic neurons of the basal forebrain. The cholinergic deficits and synaptic loss are proportional to the severity of the dementia.

A considerable amount is now known about the causes of the disease (Table 13.6). The major risk factor, apart from age, is the E4 (epsilon4) variant of the apolipoprotein E (apoE) gene. Three polymorphisms exist: apoE2, apoE3 and apoE4. Approximately 20% of the population carry one copy of apoE4 and have twice the risk of Alzheimer's disease; the 3% who are apoE4 homozygotes (i.e. two copies of apoE4) are at several-fold increased risk. Conversely, the risk is about 40% lower in people without an apoE4 allele, and those with apoE2 alleles may be at lower risk still. The effect of apoE4 is probably that it brings forward the age of onset of dementia, by about a decade (note that apoE4 is neither necessary nor sufficient for Alzheimer's disease – it is a risk factor). Many other genes of small effect probably also contribute.

Early-onset Alzheimer's disease is often familial and (unlike most cases) may be due to an autosomal dominant mutation. So far, three genes have been implicated, with several different causative mutations in each: amyloid precursor protein (*APP*), and the presenilin genes *PSEN1* and *PSEN2*. Though extremely rare, these cases helped identify the pathways involved in Alzheimer's more disease generally (see below).

Treatment with non-steroidal anti-inflammatory drugs (NSAIDs), hormone replacement therapy (HRT) or statins may be associated with a lower risk of developing dementia and Alzheimer's disease. While plausible mechanisms exists to explain these effects,

the evidence is weak, and the effects of confounding factors are likely to be important; for example, women given HRT tend to be healthier and better educated. High educational attainment and mental or physical exercise are both protective factors, perhaps by increasing '*cognitive reserve*' and supporting a 'use it or lose it' theory of brain function.

Raised plasma homocysteine is an independent, graded risk factor for developing Alzheimer's disease several years later. This may be due to its role in atherosclerotic processes, or in neurotoxicity.

The key process leading to Alzheimer's disease is abnormal metabolism of beta-amyloid, the main constituent of senile plaques, and a fragment of the amyloid precursor protein. The abnormality results in formation of insoluble forms and complexes of beta-amyloid, which accumulate and trigger a range of harmful biochemical events. This 'amyloid cascade' is promoted in various ways by the causal factors mentioned (Figure 13.2). The central role of beta amyloid is supported by findings in transgenic mice with Alzheimer's disease-causing mutations in the *APP* gene. They develop senile plaques and become cognitively impaired, unlike rodents without the gene mutation.

Abnormalities in microtubule-associated tau protein, which forms neurofibrillary tangles, may also be important, though the connection to beta-amyloid is unclear. Oxidative stress and inflammatory processes may also contribute to Alzheimer's pathology.

Table 13.6 Risk factors for Alzheimer's disease

Factor	Comments
Genetic	
Apolipoprotein E (chromosome 19)	ApoE4 allele increases risk and reduces age at onset
APP (chromosome 21); *PSEN1* and *PSEN2* (chromosomes 14 and 1)	Autosomal dominant mutations in these genes cause early-onset familial Alzheimer's disease
Other genes (chromosomes 6, 10, 11, etc.)	Identity and contribution uncertain
Down's syndrome (trisomy 21)	Alzheimer's disease occurs in middle age
Other risk factors	
Increasing age	Predominant risk factor (Figure 13.1)
Females	Slightly higher risk than men (Figure 13.1)
Homocysteinaemia	High plasma homocysteine doubles risk
Obesity or diabetes in middle age	Mechanism unclear
Head injury	Doubles risk of Alzheimer's disease
Latent herpes simplex infection	In people with an apoE4 allele
History of depression	Risk of dementia may be increased
Aluminium exposure	Controversial, probably false
Environmental – protective factors	
High educational level	'Cerebral reserve'
Physically and mentally active lifestyle	'Use it or lose it'

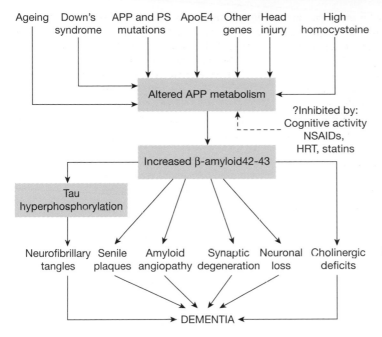

Ageing   Down's   APP and PS   ApoE4   Other   Head   High
         syndrome   mutations   genes   injury   homocysteine

Altered APP metabolism

?Inhibited by:
Cognitive activity
NSAIDs,
HRT, statins

Increased β-amyloid42-43

Tau
hyperphosphorylation

Neurofibrillary   Senile   Amyloid   Synaptic   Neuronal   Cholinergic
tangles   plaques   angiopathy   degeneration   loss   deficits

DEMENTIA

Figure 13.2 The pathogenesis of Alzheimer's disease. APP, amyloid precursor protein; HRT, hormone replacement therapy; NSAIDs, non-steroidal anti-inflammatory drugs; PS, presenilin.

Treatment of Alzheimer's disease

Treatment consists of anti-dementia medication, in addition to symptomatic treatment for behavioural and psychological symptoms (psychological support, social support and sometimes medication). *Cholinesterase inhibitors* (e.g. donepezil) are licensed for mild and moderate Alzheimer's disease. They have modest effects on cognitive symptoms, global outcome and activities of daily living. The effect is roughly equivalent to a 6-month delay in cognitive decline. They may also have benefit for behavioural symptoms. In the United Kingdom, they must be prescribed by a specialist according to specified diagnostic and severity criteria. The rationale for cholinesterase inhibitors is that they ameliorate the cholinergic deficits that occur early in the disease process; the fact they have such a modest effect probably reflects the more widespread, and progressive, disease process.

Memantine is an NMDA (*N*-methyl D-aspartate) glutamate receptor antagonist licensed for use in moderate to severe Alzheimer's disease. It can also be used if cholinesterase inhibitors are contraindicated or not tolerated. Treatment trials with NSAIDs and folic acid (to lower homocysteine) are also underway, but so far there has been no substantive evidence to support their use. Trials of HRT have been negative. Any potential preventive or disease-retarding inter-vention must take into account the fact that the pathology begins in earnest at least a decade before the first symptoms.

Vascular dementia

Vascular dementia is an umbrella term for dementia thought to be vascular in origin. One type is caused by multiple small infarcts (hence the earlier name of *multi-infarct dementia*). Others include 'small vessel disease' and Binswanger's disease (subcortical leukoencephalopathy). It is associated with risk factors for atherosclerosis and cerebrovascular disease. An overt stroke leads to dementia in 10% of cases, and in 30% after a second stroke. There is no specific treatment for vascular dementia, other than to attend to the cerebrovascular risk factors (e.g. aspirin, smoking); however, those with mixed vascular and Alzheimer's pathology may benefit from cholinesterase inhibitors. Vascular impairment acts synergistically with Alzheimer's disease to produce dementia.

Dementia with Lewy bodies (DLB)

Also called *Lewy body disease* or *Lewy body dementia*, this is the third most common form of dementia. It has a distinctive clinical appearance (Table 13.2) with visual hallucinations, parkinsonism and a fluctuating course. The overlap with

Parkinson's disease reflects their common pathology – that is, Lewy bodies (intracellular inclusions made of alpha-synuclein), but in dementia with Lewy bodies these occur predominantly in the cerebral cortex. Its aetiology is unknown, and no genes have been identified. Cholinesterase inhibitors are valuable (and may be more effective than in Alzheimer's disease). Importantly, antipsychotics should be avoided because of the risk of sensitivity reactions and increased mortality.

Parkinson's disease dementia

Although the cardinal symptoms of Parkinson's disease are motor, it is increasingly recognized as a neuropsychiatric disorder. Behavioural symptoms can include sleep disturbances, apathy, depression, anxiety and dementia – almost any psychiatric disturbance in fact! Dementia with Lewy bodies is closely related to Parkinson's disease dementia. The convention is that the latter category is used for dementia occurring more than 12 months after onset of parkinsonism. By this definition, dementia occurs in about one-third of cases of Parkinson's disease. Other cases of Parkinson's disease have a more circumscribed 'executive dysfunction' syndrome, with failures of attention and short-term memory. L-DOPA, which often dramatically improves the motor symptoms of Parkinson's disease, does not improve the dementia, but cholinesterase inhibitors may. Antipsychotics should be avoided if possible; if other treatment approaches have failed they may be used. There is modest evidence for use of quetiapine and clozapine for psychotic symptoms.

Frontotemporal lobar degeneration (FTLD)

This term embraces a spectrum of conditions affecting the frontal and temporal lobes, including *Pick's disease* (characterized by Pick bodies and Pick cells), and dementias associated with motor neuron disease. FTLD causes about 5% of dementias, more so in younger subjects. Some cases, maybe up to a half, are caused by mutations in the microtubule-associated protein tau (*MAPT*) or granulin (*GRN*, also called progranulin, *PGRN*) genes, both on chromosome 17. Others are associated with a protein called TDP-43. There is no specific treatment. Patients are very sensitive to many psychotropic drugs, which should be used with caution to treat depressive or psychotic symptoms.

Huntington's disease

Unlike most psychiatric disorders, it is entirely genetic. It is autosomal dominant, caused by a trinucleotide repeat expansion (a 'molecular stutter') in the huntingtin gene on chromosome 4. Pathologically, there is marked atrophy of the caudate nucleus, and later in the frontal lobe. The abnormal huntingtin protein is thought to be neurotoxic, though the mechanism is not clear. Predictive genetic testing is available. The psychosis and depression can be treated symptomatically, but there is no medication available for the cognitive impairment itself.

Normal pressure hydrocephalus

This accounts for up to 5% of dementia, and is the most common potentially reversible type of dementia. The term is a misnomer as CSF pressure is often increased. The clinical triad of cognitive impairment, urinary incontinence and ataxic gait is characteristic (Table 13.2), and MRI or CT scanning, showing disproportionate ventricular enlargement, may help diagnostically. The dementia is usually mild, and the other symptoms more prominent. Treatment is by ventricular shunting; 50% respond well.

Prion disease

Prion diseases are caused by an abnormal form of a protein called prion protein, and include *Creutzfeldt–Jakob disease (CJD)*. The abnormality can be inherited or acquired, because abnormal prion protein is transmissible, via blood, diet and contaminated surgical instruments. Prion disease is exceedingly rare but notable, especially in the United Kingdom, because of '*variant CJD*' (vCJD), acquired from cows with bovine spongiform encephalopathy (BSE) – prion disease in cattle – during the 1980s. One hundred and seventy-six cases of death from vCJD have been reported in the United Kingdom (August 2013). The current predictions are for hundreds more, though earlier estimates were much higher, but were not realized. Unlike typical CJD, these have occurred in young adults and present with prominent psychiatric symptoms, especially depression and personality change, which may be associated with a rapid deterioration. There may be a genetic predisposition to vCJD. Notably, the prion protein is thought to be a receptor for APP, the protein central to Alzheimer's disease. Any suspected cases of prion disease should be referred to the National Surveillance Unit in Edinburgh. There is no disease-modifying treatment for prion disease.

Alcohol-induced dementia

True alcohol-induced dementia is rare. Visuo-spatial deficits are often prominent. It is associated with atrophy of the white matter and frontal lobes. Dementia in those with alcohol dependence is more often due to Alzheimer's disease or vascular dementia rather than to the alcohol itself. Alcohol-induced dementia does not usually improve with abstinence. Note that alcohol dependence also causes amnesic syndrome (see below).

Table 13.7 Delirium versus dementia

	Delirium	Dementia
Onset	Acute	Insidious
Short-term course	Fluctuating	Constant
Attention	Poor	Good
Delusions and hallucinations	Common, simple, fleeting	Less common, more stable

Delirium

Also known as *acute confusional state* or *acute brain syndrome*. It is common on medical and surgical wards – one-third of elderly patients in hospital have an episode of delirium – so all doctors should be able to recognize and manage it. It may be helpful to review the section on the assessment of cognition and the unresponsive patient (Chapter 3).

Clinical features of delirium

Clouding of consciousness is an important diagnostic sign. It refers to drowsiness, decreased awareness of surroundings, disorientation in time and place, and distractibility. At its most severe the patient may be unresponsive, but more commonly the impaired consciousness is quite subtle. Minor degrees of impaired consciousness can be detected by problems estimating the passage of time (e.g. how long the interview has been going on), and with concentration tasks (e.g. counting from 20 down to 1). Because clouding of consciousness may not be apparent, the first clue to the presence of delirium is often one of its other features:

- Fluctuating course, worse at night.
- Visual hallucinations.
- Transient persecutory delusions.
- Irritability and agitation, or somnolence and decreased activity.
- Impaired concentration and memory.

The differential diagnosis includes dementia, especially dementia with Lewy bodies (Table 13.7), psychosis and depression. The clinical picture (especially the acute onset and rapid fluctuations), and its context, are usually sufficiently characteristic to reach a rapid diagnosis. However, differentiating delirium from dementia with Lewy bodies can be difficult in the short term, or without a good history.

Aetiology of delirium

Delirium is due to an underlying medical or pharmacological problem, so recognition of it should be followed by an urgent search for its cause (see Table 13.8 and Clinical scenarios). Medication is implicated in one-third of cases, mostly drugs with anticholinergic effects (e.g. tricyclic antidepressants) or sedatives.

Several demographic factors predict those who are at high risk of developing delirium (Table 13.9). In

Table 13.8 Common causes of delirium

Prescribed drugs
Tricyclic antidepressants
Benzodiazepines and other sedatives
Digoxin
Diuretics
Lithium
Steroids
Opiates

Other drugs
Alcohol intoxication
Alcohol withdrawal and delirium tremens
Benzodiazepine withdrawal

Medical conditions
Hypoxia, e.g. postoperatively
Infection, particularly urine and chest sepsis
Organ failure (cardiac, renal, hepatic)
Hypoglycaemia
Dehydration
Constipation
Burns
Major trauma
Pain

Neurological conditions
Epilepsy (post-ictal)
Head injury
Space-occupying lesion
Encephalitis

Table 13.9 **Predisposing factors for delirium**
Elderly
Male
Dementia
Frailty or immobility
Previous episode of delirium
Sensory impairment

these individuals, delirium can follow relatively trivial precipitants (e.g. constipation).

Management of delirium

Delirium is managed where it occurs – usually in general hospitals. Psychiatrists may be asked to assess the patient, make the diagnosis and give advice. Treatment is directed both at the symptoms and at the cause, and includes environmental and medical interventions (Table 13.10). In practice, it is important to search for a cause, and to start supportive, environmental interventions (as in Table 13.10) whilst this is ongoing. The latter may avoid the need for medication, which can complicate the problem, and which should only be used when necessary.

If sedative medication is needed, a benzodiazepine (e.g. lorazepam) is the best first-line option. This should be offered orally, and used intramuscularly (i.m.) only if absolutely necessary. Lorazepam has a quick onset of action providing immediate symptomatic relief; it is safer in older patients compared with antipsychotic medication. Lorazepam should be used as first-line treatment for alcohol or seizure-related behavioural disturbance. Antipsychotics (e.g. halop-

Table 13.10 **Management of delirium**
Environmental components
Quiet surroundings (side room), constant low lighting, clock, calendar
Regular routine
Clear simple communications
Limit numbers of staff (e.g. key nurse)
Involve family
Medical components
Monitor vital signs
Investigate and treat underlying cause (e.g. antibiotics, oxygen, stop drug)
Consider use of medication if agitation and behaviour places patient or others at risk

eridol) can be used as an alternative (again, orally first and i.m. only if necessary). They should not be used in patients with a diagnosis of, or suspected, dementia with Lewy bodies due to the risk of extrapyramidal side effects.

Occasionally, patients with delirium pose a risk to themselves, other patients or staff. If this is the case, ensure that the environment is optimized for safety, get advice from a psychiatrist about appropriate use of sedative medication and be aware that physical restraint may be needed to administer this safely. Patients with delirium may have impaired capacity. This needs to be assessed for each decision. If delirium impairs their capacity, they may be incapable of giving informed consent, and treatment under the Mental Capacity Act or common law (the doctrine of necessity) may be needed. If continuing interventions without consent are anticipated, the Mental Health Act may be required.

Q Clinical scenario: new confusion in an in-patient

Mrs White is a 78-year-old woman who presented to A&E with a fall. She had a history of dysuria and increased urinary frequency. Physical examination was normal, but bloods showed raised inflammatory markers and mild dehydration. She was admitted to hospital for treatment of a presumed urinary tract infection. Three days after admission she became acutely confused. The treating team reassessed her, but found no evidence of new or worsening infection. They noted that she had a number of risk factors for delirium, including her age, gender, current infection and reduced mobility, but realized the importance of taking a thorough history to investigate her acute confusion. Medicines reconciliation revealed that prior to admission she had been taking regular diazepam, which had been inadvertently stopped on admission. When this was restarted, her confusion quickly resolved and she was discharged back to the community.

Prognosis of delirium

Prognosis depends on the cause; whilst many people will recover in days or weeks, delirium can persist for several months. It is associated with significantly increased mortality: meta-analysis shows that in older adults (>65) who experience an episode of delirium, only 45% of individuals are still alive 2 to 4 years later. There is no good evidence that delirium progresses to dementia (although pre-existing dementia is a risk factor for delirium).

Clinical scenario: 'collapse query cause'

A 75-year-old lady is found lying on the floor and taken to hospital. She is drowsy, disorientated in time and place, distractible and unable to give any history. She thinks you are trying to kill her. She is febrile and hypotensive, but has no neurological signs or injuries. Blood tests and X-rays are performed. She is given oxygen, and antibiotics for the clinical suspicion of septicaemia. Her agitation worsens but settles with lorazepam. The GP tells you that there is no past history of note. Blood cultures grow an organism sensitive to the antibiotic. Her condition improves over 72 hours. The lorazepam is tailed off and her cognitive function returns to normal.

Other organic disorders

Dementia and delirium have been described in detail because they are common. As mentioned at the start of the chapter, there are many other 'organic' conditions, which can together present with the whole range of psychiatric disorders. The important principles, and some specific examples, are summarized here.

Organic psychiatric disorders

In classifying these disorders, the rule of thumb is to preface the psychiatric label with 'organic' and state the aetiology (Table 13.11). For example, 'Organic anxiety disorder due to thyrotoxicosis.'

Table 13.11 Organic psychiatric disorders

Syndrome	Example of cause
Organic brain syndromes	Dementia, delirium, amnesic syndrome
Organic delusional (psychotic) disorders	Systemic lupus erythematosus
Organic mood disorders	Multiple sclerosis
Organic anxiety disorders	Thyrotoxicosis
Organic personality disorders	Head injury

Each organic syndrome is very rare compared with its 'functional' counterpart, and in areas where primary care is well developed, they are frequently diagnosed within the primary care setting. However, when an organic syndrome does occur it is essential to recognize it. Detecting an organic disorder requires that you consider the possibility in every patient by taking a medical history, conducting a relevant physical examination and appropriate use of investigations. Be suspicious if aspects of the psychiatric presentation are unusual. For example, organic syndromes often produce abnormalities in unexpected functions, such as anosmia in depression due to a frontal meningioma. There may or may not be an effective treatment for the organic disorder. Regardless, the psychiatric symptoms are still treated with the appropriate pharmacological, psychological and social interventions.

As a rule, treatment response in an organic disorder is similar to that of its functional equivalent, subject to the progression of the underlying condition. For example, depression responds to antidepressants whether it is 'organic' or not. The presence of the organic disorder may, however, affect the choice of drug (e.g. avoid tricyclic antidepressants in depression following myocardial infarction).

Amnesic syndrome

Amnesic (or *amnestic*) syndrome completes the triad of conditions (with dementia and delirium) that affect memory and that always have an organic cause. Its features are:

- Selective loss of recent memory.
- Confabulation: the unconscious fabrication of recent events to cover gaps in memory.
- Time disorientation.
- Attention and immediate recall intact.
- Long-term memory and other intellectual faculties intact.

Amnesic syndrome is rare and in practice difficult to distinguish from some dementias. It is due to damage to the mammillary bodies, hippocampus and thalamus. The usual cause is alcohol-induced thiamine deficiency (*Korsakov's syndrome*), which is treated with thiamine and abstinence, and which may follow Wernicke's encephalopathy. Other causes include herpes simplex encephalitis, severe hypoxia and head injury. The memory deficits are often irreversible.

Table 13.12 **The main forms of epilepsy**

Type	Comments	Conscious level during seizure
Generalized seizures	No focal onset	
Tonic–clonic (grand mal)	The 'classic' type of seizure	Unconscious
Absence (petit mal)	Subtle and brief	Impaired
Partial seizures	Focal onset	
Complex partial (psychomotor)	Of most psychiatric significance	Impaired
Simple partial	Usually temporal lobe epilepsy	Unaffected

Epilepsy

There are several types of epilepsy (Table 13.12). Epilepsy is usually managed by neurologists, but has many psychiatric aspects. Only the latter are covered here (Table 13.13).

Relationship of psychiatric symptoms to seizures

Complex partial epilepsy was called *psychomotor epilepsy* because of the frequency of psychiatric symptoms during seizures (Table 13.14). It has also been referred to as *temporal lobe epilepsy*, though this is not always the site of the seizure focus. The risk of schizophrenia is several-fold higher in people with complex partial epilepsy, more so if the focus is in the left temporal lobe, and due to an early developmental abnormality. Psychiatric presentations can occur with other epilepsies, but are much rarer. *Absence seizures* in children produce transient lapses in concentration or simple automatisms, and can be mistaken for a behavioural disorder. Equally, a *generalized seizure disorder* can present to a psychiatrist if, for example, the person was found wandering in a post-ictal delirium.

Table 13.13 **Psychiatric aspects of epilepsy**

Category	Example
Psychiatric symptoms related to seizures	
Due to shared aetiology	Temporal lobe tumour
At start of seizure	Hallucinations during aura
During seizure	Non-convulsive status epilepticus (usually temporal lobe epilepsy) presenting as a fugue state
After seizure	Post-ictal delirium
Between seizures	Psychosis of complex partial epilepsy
Psychiatric disorder masquerading as epilepsy	Pseudoseizures
Psychiatric disorder associated with epilepsy	Common in people with epilepsy
Depression	Several times more common
Suicide	
Psychiatric problems of treatment	
Side effects of anticonvulsants	Depression with barbiturates
Seizures as medication side effect	Antipsychotics and tricyclic antidepressants

Table 13.14 **Psychiatric symptoms of complex partial seizures**
During the seizure (ictal)
Impaired consciousness
Hallucinations and other distorted perceptions: olfactory and somatic (especially epigastric)
Sense of *déjà vu*
Depersonalization and derealization
Impaired speech and memory
Automatisms and stereotyped behaviour
After the seizure (post-ictal, hours to days)
Transient, florid psychosis
Between seizures (inter-ictal)
Schizophrenia-like psychosis
Depression
Sexual dysfunction and lack of libido

Psychiatric disorders masquerading as epilepsy

Pseudoseizures (hysterical seizures or *non-epileptic attack disorder)* are a form of dissociative disorder (Chapter 10). They can be hard to distinguish clinically from a true seizure. EEG monitoring during attacks may be required to make the diagnosis. Pseudoseizures are more common in people who also have epilepsy. Other conditions that can be misdiagnosed as epilepsy include panic attacks, hypoglycaemia and schizophrenia. In children, consider temper tantrums and nightmares.

Psychological problems associated with having epilepsy

Historically, epilepsy has sometimes been attributed to demonic possession and its sufferers seen as irritable, self-centred people with criminal tendencies. Although entirely false, persisting negative attitudes, in addition to the symptoms and limitations that the illness places on patients, probably contribute to the higher incidence of psychiatric disorders and suicide in epilepsy. The most common psychiatric disorders are anxiety and depressive disorders. The suicide risk is increased five-fold, and even higher in those with complex partial seizures. Anticonvulsant treatments can compound the psychiatric problems – phenobarbitone causes hyperactivity and irritability in children; phenytoin can produce ataxia and delirium.

Head injury

In blunt trauma, the brain suffers contusions (bruises) at the point of impact; focal damage elsewhere as the brain reverberates in the skull; and diffuse axonal damage due to the shearing forces, to which the white matter is particularly susceptible. People with an apoE4 allele are at greater risk of persistent deficits following head injury.

These injuries are a major cause of organic psychiatric syndromes in young adults. They can be difficult to treat and services are greatly under-resourced. The psychiatric consequences of a head injury depend partly on the nature and location of the injury, and partly on the person's premorbid characteristics.

A wide range of psychiatric problems can follow a head injury. A head injury with loss of consciousness may produce amnesia, either *anterograde* (post-traumatic), for events after the injury, or *retrograde*. Anterograde amnesia lasting more than 24 hours predicts a poor long-term outcome, including persistent cognitive deficits. The impairment ranges from a subtle slowing of thought and distractibility through to dementia. It tends to improve in the first year, but thereafter deficits are likely to be permanent. There is no specific treatment.

Personality changes are frequent following head injury. Typically the changes are indicative of frontal lobe damage: impaired ability to plan or persevere; emotional shallowness and lability; impulsivity; and irritability. Altered sexual behaviour (in any direction) and speech also occur. Improvement is partial and slow. Mood disorder, anxiety disorders and schizophrenia are more common than expected after head injury. Left- and right-sided frontal lobe damage are associated with depression and mania, respectively.

Post-concussion syndrome describes emotional, cognitive and bodily symptoms occurring after relatively minor head injury. The symptoms are sometimes thought to be 'psychological' or even feigned, related to hopes of compensation, but may reflect subtle brain injury.

Other medical disorders associated with psychiatric disorders

Table 13.15 lists some medical disorders that often have psychiatric manifestations.

Table 13.15 Other medical disorders with psychiatric manifestations

Medical disorder	Psychiatric manifestations
Cerebral tumour	Psychiatric symptoms in 50%, more so if tumour is in frontal or temporal lobes
Cerebral abscess	May present with psychiatric symptoms
Multiple sclerosis	Mood disturbance in 25%: bland euphoria or depression Cognitive deficits in 25%: can become severe Personality change: apathy, irritability
Parkinson's disease	Depression in 50%, dopaminergic therapy may cause psychosis or dopamine dysregulation syndrome (e.g. hypersexuality, or obsessive interest in gambling or collecting)
Systemic lupus erythematosus and related vasculitides	5% at presentation, 50% at some stage: mood disorder, psychosis, delirium and seizures
HIV	Dementia in 30% with AIDS; the prevalence of psychosis is uncertain
Cushing's disease	Severe depression common; occasionally psychosis and cognitive impairment
Addison's disease	Apathy and fatigue in 80%; depression in 50%; cognitive impairment in 50%; psychosis in 5%
Hyperthyroidism	Anxiety (common), depression, mania, delirium
Hypothyroidism	Mental slowing and depressive symptoms very common; rarely 'myxoedema madness' – delirium, depression, dementia; symptoms may persist despite thyroxine replacement
Hypercalcaemia	Psychosis, delirium and mood disorders in 50%; cognitive impairment in 25%

 KEYPOINTS

- 'Organic' psychiatric disorders are those due to a recognized medical cause or pathology. Dementia and delirium are by definition organic disorders; all other psychiatric disorders can be. Hence consider an organic cause for every psychiatric presentation – epilepsy and endocrine disorders are classic culprits.

- Dementia is characterized by memory loss. It is usually progressive, though is sometimes reversible. The most common causes are Alzheimer's disease, vascular dementia and dementia with Lewy bodies.

- Delirium is an acute, fluctuating confusional state, with clouding of consciousness. It has many causes (e.g. drugs, infection) and when these are treated symptoms usually resolve rapidly.

- Treatment of organic disorders is aimed at the underlying cause *and* at the psychiatric symptoms.

 FURTHER READING

Kester MI, Scheltens P. (2009) Neurology in practice: Dementia: the bare essentials, *Practical Neurology* 9, 241–251.

National Institute for Health and Care Excellence (NICE) (2006) CG42 Dementia: a quick reference guide. Access at http://guidance.nice.org.uk/CG42/QuickRefGuide/pdf/English

National Institute for Health and Care Excellence (NICE) (2011) TA217 Alzheimer's disease – donepezil, galantamine, rivastigmine and memantine. Access at http://guidance.nice.org.uk/TA217

O'Brien JT, Burns A. (2010) Clinical practice with anti-dementia drugs: a revised (second) consensus statement from the British Association for Psychopharmacology. *Journal of Psychopharmacology.* Access at http://www.bap.org.uk/pdfs/Anti-dementia_2010_BAP.pdf

? SELF-ASSESSMENT

1 What is the most common type of dementia?
  a Alzheimer's disease
  b Vascular dementia
  c Dementia with Lewy bodies
  d Frontotemporal dementia
  e Metabolic disorders

2 Which dementia most commonly presents with a fluctuating presentation, visual hallucinations, parkinsonism and sleep disturbance?
  a Alzheimer's disease
  b Vascular dementia
  c Dementia with Lewy bodies
  d Frontotemporal dementia
  e Metabolic disorders

3 What type of drug is memantine?
  a Cholinesterase inhibitor
  b NMDA receptor antagonist
  c NMDA receptor agonist
  d Antidepressant
  e Anti-inflammatory

4 What is the first-line treatment for delirium?
  a Oral lorazepam
  b Intramuscular lorazepam
  c Oral haloperidol
  d Intramuscular haloperidol
  e Treat underlying organic cause

5 Which psychological problem is not associated with epilepsy?
  a Increased rates of anxiety disorders
  b Ataxia
  c Increased rates of depressive disorder
  d Delirium
  e Reduced rate of suicide

14

Substance misuse

Learning objectives

✓ To be able to describe key features of substance misuse, its management and its associated psychiatric disorders

---

General issues

Many substances are taken for pleasure. A substance is regarded as being *misused* (or *abused*) if it produces physical, psychological or social harm. Commonly misused substances are shown in Table 14.1. This chapter describes:

- The features of substance misuse.
- Its psychiatric consequences.
- The management of substance misuse and its associated psychiatric disorders.

Substance misuse presents in diverse ways; for example, as depression or morbid jealousy (both associated with alcohol), as an acute psychosis (amphetamines) or as haematemesis (alcoholic cirrhosis). Its various presentations, and frequency, mean that detection of substance misuse, notably of alcohol, is part of every psychiatric assessment.

Prevalence figures for misuse of substances other than alcohol are likely to be unreliable as use is frequently illegal.

- In the United States, 1.5% of adults admit to having tried heroin, 7% amphetamines, 8% LSD, 12% cocaine and 30% cannabis. A quarter of each group were regular users.
- In England and Wales (2009/10), 8.6% of adults (and 15% of pupils aged 11–15 years) had used one or more illicit drug within the last year, with cannabis being the most commonly cited drug.

- In England and Wales, the number of recorded deaths from substance misuse in 2008 was 1738, with accidental poisoning being cited as the most common cause.
- A common approach to reducing the recreational use of drugs is to make them illegal. Most countries have legal classifications based on the harmful potential of the drugs to the user and society. The classifications are not described here as they vary between countries and over time. For example, cannabis use is legal in The Netherlands and elsewhere: its legal classification is controversial in other countries. The use of alcohol, which is probably the most important cause of harm in many societies, is not legally restricted for adults in most Western societies.

Types of substance misuse

There are several categories of substance misuse:

- *At-risk consumption* – (alcohol) intake at a level associated with increased risk of harm.
- *Harmful use* – misuse associated with health and social consequences, but without dependence.
- *Dependence* – prolonged, regular use of some substances (especially alcohol, opioids, amphetamines) can lead to *dependence* (*addiction*) and *withdrawal* syndromes.
- *Intoxication* is the acute effect of the substance – being drunk (alcohol), tripping (LSD) or stoned (cannabis). Intoxication with illicit drugs may lead to an acute psychiatric presentation.

Psychiatry Lecture Notes, Eleventh Edition. Gautam Gulati, Mary-Ellen Lynall and Kate Saunders. © 2014 John Wiley & Sons, Ltd. Published 2014 by John Wiley & Sons, Ltd.

Table 14.1 **Commonly misused substances**
Alcohol
Other legal or prescribed drugs:
Benzodiazepines
Nicotine
Caffeine
Cannabis
Opioids:
Heroin
Morphine
Methadone
Stimulants:
Amphetamines
Cocaine
Ecstasy
Hallucinogens:
LSD
Phencyclidine
Solvents

Table 14.2 **Identifying motivation – the 'stages of change' model**	
Stage	**Features**
Pre-contemplation	Denial of problem
Contemplation	Consider problem and whether change needed
Decision	Decide to do (or not to do) something about it
Action	Choose strategy and implement it
Maintenance	Make progress and sustain it
Relapse	Return to earlier behaviour

Assessment of substance misuse

The principles of assessment are similar for all substances:

- Be willing and able to ask screening questions and (for alcohol) use screening tools such as the FAST, CAGE and AUDIT.
- Know the features of misuse of alcohol and other commonly used substances.
- Be aware of the psychiatric and medical conditions associated with substance misuse.
- Drug testing can be useful. Alcohol can be measured in breath or blood; most illicit drugs or their metabolites can be detected in the urine – some briefly (e.g. amphetamines), some for weeks afterwards (cannabis).

Assessment of the *motivation* of the patient to change is also important. The *stages of change model* helps to assess (and encourage) motivation (Table 14.2). People may go through many cycles of this process.

Management of substance misuse

Management is also based upon a set of uniform principles:

- Identify at-risk consumption and harmful use early, and give accurate information and advice.
- In dependency, facilitate withdrawal (detoxification) and abstinence.

- Help maintain abstinence following withdrawal.
- If abstinence is not possible, minimize harm associated with continuing use.
- Treat the complications – for example, drug-induced psychosis.
- Prevention – this largely involves population-level interventions such as pricing policies.
- Advise the person about the risks and legal requirements about driving (or operating machinery, etc.) while under the influence of alcohol or drugs.

To achieve these goals, a variety of psychological, pharmacological and social treatment methods are used.

Aetiology of substance misuse

Substance misuse has a multifactorial aetiology (Table 14.3). Together, the factors determine both the prevalence and the type of substance misused, and the nature of the misuse.

- Aetiology has been studied in most detail for alcohol. Similar factors confer vulnerability to misuse of substances in general (and perhaps to other addictions such as gambling).

Alcohol

Definitions and epidemiology of alcohol (mis)use

- In England in 2009, 69% of men and 57% of women (over the age of 16), and 18% of school pupils aged 11–15 years reported drinking alcohol on at least one day in the week prior to a survey.

Table 14.3 Aetiological and other factors associated with substance misuse

Genetic
Heritable component to vulnerability, and to subjective experiences of the substance
Genes include those related to targets of substances, and their metabolism, and those related to the personality traits associated with substance misuse

Neurobiological
Brain activity: trait differences in EEG patterns
Chemicals: abnormalities in dopamine, GABA and endogenous opioid systems
Anatomically, key site is nucleus accumbens

Psychological
Personality factors
Learned behaviour
Positive reinforcement – the drugs lead to behaviours that increase their use

Socioeconomic
Price and availability
Cultural norms and acceptability

Legal
Restrictions on sale
Penalties for possession or dealing

EEG, electroencephalogram; GABA, gamma-aminobutyric acid.

Table 14.4 Harmful effects of alcohol

Medical
Liver damage – hepatitis, cirrhosis
Cardiovascular – cardiomyopathy, hypertension
Gastrointestinal – peptic ulcer, oesophageal varices, pancreatitis
Neoplasms – liver, oesophagus
Blood – anaemia, haemochromatosis

Neurological and organic psychiatric
Blackouts
Epilepsy
Neuropathy
Delirium tremens
Wernicke's syndrome
Korsakoff's syndrome
Cerebellar degeneration
Central pontine myelinosis
Head injury (from falls)

Psychiatric
Alcoholic hallucinosis
Morbid jealousy
Alcoholic dementia
Depressive disorders
Anxiety disorders
Sexual dysfunction
Suicide

Social
Accidents
Problems with relationships
Domestic violence
Employment difficulties
Crime

- In the United Kingdom, consumption has doubled in the past 40 years – in the rest of Europe it has declined.
- *Hazardous drinking:* 24% of the population drink more than the recommended limits (21 units per week for men and 14 for women).
- *Harmful drinking:* defined as more than 50 units per week for men and more than 35 units per week for women.
- *Dependent drinking* (see below): 9% of men and 4% had features of alcohol dependency.
- A low intake of alcohol may be beneficial: up to 2 units per day is associated with a moderate protective effect against heart disease in men aged over 40 years. As intake increases, however, there is an escalating morbidity and mortality (Table 14.4). This produces a so-called J-shaped curve when mortality is plotted against alcohol consumption.
- Alcohol use disorders account for 4% of the global burden of disease, and have many other direct and indirect health costs; estimated to be £21 billion pounds annually in the United Kingdom. In England and Wales, there were 6584 deaths related directly to alcohol in 2009.

Clinical features of alcohol misuse

Dependence

The diagnosis of alcohol dependence (alcoholism) is made if three or more of the following are present:

- Feeling compelled to drink.
- Primacy of drinking over other activities – for example, eating, family life, work, health.
- Increased tolerance to alcohol – being able to drink quantities that would incapacitate others.
- Relief drinking – drinking to stop or prevent withdrawal symptoms.
- Stereotyped pattern of drinking.
- Reinstatement after abstinence – unable to give up alcohol for long.
- Drinking despite awareness of harmful consequences.
- Withdrawal symptoms.

Withdrawal and delirium tremens

The main features of alcohol withdrawal are:
- Tremulousness ('the shakes').
- Agitation.
- Nausea and retching.
- Sweating.
- Overwhelming desire to drink (craving).
- Withdrawal symptoms are relieved by alcohol. If untreated, the symptoms may last for several days. Transient misperceptions and hallucinations may occur.
- Withdrawal symptoms often occur on waking as the blood alcohol concentration falls during sleep.
- The most severe form of withdrawal (5% of cases) is *delirium tremens* (the 'DTs'), a potentially fatal condition (Table 14.5).

Wernicke's syndrome

An acute encephalopathy presenting with delirium, ataxia, nystagmus and ophthalmoplegia, occurring in the severely alcohol dependent, usually in the context of withdrawal. It is due to thiamine deficiency and requires urgent treatment. It may progress to Korsakoff's syndrome, which presents with cognitive deficits and confabulation.

Harmful alcohol use

About 20% of patients attending GPs drink hazardously (i.e. above the recommended limits) – most of

---

Table 14.5 Features of delirium tremens
Onset 24–48 hours after stopping heavy, prolonged drinking
Delirium
Visual hallucinations
Delusions, usually persecutory and transient
Fear and agitation, sometimes aggression
Coarse tremor
Seizures
Autonomic disturbance (sweating, fever, tachycardia, hypertension)
Insomnia
Dehydration and electrolyte disturbance
Lasts 3–4 days, followed by exhaustion and patchy amnesia for the episode

---

these are 'asymptomatic' and most go undetected. Detection can be improved by:

- Asking about alcohol intake during all medical and psychiatric assessments, including use of FAST, CAGE or AUDIT questionnaires. CAGE (Cut down, Annoyed, Guilty, Eye Opener) is a quick four-question screen. The AUDIT (Alcohol Use Disorders Identification Test) has 10 questions and takes 2 minutes; its strength is that it would assess hazardous, harmful and dependent drinking. FAST is a four-item test and can be completed in as little as 15 seconds, thereby making it valuable in areas such as busy A&E departments. A printable version can be accessed on the NICE website (link included at the end of this chapter).
- Following up on comments suggesting that a patient thinks he or she drinks too much.
- Unexplained macrocytosis or abnormal liver function tests.
- Noting the presence of one or more of the psychiatric or social consequences of harmful alcohol use (Table 14.4).

Associated medical disorders

If alcohol misuse has led to a medical disorder, then psychiatric or social impairments (Table 14.4) are likely. Assess and take appropriate action. If an alcohol-related psychiatric disorder is present, check for physical symptoms and signs of alcohol dependency.

Associated psychiatric disorders

Alcohol misuse is associated with an increased risk of, and worse prognosis for, most psychiatric disorders. These are covered in the respective chapters.

- In *alcoholic hallucinosis*, a heavy drinker experiences recurrent auditory hallucinations, usually of a threatening or derogatory nature. The hallucinations occur in clear consciousness (cf. withdrawal hallucinations). The syndrome is an example of a drug-induced psychosis.
- About 10% of people who are alcohol dependent commit suicide.

Management of alcohol problems

The focus in this section is on clinical rather than on population-based interventions.

- Figure 14.1 gives an algorithm for management of hazardous, harmful, and dependent drinking.

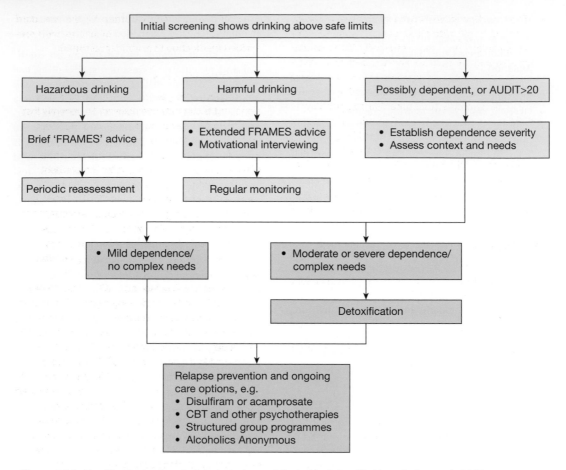

Figure 14.1 Algorithm for treatment of alcohol misuse. Adapted and simplified from Parker et al., 2008.

Management of hazardous and harmful alcohol use

A brief intervention in primary care is usually sufficient if someone is drinking more than the safe limits but is not dependent and has no specific medical or psychiatric disorder. The components are:

- Assess accurately the amount consumed (use diaries, informants).
- Assess the nature and extent of harm (e.g. liver function tests, work record).
- Provide brief advice of the hazards of excess alcohol intake. Tailor advice to the individual, and reinforce with written information. Advice should be given in a non-judgemental manner.
- Review progress. If problem drinking persists, or is in the harmful range, consider extended brief intervention and/or motivational interviewing.

The FRAMES acronym covers the main approach to giving advice about drinking:

- Structured *Feedback* on risk and harm.
- Emphasis on the patient's *Responsibility* for change.
- Clear *Advice* to make a change in drinking.
- Discuss a *Menu* of options for making change.
- Express *Empathy* and be non-judgmental.
- Reinforce the patient's *Self-efficacy*.

Treatment of alcohol dependence

The first requirement is detoxification ('detox', 'drying out'), which is controlled withdrawal, using a reducing course of a benzodiazepine in place of alcohol. This should always be done as part of a care plan that includes after-care and relapse prevention.

- *Mild dependence* – withdraw at home without drugs or with small doses of benzodiazepines.

- *Moderate dependence* – can usually facilitate withdrawal at home with a reducing regimen of chlordiazepoxide over 5 days, especially if the patient has a supportive network and an absence of physical complications or proneness to seizures. Advise the patient to drink plenty of non-alcoholic liquids. Prescribe vitamins (thiamine 300 mg per day) – deficiencies are common and withdrawal may precipitate Wernicke's syndrome. Consider parenteral thiamine if risk of Wernicke's syndrome is judged to be high as oral thiamine has limited bioavailability.
- *Severe dependence, or history of complications such as DTs, cognitive impairment, etc.* – may need higher doses of chlordiazepoxide, and/or in-patient treatment. Give parenteral thiamine routinely.

Maintaining abstinence

Various strategies are used to prevent relapse following withdrawal from alcohol. None has been shown to be very effective.

- Aim for abstinence where possible – it has a better long-term outcome than controlled drinking.
- Regular liver function tests and breath alcohol measurements help monitor progress.
- Encourage attendance at groups run by local community alcohol services or Alcoholics Anonymous.
- Consider disulfiram (Antabuse), acamprosate or opioid antagonists. Disulfiram works through negative reinforcement as it causes undesirable symptoms when alcohol is consumed alongside it; acamprosate leads to a reduction of craving, and opioid antagonists work via the autonomic nervous system.
- Psychological interventions include cognitive behavioural therapy (CBT), social skills training, problem solving and motivational interviewing (helping them make the decision to change their behaviour).
- About 50% of patients will return to drinking again within 6 months of abstinence.

Treatment of associated medical disorders

Many of the medical syndromes arising from alcohol misuse can present as emergencies (e.g. Wernicke's encephalopathy, bleeding varices), and the admission provides an opportunity for psychiatric intervention. Look out for withdrawal symptoms occurring during hospitalization.

Treatment of associated psychiatric disorders

The principles are:

- Reduce intake to safe limits, since continuing alcohol misuse acts as a perpetuating factor.

- Treat the psychiatric disorder in the standard manner. Check for interaction of alcohol with prescribed medication (e.g. antidepressants).

 Clinical scenario

Mr Campbell is 45-year-old gentleman who lives alone and is currently unemployed. He recently lost his driving licence due to drink-driving. However, he continued driving his car and got into a road traffic accident, which has resulted in a fracture of the bones of his lower leg. After the accident he was admitted to a trauma unit, awaiting surgical reduction of the fracture. Twelve hours after admission he gradually became anxious, intolerant of bright light, restless and tremulous. He complained of nausea, visual disturbances, headache and sweating. On examination he was apyrexial but slightly tachycardic with clammy trembling hands. A screening CAGE questionnaire noted that he had been drinking alcohol first thing in the morning to relieve 'hangover' from the previous day for some months. He had been drinking over10 units a day, and on completing an Alcohol Users Disorders Identification Test (AUDIT), moderate alcohol dependence was noted. He was diagnosed with an alcohol withdrawal syndrome and prescribed a 5-day reducing regimen of chlordiazepoxide. After receiving the first dose of chlordiazepoxide his symptoms of anxiety, restlessness and tremor significantly subsided and the subsequent doses relieved the rest of the symptoms. In view of malnourishment, he was also prescribed a course of parenteral thiamine therapy for prophylaxis of Wernicke's encephalopathy. Following the orthopaedic surgery, on his discharge from hospital he was advised to continue with oral vitamins and see his GP with a view to receiving psychological interventions (motivational interviewing) aimed at abstinence from alcohol consumption in the future.

Cannabis

Epidemiology and pharmacology

Cannabis is derived from the hemp plant *Cannabis sativa*. The main psychoactive ingredient is Δ^9-tetrahydrocannabinol (THC), which acts on endogenous cannabinoid receptors in the brain. Cannabis also contains cannabidiol, which to some extent antagonizes the effects of THC.

- The THC content of cannabis varies, and is rising over time in material supplied to the United Kingdom.

- Usually smoked.
- *Marijuana* is the dried flowers and leaves of the cannabis plant; *hashish* is the dried resin.
- It is the most widely used illicit recreational drug. Used for millennia for medical and religious purposes, its use as a recreational drug has increased dramatically over the past 40 years particularly in adolescents and young adults.
- Used by an estimated 150–200 million adults worldwide. In England and Wales, 6.6% of adults and 8.9% of pupils aged 11–15 years report use of cannabis within the last year.
- 10% of those using the drug become daily users.

The effects of cannabis are shown in Table 14.6.

Adverse health effects

- Difficult to untangle causality because users of cannabis are more likely to smoke and drink alcohol.
- Anxiety and panic – especially in first-time users.
- Paranoid ideation – especially in first-time users – and occasionally delirium.
- Increased risk of road traffic accidents.
- Increased risk of using other, more harmful, drugs.
- Possible increased risk of respiratory illness.
- Possible mild long-term cognitive impairment in heavy and regular users.
- May provoke angina in people with heart disease.
- Cannabis does not cause dependence or withdrawal, though some tolerance occurs (and use may become so ingrained as to warrant the term 'psychological dependence').
- Early and heavy use of cannabis increases risk for schizophrenia.
- Continued use in schizophrenia is associated with a worse treatment response.

Treatment

Cognitive behavioural therapy may reduce cannabis use, but there are high rates of reuse within 6–12 months.

Table 14.6 Effects of cannabis

Dose-related impairment in reaction time, information processing, coordination, motor performance, attention
Exaggeration of pre-existing mood
Mellowness and increased enjoyment of aesthetic experience
Distortion of sense of space and time
Reddening of eyes

Opioids

Epidemiology and pharmacology

- Opioids mimic endogenous endorphins and enkephalins and activate opioid receptors.
- They include naturally occurring substances (morphine and codeine) and synthetic opioids (heroin and methadone).
- Highly addictive.
- Heroin is most commonly misused because it causes euphoria – estimated 100 000 regular users in the United Kingdom.
- There are several modes of use:
  - Intravenous injection ('mainlining'). It is associated with a high risk of infections, thrombosis and phlebitis. Hepatitis B and C, and HIV, should be suspected and testing performed (with informed consent and appropriate counselling) in anyone who has injected drugs.
  - Inhalation – 'chasing the dragon': the opiate is melted on metal foil and then inhaled as it vaporizes.
  - 'Snorting' – the opioid is cut into a fine powder and then sniffed.

The effects of opioids are shown in Table 14.7.

Adverse health and social effects

Opioids have many serious adverse effects.

- They cause high levels of morbidity and mortality – the mortality rate is 12 times that of the general population; most deaths occur in males.
- Different routes have a major influence on bioavailability, speed of onset, severity of dependence and

Table 14.7 Effects of opioids

Euphoria
Analgesia
Drowsiness
Respiratory depression
Cough reflex suppression
Nausea and vomiting
Bradycardia and hypotension
Lowering of body temperature
Pupillary constriction
Constipation

rates of physical complications. Intravenous injecting has the highest risk of overdose and complications.

- Risk of transmission of blood-borne viruses – HIV, hepatitis B and C.
- Psychiatric comorbidity, including misuse of other substances. The suicide rate is increased 14-fold.
- Major negative social effects.

Clinical features

Dependence

Tolerance to all opioids rapidly develops. Because of this (and because of batch-to-batch variation in purity), overdose is common and frequently fatal due to respiratory depression.

- Tolerance makes pain management in an opioid user difficult as higher doses may be required.
- High risk of overdose after detoxification – for example, released prisoners.

Withdrawal

Stopping opioids leads to an extremely unpleasant withdrawal syndrome called 'cold turkey' (Table 14.8). The onset is usually within 8–12 hours of the last dose (longer after methadone), peaking 24–48 hours later and subsiding over 10 days. Though severe, opioid withdrawal is rarely life threatening.

Management

Rapid detoxification and abstinence

- In-patient detoxification is more effective than out-patient detoxification – probably because many opioid-dependent people live in chaotic environments (often with other users). Information is given about the nature and course of withdrawal symptoms.

Table 14.8 Features of opioid withdrawal
Craving
Restlessness and insomnia
Myalgia
Sweating
Abdominal pain, vomiting and diarrhoea
Dilated pupils, running nose and eyes
Tachycardia
Yawning
'Goose bumps'

- Prescribe reducing doses of a substitute drug, methadone linctus, which reduces the severity of the withdrawal symptoms. Clonidine (works on the alpha-2 receptor) and naltrexone (an opioid antagonist) are also used.
- Post-withdrawal abstinence programmes vary from specific relapse-prevention therapies to residential houses where a network of ex-users helps the recovering addict overcome the craving.
- Even when withdrawal is achieved, the relapse rate is high (40% at 6 months; the majority at 1 year).

Harm reduction and maintenance therapy (substitution treatment)

In maintenance therapy for opioid dependence, the priority changes from abstinence to reducing the harm from ongoing opioid use. The first aim is to make services acceptable to users in order to engage them in treatment. Then, the aims are to:

- Reduce injecting.
- Stabilize drug use and lifestyle.
- Reduce criminal behaviour by avoiding need to obtain expensive drugs.
- Reduce the death rate.

Motivational interviewing and contingency management may be helpful when combined with pharmacological management.

The harm reduction approach is pragmatic and includes a range of initiatives such as free needles and syringes and public education. A central feature is *substitute prescribing*. Oral methadone is prescribed to prevent the need for intravenous injections. Oral buprenorphine is an alternative to methadone with a less sedating effect and a relatively better safety profile if taken in overdose. Long-term use of oral substitute drugs is usual.

- Substitute prescribing does not suit all opioid users. It is best targeted at those whose social functioning and health have already been seriously affected by drug use, and where abstinence is an unrealistic goal.

Management of overdose

Early recognition and treatment is vital.

- Patient is unconscious, with pinpoint pupils, bradycardia, hypotension and shallow breathing or snoring. Check for respiratory arrest.
- Place in recovery position. Naloxone (opioid antagonist) can be administered subcutaneously, intravenously or intramuscularly – and may need to be repeated. The endpoint of naloxone therapy should be the restoration of adequate spontaneous ventilation.

Clinical scenario

Mr Ryan, a 20-year-old man, was released after a 9-month prison sentence for robbery and drug dealing. He was well known to the local police as an intravenous heroin user. Whilst in prison he did not engage with the Addiction Service and did not have access to opioids or any illicit substances. On release from prison he decided to 'celebrate' with his brother, also an intravenous drug user, by having a drug party at home. Before his last imprisonment Mr Ryan had been regularly injecting at least 2 grams of heroin a day and felt that was just about enough to induce a euphoric state. Mr Ryan thought that injecting his usual 2 grams of heroin would produce the desired effect. He could not wait for the arrival of his brother and after drinking some alcohol decided to inject the heroin alone. However, after having injected the usual 2 grams he slumped into an unconscious state with slow shallow breathing. He vomited, aspirated his vomit and finally stopped breathing. When his brother arrived home and found Mr Ryan unresponsive he took him in his car to the nearest A&E department where he was pronounced dead on arrival. His brother when talking to you expressed his disbelief and surprise as he knew that 2 grams of heroin was Mr Ryan's 'usual' dose. You explained to Mr Ryan's brother that tolerance develops rapidly in heroin users but the same reverses on prolonged abstinence from opioids (such as abstinence in prison) and therefore overdose on 'going back to the usual dose' was common. Death usually occurs due to respiratory suppression, particularly when heroin is taken with other respiratory depressants such as alcohol. You explained that naloxone, if it were administered promptly, would have rapidly reversed the CNS and respiratory depression and saved Mr Ryan's life. You gave Mr Ryan's brother advice on safe injecting before he left the hospital.

Stimulants

Amphetamines

Amphetamines ('speed', 'whizz') may be taken orally, snorted or injected. They produce symptoms similar to those of hypomania: elevated mood, over-talkativeness, increased energy and insomnia. Pulse and blood pressure increase, pupils dilate and mucous membranes become dry.

- *Dependence* occurs. Regular users develop depression and mood swings. The withdrawal syndrome can be severe (a 'crash'), with agitated depression, lethargy, suicidal thoughts and craving.
- Treat intoxication or psychosis with benzodiazepines and antipsychotics; treat depression with tricyclic antidepressants (TCAs).
- Prolonged use can lead to *paranoid psychosis*, which can last for months after use has ceased.
- Amphetamines are used clinically for attention deficit hyperactivity disorder and narcolepsy.
- Amphetamines are potent dopamine enhancers – they inhibit its reuptake and stimulate its release. Noradrenaline (NA) and serotonin (5-HT) are also enhanced.
- '*Crystal meth*' (D-methamphetamine hydrochloride) is a particularly addictive form of amphetamine that reaches high brain concentrations when smoked. It is associated with frequent and severe psychiatric symptoms, and withdrawal reactions.

Cocaine

Cocaine produces similar effects to amphetamines, but the features tend to be more dramatic.

- Cocaine is either snorted, or smoked in the form of 'crack' or 'freebase' (cocaine processed to remove the hydrochloride), which increases the intensity of the effect.
- Cocaine misusers often also misuse opioids and alcohol.
- Acute cocaine intoxication can mimic mania or psychosis. Cocaine-related violent behaviours can occur in over half of those who present with such induced psychiatric symptoms.
- '*Formication*' or 'cocaine bugs' refers to delusions of infestation, which can lead to numerous scabs from picking at the skin. Also seen with crystal meth.

3,4-Methylenedioxymethamphetamine (MDMA, ecstasy)

Ecstasy is a synthetic amphetamine analogue with mild stimulatory and hallucinogenic effects. It is widely used in Britain – 30% of teenagers say they've tried it. Tolerance occurs and the best experience is said to be the first. Though safer than amphetamines or cocaine – probably much safer – there is concern about its harmful effects:

- Adverse reactions – hyperpyrexia and acute renal failure due to dehydration, as well as water intoxication in users who overcompensate. There are very rare, but well-publicized, fatalities.

- Can cause acute psychosis – prevalence unknown.
- The drug is neurotoxic to 5-HT fibres (at least in monkeys), and chronic users have lowered central 5-HT levels and some cognitive deficits. There is, therefore, concern that depression and impulsivity may be a long-term consequence, although no good evidence of this has emerged.

Management of stimulant misuse has a very limited evidence base. Use the same approaches as for opioids. Antipsychotics and benzodiazepines are used to treat acute agitation and psychosis.

Hallucinogens

Hallucinogens alter perception, producing *psychedelic* experiences. They are taken orally. LSD (lysergic acid diethylamide) is the main synthetic hallucinogen; similar effects can be achieved using magic mushrooms. Agonism at $5\text{-}HT_2$ receptors is a likely common mechanism.

Lysergic acid diethylamide (LSD)

The 'trip' starts about 2 hours after consumption, lasts 8–12 hours and consists of distorted sensory perception, alteration of the sense of time and scale, and changes in body image (e.g. out-of-body experiences). The effects can be very intense – and occasionally terrifying (a 'bad trip').

- Hallucinogens rarely cause dependence or withdrawal. They are associated with *flashbacks* when the sensations of a trip are re-experienced long afterwards.
- Emergency psychiatric referral may occur because of the panic or agitation associated with a bad trip. Reassurance, reorientation and 'talking down' are necessary. Sedation as required with benzodiazepines. The person may also come to harm from responding to the hallucinations.

Other substances

Phencyclidine

Phencyclidine (PCP, 'angel dust') and ketamine ('special K') are volatile anaesthetics that in smaller doses produce a sense of drunkenness, hallucinations, disorientation and agitation. The picture resembles schizophrenia. Complications include nystagmus, tachycardia, hypertension and seizures.

- Usage is common in the United States but still rare in the United Kingdom.
- The drugs are antagonists at NMDA glutamate receptors.
- When managing PCP intoxication or psychosis, avoid chlorpromazine. The medical complications may need treatment.

Solvents

Solvent misuse (of glue, aerosols, petrol, etc.) is mainly an adolescent male group activity. The effects are rapid in onset and short-lived – euphoria, disinhibition, blurred vision, ataxia.

- Solvent use comes to medical attention when complications arise – cardiac arrhythmias, inhalation of vomit, coma. Chronic damage to the liver and brain can occur.

Anabolic steroids

Anabolic steroids are misused mainly by male athletes and bodybuilders. They produce a range of psychiatric effects that can be severe and persistent – euphoria, depression, aggression ('road rage') and hyperactivity. A form of dependency may result in some users. Clinical suspicion may be raised by the physical appearance.

Benzodiazepines

Benzodiazepines are taken illicitly, often as part of multiple drug misuse and as an opioid substitute. It can sometimes be difficult to decide whether symptoms and side effects are attributable to the benzodiazepine or to the other drugs being used. Iatrogenic benzodiazepine dependence can be difficult to manage but principles of management involve changing to a drug with a longer half-life and then reducing dosage in small steps.

Nicotine and caffeine

Both nicotine and caffeine are addictive – ask any smoker or serious coffee drinker. Each has its own acute actions and side effects, but psychiatric problems are rare.

- Psychiatric patients smoke more than the population average – 90% of people with schizophrenia do so. For unknown reasons they have a lower incidence of lung cancer than other smokers.

- Abstinence rates after nicotine dependence (30% at 6 months) are worse than for opioids, cocaine and alcohol.

'Legal highs'

A recently growing problem is the availability of designer drugs on the open market; the regulation of these is problematic as there is a lack of legislation restricting some of these substances. Some may be herbal preparations but sprayed with cannabinoids, others may mimic ecstasy. The use of these drugs is not picked up by routine drug testing carried out within services either so they are difficult to monitor for, but may have serious health consequences. One such drug, methoxetamine (or 'mexxy'), was banned in the United Kingdom in 2012.

KEYPOINTS

- For each substance, consider: What are its acute effects? Does it cause dependence and withdrawal? What are the associated psychiatric, medical and social complications?
- Dependence is a combination of physical and psychological effects. It is common in people who regularly use alcohol, opioids or stimulants. Withdrawal occurs if the substance is withheld.

- Substance misuse is widespread. Those in treatment are a small and unrepresentative fraction.
- Substance misuse is often comorbid with psychiatric disorders. Both need to be treated. The combination worsens prognosis.
- Alcohol produces a wide range of psychiatric, medical and social problems. Enquire about alcohol intake and consider a role for alcohol misuse in all patients.
- Management of substance misuse includes psychological, pharmacological and social components. The prognosis for persistent abstinence after being dependent on any substance is poor.

 FURTHER READING

Health Development Agency (2002) Manual for the Fast Alcohol Screening Test (FAST). Access at www.nice.org.uk/nicemedia/documents/manual_fastalcohol.pdf

Parker AJR, Marshall EJ, Ball, DM. (2008) Diagnosis and management of alcohol use disorders. *British Medical Journal*, 336. Access at www.bmj.com/content/336/7642/496

National Institute for Health and Care Excellence (NICE) (2007) CG51 Drug misuse: psychosocial interventions. Access at www.nice.org.uk/cg51

SELF-ASSESSMENT

1 A 20-year-old man who reports being an opiate user is seen in general practice. He complains of feeling nauseous, suffering with diarrhoea, watering eyes, a runny nose and describes experiencing abdominal cramps. You see him constantly yawning. His pupils are dilated, his skin is clammy and looks like 'goose flesh'. Which is the most appropriate first-line treatment?
  a Lofexidine
  b Naloxone
  c Naltrexone
  d Methadone
  e Buprenorphine

2 A 25-year-old female is brought to A&E with hyperthermia and tachyarrhythmia after a party. She is excited, restless and fidgety, constantly picking at the skin of her arms. Which of the following diagnoses is the best explanation for her presentation?
  a Heroin intoxication
  b Cannabis intoxication
  c Ketamine intoxication
  d Cocaine intoxication
  e Cocaine withdrawal

Personality disorders

Learning objectives

✓ To understand the concept of personality and when it becomes a disorder

✓ To be able to describe the relationship between personality disorder and other psychiatric disorders

✓ To learn about the classification of personality disorders

✓ To be able to describe broad principles in the management of personality disorder

---

Personality and personality disorder

Personality describes the characteristic behavioural, emotional and cognitive attributes of an individual. Thus we talk about an aggressive man, a nervous woman, and so on. Such traits are usually apparent by mid-adolescence and once established remain fairly stable. However, at times of stress these traits can become accentuated (decompensation) and it is at these times that they may be encountered in psychiatry. Personality is relevant to all areas of medicine as it forms a major part of the contextual understanding of a case. Psychiatrists are particularly interested in personality as it interacts with psychiatric disorders in many ways. It is only when certain personality traits are extreme enough to cause problems for the person or others that a personality disorder is defined. A formal definition is given in Box 15.1.

People with personality disorder come into contact with medical and psychiatric services either because they are concerned about themselves or, more commonly, because others are concerned or affected by their actions. For example:

- A trainee doctor who cannot get on with his team and repeatedly appears to ignore feedback regarding his overconfidence.
- A man who has lived with his parents throughout his adult life who when they die is unable to make decisions and wants others to do so for him.
- A young woman who takes impulsive overdoses each time a boyfriend leaves her.

 Box 15.1 Definitions of personality disorder

- ICD-10: '… a severe disturbance in the characterological constitution and behavioural tendencies of the individual, usually involving several areas of the personality, and nearly always associated with considerable personal and social disruption.'

DSM-IV and DSM-5: 'an enduring pattern of inner experience and behaviour that deviates markedly from the expectations of the individual's culture, is pervasive and inflexible, has an onset in adolescence or early adulthood, and leads to distress or impairment.'

A personality disorder may also be detected during the assessment or treatment of a psychiatric disorder – though it is very important to bear in mind that

---

Psychiatry Lecture Notes, Eleventh Edition. Gautam Gulati, Mary-Ellen Lynall and Kate Saunders. © 2014 John Wiley & Sons, Ltd. Published 2014 by John Wiley & Sons, Ltd.

the person's behaviour and self-description may be modified by the illness and consequently give a misleading impression about their 'normal' personality. Caution should be exercised when diagnosing personality disorder in this context.

Personality disorder and psychiatric disorder

The interaction between personality (disorder) and psychiatric disorder is important and manifold (Figure 15.1):

- Personality disorder can *predispose to* psychiatric disorder.
- Personality disorder can *coexist with* psychiatric disorder (a type of comorbidity). This worsens prognosis.
- Personality disorder can be *mistaken for* psychiatric disorder, and vice versa. For example, someone with a depressive disorder may give the impression that they have a personality disorder; a person with borderline personality disorder may be misdiagnosed as having a bipolar disorder.
- Personality can be *affected by* psychiatric disorder. For example, the deterioration in personality in chronic schizophrenia.
- Personality can have a *pathoplastic* effect on psychiatric disorder – that is, it can modify the clinical features even if it has no direct causal role.

Key aspects of personality disorder

Diagnosis

Diagnosis of personality disorder is based on a marked deviation of one or more aspects of personality. Common to all personality disorders are the following features:

- The personality attributes cause distress or dysfunction for the individual or those he or she interacts with.
- The dysfunction occurs across a range of situations.
- The characteristics are pervasive, stable and recognizable since late adolescence.

It often useful to seek a corroborative informant particularly if a comorbid mental illness is present.

The specific personality disorders are diagnosed according to the domain(s) of personality that are most affected, and the most prominent behaviours.

Classification

Personality disorder in ICD-10 is divided into 10 types. However, the validity and reliability of these categories is limited. Most patients seem to fit several descriptions or none of them. A simpler option, from DSM-IV and DSM-5, is to use three clusters, which encompass the individual categories (Table 15.1).

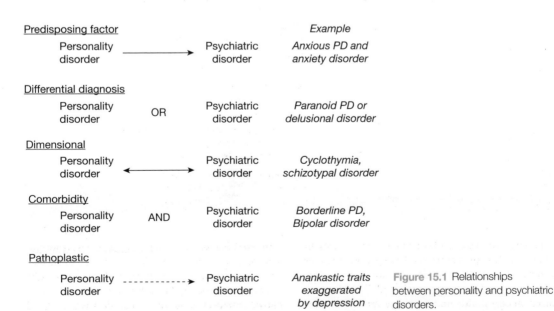

Figure 15.1 Relationships between personality and psychiatric disorders.

Table 15.1 **Classification and features of personality disorders**

Cluster and subtype	Main features
Cluster A (eccentric)	Aloof or suspicious, solitary
Paranoid	Suspicion and distrust of others Sensitivity to criticism Bears grudges Self-importance
Schizoid	Emotionally cold and detached Introspective Social isolation Lack of *joie de vivre*
Cluster B (dramatic)	Emotionally labile and intense
Dissocial (= psychopathic, antisocial)	Callous Unstable, transient relationships Low frustration threshold Irritable and impulsive Failure to learn from experience Failure to accept responsibility Lack of guilt Tend to be young men
Borderline (= emotionally unstable)	Multiple, turbulent relationships Impulsivity Recurrent emotional crises Variable, intense mood Stress-related psychotic-like symptoms Tend to be young women
Histrionic	Exaggerated, theatrical displays of emotion Attention seeking Vain Suggestible Shallow, labile mood Crushes and fads
Narcissistic	Grandiose self-importance Exaggerates achievements and abilities Exploits others Arrogant Expects special praise and respect
Cluster C (anxious)	Timid, dependent, low self-esteem
Anankastic (= obsessional)	Excessive orderliness Preoccupation with detail Inflexible and dogmatic Humourless
Anxious (= avoidant)	Persistent tense and apprehensive feelings Avoid personal contact Fear of criticism or rejection
Dependent	Encourage others to make decisions Excessive need to be taken care of

In practice, both categories and clusters are used by clinicians. The proposals for DSM-5 had included significant changes in the classification scheme, with a move towards a 'prototypic' model of diagnosis based on personality traits and how strongly they are expressed, rather than symptom checklists. However, lack of agreement within the personality disorders working-group meant that the criteria for personality disorders were not updated. Instead, a possible alternative classification for these disorders was outlined for evaluation and research purposes in Section III of DSM-5.

Personality traits and personality disorders are, in reality, *dimensional* – that is, they exist on a continuum and merge into each other (and into psychiatric disorders). Consequently, any categorical classification (limiting to either the presence or absence of a disorder or trait) can be problematic. The two diagnostic systems do not always agree as to what should be classed as a personality disorder. For example schizotypal disorder is classed as axis 1 in ICD and axis 2 (personality disorder) in DSM-IV.

Epidemiology

Estimates of the prevalence of personality disorders vary widely – for example, from 2% to 15% in the general population. A recent large survey of British households found:

- A personality disorder was found in 4.4% of people. Of these, half met the criteria for two or more disorders.
- The most common were obsessive-compulsive, avoidant, schizoid and borderline.
- No cases of histrionic or narcissistic personality disorder were seen.
- Personality disorders frequently coexist with psychiatric disorders.

The prevalence of personality disorder is much higher in specific populations. For example:

- Prisoners: over 50% of men and 30% of women, with most being antisocial personality disorder.
- Psychiatric patients: about 50%.
- Patients with substance misuse or eating disorder: 70%.

Aetiology

Very little is known about the aetiology of personality disorders, partly because so little is understood about the determinants of normal personality. Most current research focuses on borderline and dissocial personality disorder, largely because they cause the greatest clinical and forensic difficulties (see below).

- Patterns of childhood behaviour, even as young as infancy, predict personality and personality disorders, albeit only weakly, emphasizing the early origins and stability of personality characteristics.
- Upbringing and childhood experiences have major influences on our personality for better and worse. Adverse childhood events, including sexual and

physical abuse, are important risk factors for personality disorder.

- There is a moderate genetic contribution to personality traits (e.g. 35–50% heritability for neuroticism and extraversion) and to some personality disorders, especially anankastic and dissocial types.
- Aggressive behaviour may be slightly more common in men with sex chromosome abnormalities (especially XYY), but much less so than sometimes portrayed.

Specific personality disorders

Refer to Table 15.1 for key features of each personality disorder, and a comparison of clusters and subtypes.

Cluster A personality disorders ('eccentric')

People with cluster A personality disorder (especially schizoid type) by their nature tend to avoid services, and usually present (as with Dr E in the Clinical scenario) when their suspiciousness or persecutory beliefs lead them to behave in a way that concerns others (e.g. making accusations or threatening retribution for a perceived wrongdoing). The key issues are:

- To distinguish the personality disorder from a psychosis, especially chronic delusional disorder. Paranoid personality disorder is a risk factor for development of a psychosis.
- To decide if there is a significant risk of harm to the person or others.
- To decide what, if any, treatment should be given for the personality disorder. Low-dose antipsychotics may be tried, with appropriate consent, but compliance is likely to be poor. Similarly, social interventions may be offered, but isolation is rarely perceived as a problem. Psychotherapy is said to be ineffective, even harmful, and is contraindicated.

Cluster B personality disorders ('dramatic')

There is considerable overlap between the individual disorders in this cluster. In practice, the only widely used categories are borderline (for women) and dissocial (for men).

Borderline personality disorder

Miss D (see Clinical scenario) fits the typical profile of borderline personality disorder. There may be frequent presentations for a variety of reasons:

- Following an overdose or self-cutting.
- With depressive or 'quasi-psychotic' symptoms or suicidal ideation. The psychiatric presentation and subjective description is often dramatic, yet somewhat out of keeping with the objective impression.
- With a dramatic plea or demand for help of some kind (e.g. admission, medication).
- The diagnosis of 'borderline personality disorder' is sometimes applied loosely and pejoratively, especially to young women who self-harm, abuse alcohol, have eating difficulties and have chaotic lifestyles. Use the label carefully, sticking to the principles outlined here.

Borderline personality disorder is under active research investigation at present.

- The key neuropsychological deficits are thought to be *affective instability* and *impulsivity*.
- Brain imaging suggests frontal lobe dopaminergic and serotoninergic function may be important.
- There is an association of borderline personality disorder with childhood sexual abuse, post traumatic stress disorder and bulimia nervosa. However, these associations are neither as strong nor as specific as sometimes claimed.

Dissocial (psychopathic, antisocial) disorder

In practice, most general psychiatrists rarely treat people with dissocial personality disorder (with or without consent) as no interventions have been shown to be effective. Admission is usually avoided, as it is often disruptive for other patients. The main goal is to exclude other diagnoses that may be more treatable. Forensic psychiatrists, on the other hand, have some expertise in assessing and managing the disorder.

- The Mental Health Act is sometimes used to admit people with dissocial personality disorder who have committed serious crimes to secure psychiatric hospitals either from court or prison. This is controversial, affected by societal and financial influences. In hospital, prolonged psychotherapy or antipsychotic drugs may be tried although the evidence base for the effectiveness of treatment is very limited. Treatment programmes exist within the criminal justice system and are increasingly being viewed as the most appropriate to offer.
- The problems of dissocial personality disorder are often worsened by drugs and alcohol.
- The whole range of genetic, developmental, psychological and social factors are thought to be involved in the origins of dissocial personality disorder. A few people have temporal lobe EEG abnormalities. *Minimal brain dysfunction* refers to the view that the disorder results from minor brain injury or delayed maturation.
- As with borderline personality disorder, the core neuropsychological deficits are thought to involve impulsivity and decision-making, and relate to abnormalities in the regulation of frontal lobe activity by dopamine and serotonin (5-HT).

Cluster C personality disorder ('anxious')

This cluster rarely presents clinically, and there is little information about how to manage it. If it does, set realistic goals for treatment, try to enhance self-esteem and avoid escalating contact, which simply fosters dependency.

- The diagnosis is usually made in someone who presents with a depressive disorder or anxiety disorder. Cluster C personality disorder is a risk factor for both.

 Clinical scenario

Miss D is 22 and has taken an impulsive overdose. She felt bored and angry with her boyfriend and various others. She has repeatedly self-harmed since early adolescence in response to minor life events – particularly when she feels abandoned. She reports having been sexually abused by her stepfather. Her lifestyle is chaotic and she misuses alcohol. Previous attempts to offer help have been thwarted by her failure to keep appointments. Her one enduring pleasure in life is looking after horses. Two days later she discharges herself; her boyfriend sent her some flowers and she is planning to marry him.

Key features: impulsivity, sensitive to rejection, emotional instability.

Positive attributes: the care of animals. Has done unpaid work for an animal charity.

Cluster: B (dramatic)

Subtype: emotionally unstable (borderline) personality disorder.

Clinical scenario

Dr E is a 60-year-old scientist who has accepted psychiatric referral under protest. He is unmarried and has had several brief, unsatisfactory relationships. He feels strongly that he has been denied the acclaim he deserves and is currently complaining bitterly to his head of department after unsuccessfully applying for promotion. He alleges that other workers steal his ideas. He does not mix with his colleagues and is uneasy in social gatherings.

Key features: socially isolated, suspicious, tendency to exaggerate self-importance.

Positive attributes: his research eminence shows a high level of functioning.

Cluster: A (eccentric)

Subtype: paranoid personality disorder.

Management

The traditional view has always been that personality cannot usually be modified to any significant degree in adults, but there is an increasing evidence base that some treatments are effective, particularly for cluster B personality disorders. Management can be difficult and it is not uncommon for clinicians to oscillate between over-reacting and failing to intervene, particularly for cluster B disorders.

The broad principles of management are:

- Help the person to avoid situations that cause problems such as intoxication or confrontations.
- Help them to find a lifestyle that suits their strengths and minimizes the effects of their personality difficulties.
- Be consistent in managing crisis presentations. Admissions are rarely helpful and may reinforce the behaviour. A consistent, limited and community-based approach is usually better.
- Careful differentiation, as far as is possible, from mood disorders and psychosis. Bear in mind the symptom profile and the onset and course.
- A written care plan. Ensure good communication between the agencies involved to avoid 'splitting' (disagreements between staff induced by the patient – people with these personality traits induce a range of strong feelings).
- Respond to threats consistently and do not reinforce manipulative behaviour.
- Clear boundaries should be agreed about unacceptable behaviour and about the nature of care that will be provided. For example, recurrent psychiatric admission is probably not helpful.

- A psychotherapeutic assessment should be considered.
- Treat any coexisting psychiatric disorder.
- Treat any coexisting substance misuse.
- For borderline personality disorder a very intensive and specific form of psychotherapy, *dialectical behaviour therapy*, is effective in decreasing self-harm. *Cognitive analytical therapy* is also advocated. Group therapy in *therapeutic communities* may occasionally be helpful.
- There are no licensed medications for the treatment of personality disorder although in practice patients are often given medication trials on an off-licence basis to reduce distress or for help with symptoms.

Prognosis

The fact that personality disorders are considered to be lifelong and stable implies that prognosis is uniformly bad. In fact, considerable fluctuations do occur, and improvement is often observed by middle age. Some clinicians distinguish:

- Mature personality disorders (equating to cluster A), which are first recognizable in late adolescence and which remain stable or worsen with age.
- Immature personality disorders (clusters B and C), which have an onset in childhood and which mellow with age.

Personality disorder is associated with an increased mortality rate. It also worsens outcome of co-morbid psychiatric disorder, and increases the risk of violence when comorbid with psychosis.

Problems with the concept of personality disorder

The concept of personality disorder has been controversial. Arguments include:

- It isn't a 'disease'. It medicalizes individual differences and implies they can and should be treated by doctors.
- Its diagnosis is unreliable.
- One man's personality disorder is another man's virtue. Many famous people meet the criteria for personality disorder, yet the traits are either tolerated because of, or are actually the basis of, their success.

- The term is pejorative: the label is applied to patients whom doctors don't like or find hard to manage, or is used as a justification to avoid trying to help.
- There is no clear distinction to be made between personality disorders and psychiatric disorders.

Some of these arguments raise issues that go well beyond the boundaries of psychiatry. Given the current state of knowledge, psychiatrists must at least ensure that they use the term 'personality disorder' as reliably and usefully as possible.

- Always be wary of diagnosing personality disorder solely on the basis of behaviour during an episode of psychiatric illness. Illness can affect how personality is expressed.
- Personality disorder interacts with psychiatric disorder in several ways: as a predisposing factor, a pathoplastic factor, a prognostic factor, a comorbid disorder and as a differential diagnosis.
- Focus treatment on helping the person modify their circumstances, removing exacerbating factors and reinforcing positive behaviours. Medication has a very limited role. Specific psychotherapies may help borderline personality disorder.

 KEYPOINTS

- Personality is the combination of persistent and relatively stable emotional, cognitive and behavioural traits that characterize each of us. A personality is deemed disordered if these traits are excessive or deficient, and cause problems for the individual or for those around her or him.
- Personality disorders are classified pragmatically into three clusters: eccentric, dramatic and anxious. Important specific types are paranoid, dissocial (psychopathic) and borderline.

 FURTHER READING

National Institute for Health and Care Excellence (NICE) (2009) CG78 Borderline personality disorder: treatment and management. Access at http://www.nice.org.uk/cg78

National Institute for Health and Care Excellence (NICE) (2009) CG77 Antisocial personality disorder: treatment, management and prevention. Access at http://guidance.nice.org.uk/CG77

 SELF-ASSESSMENT

1 A 23-year-old woman presents with severe mood swings, impulsive behaviour and alcohol misuse. She has taken four overdoses in the past 2 months, many in the context of relationship breakdowns. She has ongoing suicidal ideation. You are asked to assess her. What else would you need to do to confirm a diagnosis of borderline personality disorder?

a Enquire about dissociative symptoms.
b Explore whether she has had abusive experiences in her childhood.
c Establish the presence of a family history of bipolar disorder.
d Take a corroborative history from a friend or family member to confirm the pervasive nature of the symptoms.

2 A 45-year-old man is referred to you following the death of his mother 1 year ago. He feels unable to cope. He has never moved out of the family home and has never worked. He appears unable to make decisions and is requesting that he is taken into residential care although he has no physical ailments. What is the most likely primary diagnosis?

a Delayed grief reaction.
b Adjustment disorder.
c Dependent personality disorder.
d Normal bereavement.

Childhood disorders

Learning objectives

✓ To be able to describe the prevalence and presentations of common psychological problems in children and to develop a framework for assessing these

Principles of child psychiatry

Interviewing children

When interviewing a child, the objectives are the same as with adults: to establish rapport, make a diagnosis, understand its context and plan treatment. However, for several reasons, the nature of the interview differs, especially with young children:

- The child may not understand the question or be unable to express him or her self.
- The range of disorders being sought, and hence the diagnostic focus, is different.
- Parents determine when and how the child presents.
- Family factors contribute to many disorders – so more attention is paid to the family environment. Child psychiatry interviews have several features:
- Parents are present but child and parents are often seen separately for part of the interview once rapport has been established.
- The interviewer must be able to jump from one topic to another as led by the child.
- Assessment may start with play and gentle conversation to gain trust.
- Much information comes from the child's appearance and behaviour.
- Significant others (e.g. teachers, siblings) provide key parts of the history.
- More than one session may be needed to complete the interview.

By adopting these strategies, the interviewer aims to collect information about the topics in Table 16.1.

In addition a physical health history and neurological examination may be indicated. To complete the assessment, background information is sought from relevant sources, such as teachers, social services, general practitioners or community paediatricians.

- Get parental consent at each stage, unless abuse is suspected, in which case the duty of care to the child may over-ride this principle.

Classification

The major childhood psychiatric disorders are shown in Table 16.2. A multiaxial scheme is often used to record the diagnostic information because of the importance of developmental stage, overall abilities and social circumstances:

Axis I: psychiatric disorder(s) present.

Axis II: developmental stage and delays.

Axis III: intellectual level.

Axis IV: medical problems.

Axis V: abnormal social situations.

Learning disability in children is covered in Chapter 17.

Epidemiology

Transient symptoms and behavioural disturbances are common in children of all ages. As in adults, making a psychiatric diagnosis requires a persistence and

Psychiatry Lecture Notes, Eleventh Edition. Gautam Gulati, Mary-Ellen Lynall and Kate Saunders. © 2014 John Wiley & Sons, Ltd. Published 2014 by John Wiley & Sons, Ltd.

Table 16.1 Topics for the child psychiatric interview

Presenting problem
Onset, duration, factors affecting it
Associated problems and symptoms
Recent life events
Parents' and child's explanation for it

Developmental milestones
Motor, e.g. sitting, walking
Social, e.g. smiling
Emotional, e.g. attachment behaviour
Cognitive, e.g. talking, reading
Other, e.g. toilet training

Emotional profile
Temperament
Problem behaviours
Likes and dislikes

Family
Relationship with parents and siblings
Problems at home
Separations from parents
Parental and sibling health and personalities

Schooling
Educational record
Attendance
Relationship with peers

General health
Hospital admissions
Previous psychiatric history
Sleep pattern and problems

Observation of child
General appearance
Interactions with interviewer and family members
Attention and concentration
Prevailing mood and range of emotions expressed
Language and motor skills

Table 16.2 Classification of childhood psychiatric disorders

Emotional disorders (neuroses)
Anxiety disorders
Somatoform disorder

Behavioural disorders
Conduct disorder
Attention deficit hyperactivity disorder (ADHD)

Depressive disorder
Developmental disorders
Autism and other pervasive developmental disorders
Specific (e.g. specific reading disorder)

Miscellaneous conditions
Enuresis
Encopresis
Selective mutism
Tics

Aetiology

The same broad range of aetiological factors operate in childhood as in adulthood (Table 16.3).

- There is a probable genetic component to most disorders.
- The major environmental factors are the family and social circumstances.
- Genes and environment are not independent factors, but interact to determine risk.

Management

Management of children with psychiatric disorders is based upon several principles:

- Take the child's developmental stage and overall level of functioning into account.
- Most problems are treated initially with advice, support and behavioural interventions.
- Involve the family and school.
- Avoid removal from school or home wherever possible.
- Medication is used less frequently than in adult psychiatry, though can be helpful in ADHD, anxiety and depression when other interventions have had limited effect; adolescents with bipolar disorder or psychotic disorders typically require psychopharmacological management with careful attention to side effects.
- Further details are discussed in the sections describing the specific disorders.

pervasiveness of symptoms, and evidence of difficulty in functioning in the home or school environment, or both. The major epidemiological features of childhood psychiatric disorder are:

- Prevalence at age 10 is 7% in rural areas and 13% in urban areas. At age 14 the prevalence is higher. (These numbers come from a classic, though dated, UK study.)
- Boys are affected more often than girls for many diagnoses, such as attention deficit hyperactivity disorder and autistic spectrum disorder.
- The most common diagnoses are emotional disorders and conduct disorders.
- Disorders are more common in children with learning disability, epilepsy and chronic physical illnesses.

Table 16.3 Causative factors in child psychiatry

Factor	Examples
Genetic	Autism shows high heritability
Environmental	
Family factors	
Parenting styles	Harsh, critical style associated with conduct disorder
Parental conflict	Increased risk of emotional or conduct disorder
Parental psychiatric disorder	Increased risk of eating disorder
Social factors	
Deprivation	Increased risk of conduct disorder
Bullying	School refusal
Other factors	
Prematurity	Increased risk of developmental delay and behavioural disorders
Medical disorder	Epilepsy increases risk of most disorders
Physical abuse	Increased risk of emotional and behavioural disorders

- Psychodynamic approaches continue to have an important role in some child and adolescent services.

Prognosis

Childhood psychiatric disorders have a variable outcome, in part because of the influence of the child's ongoing development and experiences. The basic pattern is summarized in Table 16.4.

Emotional disorders

Emotional disorders refer to the neuroses as described in Chapter 10. In children, the disorders are in many ways similar but there are important differences too:

- 'Emotional disorder', not neurosis, is the usual term.

Table 16.4 Prognosis of psychiatric disorders in childhood

Category	Long-term outcome
Emotional disorders	Good, two-thirds resolve in a 4-year period
Mood disorder	Variable, half have depressive disorder in adulthood
Behavioural disorders:	
Conduct disorder	Poor, often leads on to personality disorder or substance misuse
Attention deficit hyperactivity disorder (ADHD)	Variable, some cases resolve, or young people find a 'niche' where symptoms are less problematic; others require medication in adulthood
Developmental disorders:	
Autism	Lifelong; severe cases may require intensive support throughout adulthood; able individuals may find a career 'niche' and succeed, and some may learn social skills by technique rather than instinct and function well
Other conditions:	
Enuresis	Good
Tics	Usually transient (unless Tourette syndrome)
Selective mutism	Variable, may have persistent communication problems

- Some subtypes are different (e.g. separation anxiety).
- Medication is rarely used but may have a role where psychological approaches are challenging or have not worked.
- Equal male to female ratio (cf. 1:2 in adults) until puberty.
- Many affected children recover fully.

Anxiety disorders

Crying when mum goes out, or becoming fearful of spiders, are normal anxieties that children may experience at particular developmental stages, especially at times of stress and transition. They must be distinguished from persistent, significant symptoms warranting a diagnosis of anxiety disorder. The latter affects 5% of children at some time. As in adults, anxiety manifests with behavioural, psychological and physical symptoms (Table 16.5).

Separation anxiety

Among 5–11-year-olds, 3–4% have excessive anxiety when faced with separation from parents or others they are attached to. The child clings to the person and tries to avoid being separated from them. Sleep disturbance may occur. Older children may describe being fearful that the person will be harmed or will not return. Separation anxiety often begins at times of stress, such as after the death of a loved one or the family pet. Some parents are noted to be overprotective. Management includes:

- Working with the family to explain and reassure.
- Identification and resolution of stressors.

Table 16.5 **Symptoms of anxiety in children**

Behavioural
Clinging to parent (or other carer)
Unwilling to leave house
Unwilling to go to bed
Actions designed to avoid feared event (e.g. hiding)

Psychological
Feeling worried
Nightmares

Physical
Abdominal pain
Headaches

- Ensuring the parents are not reinforcing the problem (e.g. by appearing anxious when about to leave the child).
- Use of specific interventions for secondary problems that develop, such as school refusal.

Somatoform disorder

Children readily develop somatic symptoms, especially when under stress. Non-specific abdominal pain and headaches are the most common and may lead to a paediatric referral. As in adults, *somatoform disorder* describes bodily symptoms that are unexplained by a medical condition. The assessment of these requires:

- Exclusion of a medical disorder that fully explains the symptoms.
- Exclusion of other diagnosable emotional or depressive disorders.
- Identification of likely precipitating and perpetuating factors. For example, the child may be unhappy at home, or worried about a sick sibling.

Management is aimed at avoiding reinforcing the symptoms (e.g. by teaching the parents how not to do this inadvertently) and at tackling the underlying stressors. The prognosis is variable. Some children proceed to somatoform disorder as adults.

Other emotional disorders

Obsessive-compulsive disorder in children is rare clinically, and has a prevalence of 1 in 400 in British 5–15-year-olds. It is sometimes associated with *Tourette syndrome* (see below). A subset of cases may result from a streptococcal infection causing an immune reaction, though this remains controversial.

- There is good evidence that antidepressants (clomipramine, fluoxetine) and psychological (cognitive behavioural) therapy are effective in OCD. Nevertheless, the prognosis in severe cases is quite poor.

Children also suffer from the other emotional disorders seen in adults (Chapter 10). For example, they can get *specific phobias* or develop emotional disorders following particular stresses (*adjustment reactions*).

- *Chronic fatigue syndrome* is also now well recognized in children. As in adults, its aetiology and management remain controversial. Pending better

Table 16.6 Assessment of suspected school refusal

Why is the child absent from school?
- School refusal
- Truancy
- Parents keeping child at home
- Physical illness

What does the school refusal reflect?
- Reluctance to leave home (i.e. secondary to separation anxiety)
- A specific fear relating to the school environment (e.g. of getting there, or being bullied)
- A more generalized disorder (e.g. social phobia, depressive disorder, undiagnosed autism spectrum disorder)

What other factors are relevant?
- Recent life events (e.g. bereavement)
- Recent events at school (e.g. change of class)
- Parental characteristics (e.g. overprotective)

Table 16.7 Distinguishing school refusal from truancy

School refusal	Truancy
Younger (<11 years old)	Older (>11 years old)
Underlying emotional disorder	Underlying conduct disorder
Good school record	Poor school record
Good prognosis	Poor prognosis
Parents overprotective	Poor parental supervision

evidence, treatment is based on the same principles of graded return to activities and cognitive behavioural methods, with the close involvement of the family.

School refusal

School refusal is not a psychiatric disorder, but it is a common cause of referral to a child psychiatrist and is frequently attributable to an emotional disorder. Its assessment is summarized in Table 16.6.

- Exclude truancy and parental behaviour as causes for the absence from school. The characteristics of school refusal and truancy are different (Table 16.7).

School refusal is usually due to separation anxiety, often provoked by recent events at home or at school. In older children, school refusal may reflect bullying; it can also herald a more pervasive problem such as social phobia or depressive disorder.

Management of school refusal is aimed at a rapid return to school before avoidance is too ingrained. Sometimes a graded re-exposure is needed. Address any specific fears or stresses, and treat any associated psychiatric disorder.

The prognosis in younger children is good. In older children, the problem may become prolonged and other psychiatric problems emerge. It may recur at times of transition (e.g. moving schools). There is a slightly increased risk of anxiety disorder in adulthood.

Mood disorders

The existence of mood disorders in prepubertal children used to be disputed. It is now clear that they occur, even in young children.

- Prevalence estimates are variable. They increase dramatically after puberty, when the higher rate in females first appears.
- The occurrence of bipolar mood disorder prepubertally is more controversial; although some United States-based research groups argue for its existence, other groups counter that diagnostic criteria are too loosely applied.

When evaluating mood and mood disorder in a child, apply the same principles as in adults:

- Symptoms should be present for at least 2 weeks and associated with distress and dysfunction.
- If there are also symptoms of an emotional disorder, attempt to distinguish the primary diagnosis.
- Children, especially adolescents, may present in crisis or after self-harm, with isolated or transient depressive symptoms, which (as in adults) are better viewed as an adjustment reaction than as a depressive episode.
- Childhood depressive disorders are classified in a similar way as adults (Chapter 9).
- As in adults, depression, especially in postpubertal children, carries an increased suicide risk. In severe cases, psychotic symptoms may occur.
- The main difference from adults concerns young children, who may not experience depression in the same way or be unable to articulate their feelings. Much diagnostic attention must therefore be placed on their appearance and behaviour both

in the interview and elsewhere (e.g. school work, activities, sleep pattern).

The aetiology of childhood depressive disorder involves the same mixture of genes, life events and unknown influences as prevail in adult cases.

Management includes support, monitoring and reducing stressors.

- Psychological approaches including CBT and family therapy, rather than medication, are first line; occasionally medication is used instead of therapy if symptoms are too severe to permit engagement with therapy, or if the young person has additional complexities such as autism spectrum disorder, which limit the ability to engage with psychological approaches. Despite a relative lack of evidence, various SSRIs were prescribed to children and adolescents, but their use is now very restricted because of concern that they may increase suicide risk. Only fluoxetine is currently allowed (in the United Kingdom) for use in under-18s as it appears to have some benefit and a low likelihood of increased suicidality.
- Admission may be needed for severe or psychotic depression. ECT is very rarely used.

The prognosis of childhood depressive disorder is variable. The condition may become chronic, and half go on to suffer from depressive disorder in adulthood.

Behavioural disorders

Behavioural disorders are diagnosed in children who have persistent problematic and antisocial behaviour. The main distinction is between behavioural problems that result mainly from hyperactivity (ADHD) and those that do not (conduct disorder) – though in practice the boundary is often hard to determine.

- Neither label should be applied unless the diagnostic criteria are met – all children are 'naughty' and 'hyper' from time to time; children with diagnosable difficulties show problems persisting across time and across contexts.

Conduct disorder

Conduct disorder is the most common psychiatric disorder of childhood and adolescence. Prevalence estimates range from 1% to 15%. It occurs mainly in boys (sex ratio 5:1). Conduct is disturbed and antisocial well beyond the range of misbehaviour normally observed for that age group (Table 16.8). Diagnosis is usually made after age 7, though problems have often

Table 16.8 Clinical features of conduct disorder

In pre-school children
Aggressive behaviour
Poor concentration

In mid-childhood
Lying
Stealing
Disruptive and oppositional behaviour
Bullying

In adolescence
Stealing
Truancy
Promiscuity
Substance misuse
Vandalism
Reckless behaviour

been apparent much earlier. The term *oppositional defiant disorder* may be used for these younger children.

- A distinction is sometimes made between *socialized conduct disorder*, where the activities occur within a peer group, and *unsocialized conduct disorder*, where the child acts in isolation.

In adolescence, conduct disorder has a strong relationship with juvenile delinquency and substance misuse. There is often repeated police contact and convictions for theft, criminal damage or assault. Conduct disorder is associated with a variety of indices of social deprivation and poor parenting (Table 16.9). There is also a small genetic contribution.

Table 16.9 Factors associated with conduct disorder

Family factors
Parental personality disorder
Paternal alcoholism
Parental disputes and violence
Harsh, inconsistent parenting
Being in care early in life
Large family size
Social factors
Inner cities
Deprivation and overcrowding

Individual factors
Brain damage
Epilepsy
Specific reading disorder

The long-term prognosis is poor; 50% of cases progress to dissocial personality disorder, and persistent substance misuse and criminality are common. Those who form stable relationships have a better outcome. There is no standard therapeutic approach, and a mixture of attempts to shape and reward behaviour is used, with varying degrees of evidence:

- Family-focused treatments seek to identify and remedy causes for the behaviour, improve the home environment, and include teaching parents how to cope with the behaviour and reduce conflict ('parental training').
- Praise and rewards for positive behaviour.
- Setting out clear rules and commands, with consistent and calm responses to unwanted behaviour.
- Anger management.
- 'Problem-solving skills training' is a recent approach that focuses on the child rather than the parents. It is based on evidence that children with ADHD are poor at problem-solving and interpersonal skills.
- Structured outlets for energies and behaviours (e.g. youth clubs, car workshops).
- Tackle associated problems such as truancy and substance misuse.
- Stimulant medication may have good results especially if there are coexistent ADHD symptoms.
- Residential care is occasionally unavoidable.

Cases of conduct disorder without additional psychiatric disorders are not usually managed by specialist Child and Adolescent Mental Health Services.

Attention deficit hyperactivity disorder (ADHD)

The clinical features are shown in Table 16.10. As with conduct disorder, the diagnosis requires that the problem is both persistent and extreme. In Britain, the prevalence is 2%; three-quarters are boys. In the United States, where less stringent criteria are used, prevalence and treatment rates are correspondingly higher.

- *Hyperkinetic disorder* is sometimes used interchangeably with ADHD. Strictly, it refers to a severe subgroup of ADHD in which all three core signs (inattention, hyperactivity and impulsiveness) are present, pervasive and with onset before age 7.
- ADHD is often comorbid with conduct disorder, anxiety, depression, tic disorders and pervasive developmental disorders.

The aetiology of ADHD is multifactorial:

- There is a significant genetic contribution (heritability ~70%), including genes affecting dopamine and

Table 16.10 Features of attention deficit hyperactivity disorder (ADHD)

Core features
Hyperactivity
Poor attention and concentration
Impulsivity
Present for at least 6 months
Evidence of impaired functioning in two or more settings
Onset by age 9, usually by 5

Other features
Distractibility
Poor at planning and organizing tasks
Learning difficulties
Clumsiness
Low self-esteem
Socially disinhibited
Unpopular with other children
Non-localizing neurological signs
Conduct disorder coexists in 50%

serotonin functioning in the brain. Families also show increased rates of depressive disorder, learning difficulties, alcoholism and dissocial personality disorder.
- A neurodevelopmental abnormality is suspected, on the basis of the soft neurological signs and learning difficulties, and from brain imaging and EEG findings.
- There is an association with social deprivation, though less striking than for conduct disorder.
- Other risk factors include maternal smoking and alcohol intake.
- Many parents blame food allergy, but this is rarely substantiated when investigated properly.

The management of ADHD involves:

- Support and psychoeducation for the child and family.
- Specific educational approaches, including attention to associated learning difficulties.
- Firm adherence to behavioural principles (to reward good behaviour and discourage hyperactive behaviour).
- Psychostimulants (e.g. methylphenidate, atomoxetine) have an important role and are recommended in UK guidelines as part of a comprehensive treatment programme for severe symptoms. This seemingly paradoxical treatment originated from the (incorrect) belief that there is a failure of cortical arousal in ADHD. Their main neurochemical effect is to increase dopamine in the synapse. Side effects are insomnia, poor appetite and headaches. Concerns about addiction have not been borne out in

practice. Breaks in treatment can be helpful if there are significant concerns about growth or appetite.
- Dietary restriction (e.g. of food additives or colourings) is not generally recommended.

ADHD has a variable prognosis. Gradual improvement typically occurs in adolescence, and one-third of cases resolve. The rest have residual hyperkinetic features, especially in those with learning difficulties or conduct disorder. Dissocial personality disorder and substance misuse sometimes develop. It is unclear how long treatment should continue into adulthood.

There is increasing interest in ADHD in adulthood, but no consensus on its diagnostic status or management.

 Clinical scenario

Harry is a 7-year-old boy whose head teacher has made a referral to Child Mental Health Services. He is always moving around the classroom, and forgets and loses his possessions very frequently. His parents report he is boisterous at home and has always been a 'livewire'. He has injured himself on several occasions by climbing and jumping off furniture in the home. You use questionnaires with his parents and teacher to assess symptoms of possible attention deficit hyperactivity disorder, and a colleague spends a morning at school without Harry's knowledge to conduct a 'school observation'. They speak to the Special Educational Needs Coordinator (SENCO), class teacher, and teaching assistant, who all view Harry as being a bright boy whose difficulties concentrating are stopping him from achieving his potential. You make an ADHD diagnosis and discuss the possibility of stimulant medication (methylphenidate) with his parents. They are concerned when you talk about possible effects on heart, blood pressure and appetite, but when you explain the monitoring plan in detail they decide to try the medication. Harry starts a low dose of long-acting methylphenidate. After 1 month, you meet Harry and his parents and notice he is able to sit on the chair to talk to you for several minutes before he goes to play with the toys. School and parents feel he is focusing much better and is less often in trouble. You agree to continue on the low dose and meet with Harry regularly to check his cardiovascular health and growth.

Developmental disorders

Developmental disorders can be *pervasive* or *specific*. The former, typified by *autism*, affect many aspects of psychological and neurobiological development; in the latter, there is impairment in only one domain (e.g. reading) relative to overall development.

- The abnormality is thought to be directly related to aberrant brain development.
- Their course lacks the fluctuations of most psychiatric disorders.

Pervasive developmental disorders

Current classification divides this category into several distinct disorders, as outlined here. However, the concept of *autistic spectrum disorders* is increasingly being used, recognizing that all share core impairments in social interactions, language and communication, and the child's range of interests and activities.

Autism

Autism is a syndrome characterized by a failure to develop normal communication, especially social and emotional communication. Autistic children have a delayed, restricted and unusual use of language. They seem oblivious to non-verbal cues and emotional expressions, with difficulties interacting with others. They demonstrate a limited range of solitary, repetitive behaviours and show excessive anxiety when routines are changed. Many also have a degree of learning disability. The features are summarized in Table 16.11.

- Very few autistic children (and adults), called *savants*, have remarkable abilities in discrete areas, such as complex mental arithmetic (as in the film *Rain Man*).

Table 16.11 Features of autism

1 in 100 children from surveys
80% are boys
Age of onset <3 years

Core features (the 'autistic triad')
Lack social reciprocity('aloof')
Impaired language and communication
Solitary, repetitive behaviours

Associated and comorbid features
Learning disability in 75%
Coordination difficulties
Sensory hypersensitivity or hyposensitivity
Epilepsy in about 25%
Mannerisms and rituals
Hyperactivity (40%)
Anxiety
Sleep disturbance
Hypotonia

The diagnosis is made based on a careful history and observations. Various checklists and structured interviews are also used.

- The differential diagnosis of 'classical' autism comprises other disorders with autistic features such as Asperger's and Rett's syndromes (see below), and fragile X syndrome and tuberous sclerosis complex (Chapter 17). These other disorders account for only about 10% of autism-like conditions. The term *autism spectrum disorder* is increasingly used in healthcare and education.
- Remember other causes of a failure to develop communication that may be mistaken for autism, such as specific language disorder and deafness. The aetiology of autism is strongly genetic.
- Many known or suspected autism susceptibility genes exist, including neuroligins 3 and 4, and other genes that probably converge upon synaptic development. There may also be microscopic structural abnormalities of the chromosomes, called *copy number variation* (CNV). The genetic basis of autism overlaps with that of schizophrenia.
- No confirmed environmental risk factors are known.
- Though there is clearly now greater awareness and/or a loosening of the diagnostic category, it remains uncertain whether there has been a genuine rise in the prevalence of autism.
- MRI scans show increased brain size early in life, suggestive of an aberrant growth trajectory. Neuropathological studies suggest cellular alterations in several brain areas, notably Purkinje cells in the cerebellum, also the brainstem and hippocampus. Neurochemically, excess 5-HT (serotonin) function affecting neurodevelopment has been postulated.
- Psychologically, the main hypothesis is a failure to develop a '*theory of mind*' – that is, the ability to attribute mental states and beliefs to others. This is thought to underlie the behaviour and lack of social engagement that characterize autism.

The prognosis is poor in classical autism. Speech eventually develops in some, but communication remains limited and the core abnormalities rarely improve. Seizures can occur later in childhood. Most autistic children need special schooling and residential care, and only a minority are ever able to live independently. Those with high-functioning autism may gradually make some improvements in their social interaction skills by different routes, and may find a suitable niche that allows them to make the most of their strengths.

There is no specific, evidence-based treatment for autism. The main components of management are:

- Make the diagnosis, and support the family in understanding autism and its implications.
- Consider interventions that are aimed to improve socialization, communication and behaviour.
- Provide appropriate education and, if required, accommodation.
- Deal with associated medical problems (e.g. epilepsy).
- Treat the anxiety.
- Medication is sometimes used, despite very limited evidence. For example, SSRIs for repetitive behaviours, or atypical antipsychotics for severe aggression.

Asperger's syndrome

Asperger's syndrome is similar to autism, with abnormalities in social communication and repetitive, isolated behaviours. However, language is not delayed. The child, usually a boy, prefers his own company and often has intense interests. Unlike autism, intelligence is normal, and seizures are not a feature. The prevalence is uncertain, with estimates from 1 to 50 per 10 000.

- The aetiology is unknown. It may or may not be causally related to autism.
- Asperger's syndrome persists into adulthood, and sometimes first presents at that time, when it may be mistaken for schizotypal or schizoid personality disorder, or schizophrenia.

Rett's syndrome

Rett's syndrome is a rare, progressive and severe disorder occurring almost exclusively in girls. The main features are autism, learning disability, seizures, loss of speech and skilled movements, and irregular breathing. It is usually caused by sporadic mutations in the *MECP2* gene on the X chromosome, and is fatal by early adulthood. Unusual hand-wringing movements are a classical feature.

Specific developmental disorders

Specific developmental disorders are conditions in which there is marked delay in one area of development relative to the child's overall IQ. The most common problem is with reading (80% of cases), but also disorders selectively affecting arithmetic, language or motor skills. Though the disorders are not really 'psychiatric', they are often referred to (or detected by) child psychiatric services because of associated emotional or behavioural difficulties.

- Specific speech and language disorder is related to the *FOXP2* gene.

Specific reading disorder

In specific reading disorder, reading skills are significantly (>2 standard deviations) below that predicted by the child's overall performance. Visual impairment or lack of education must be excluded as the cause. It affects 2–10% of 10-year-olds, and is four times more common in boys than in girls.

- It is associated with conduct disorder in one-third of cases, also with ADHD, low socioeconomic status and a disturbed family background. The direction of causality between these factors is unclear.
- Assessment should be by an educational psychologist using standardized tests.
- Management involves enhancing self-esteem and appropriate expert educational help.
- Nutritional supplements (fish oils) are being advocated by some researchers and families.
- Prognosis is poor, with reading abilities often remaining well below average.

Other conditions

Enuresis

Enuresis is urinary incontinence after the age at which bladder control is expected (*primary enuresis*; must be at least 5 years old) or after previous normal continence (*secondary enuresis*). It usually presents as bedwetting in the first half of the night (*nocturnal enuresis*). It affects 15% of 5-year-olds, 2% of 10-year-olds and 1% of 14-year-olds. Boys outnumber girls 3:1.

- Enuresis can cause great distress, affect self-esteem, interfere with normal activities (e.g. sleepovers) and can lead to bullying or intolerant parenting.

In the assessment, exclude urinary tract infection (UTI), diabetes or neurological disorder. Enuresis may be a sign of sleep apnoea. Search for recent stressors and symptoms of emotional disorder (twice as common as expected in those with enuresis). There is often a history of enuresis in male relatives. The management of enuresis includes:

- Reassurance, explanation and limiting fluid intake in the evening.

- Treatment of associated psychiatric or medical disorder.
- Behavioural methods are the main treatment. A *star chart* is best for younger children; they are rewarded for achieving a realistic target (which may not be a 'dry bed' initially) with stars or other suitable token. An *enuresis alarm* ('pad and buzzer') is a moisture-sensitive pad worn by the child. When urine is passed, a buzzer goes off, which wakes the child in time to go to the toilet to finish. He or she also participates in changing the sheets. An alarm is usually effective if persisted with for several weeks, especially in children over 7 years old.
- Pharmacological methods are sometimes used, though behavioural methods are preferred. Intranasal desmopressin is the usual first-line drug, with moderate success and few side effects. The tricyclic antidepressant (TCA) imipramine is licenced for enuresis from the age of 6, but is of limited efficacy, is potentially dangerous and not usually recommended. Relapse is common with both methods.

The prognosis is good, though a few boys remain enuretic into adulthood.

Encopresis

Encopresis is the passing of faeces in an inappropriate place after age 4. As with enuresis, it can be primary or secondary. Children may soil their pants, pass faeces in hidden places or occasionally smear them. At assessment, exclude physical problems (e.g. constipation, Hirschsprung's disease) and learning disability.

- There is often a history of inadequate or harsh toilet training combined with recent stresses and emotional disorder in the child.

Management is by reassurance, help with associated problems and ensuring that the parents do not become punitive. The standard behavioural manoeuvre is to toilet the child after each meal, and to reward her or him for staying there, for producing a motion and for not soiling. Most encopresis cases resolve with treatment within a year. Occasionally it persists into adolescence.

Tics

Tics are involuntary, rapid, spasmodic movements, usually repeated blinking and grimacing. They are common, especially in young boys, and may begin after an emotional upset. They are generally transient and need no specific treatment. However, some tics become severe, prolonged and incapacitating.

The main tic disorder is (*Gilles de la*) *Tourette syndrome*, in which tics are accompanied by vocal grunts and sometimes by stereotyped phrases, movements or expletives (*coprolalia*). Obsessive-compulsive and ADHD symptoms often occur. Boys are affected more than girls (3:1). The incidence is usually considered to be around 1 in 2000, but much higher figures exist.

Mild cases need no treatment. Troublesome tics are controlled by low-dose antipsychotics. Obsessional and hyperactivity symptoms can be treated as appropriate. Though the tics tend to diminish in adulthood, some symptoms persist.

- Tourette syndrome has a genetic basis, which overlaps with that of OCD. Autoimmune processes may also contribute. Abnormalities in basal ganglia pathways and the dopamine system are implicated.

Selective mutism

In selective (also called elective) mutism, children refuse to speak although able to do so. Speech is usually normal in one setting (e.g. at home) but absent elsewhere. Non-verbal communication is preserved. Onset is from 4 to 8 years old. Affected children tend to be shy, anxious and isolated in most settings, though can sometimes be aggressive and disturbed at home. The disorder is rare, and unusually it is more common in girls than boys. It may be associated with overprotective parenting and maternal depression.

- Selective mutism is increasingly being viewed as an anxiety disorder.
- There is no specific treatment; a range of behavioural interventions may be tried.
- Selective mutism can persist for several years, and residual social anxiety and communication problems are common.

Sleep disorders

Children, like adults, can suffer from sleep problems secondary to psychiatric disorders, and from sleep disorders. The sleep disturbance can impair the child's behaviour and development, and affect the whole family. A sleep history is part of the assessment (Table 16.1).

- Childhood sleep disturbance is particularly common in those with learning disability (Chapter 17) and autism.

Psychoses in childhood and adolescence

Schizophrenia may begin in adolescence, and occasionally in younger children. *Bipolar disorder* can also start in adolescence.

- The disorders are treated in a similar fashion to adult-onset cases, and are one of the few clear indications for medication in child psychiatry. The prognosis of childhood-onset psychosis is poor.

Special groups

Toddlers

Toddlers are notorious for *temper tantrums*. Reassurance that this is normal, and simple advice on setting limits, are usually all that is needed. Consistency in the parents' response to the behaviour is crucial. Self-help books are available.

Sleep disturbances are common, either refusal to settle or night-time waking due to night terrors and *nightmares*. Use reassurance and a consistent bedtime routine. Psychiatric referral is rare, though occasionally the disturbances herald an emotional or behavioural disorder.

Teenagers

Contrary to the stereotype, neither emotional turmoil nor delinquency is normal for teenagers. Persistently withdrawn, disruptive or bizarre behaviour should be assessed to exclude psychiatric disorder. Diagnostically, adolescents get the tail end of childhood disorders and the early onset of adult disorders (Table 16.12), so the clinician must know about both, and the continuities between them. This has led to *adolescent psychiatry* as a subspecialty.

Table 16.12 Important psychiatric disorders of adolescence

Conduct disorder
Eating disorder
Substance misuse disorders
Depressive disorder
Anxiety disorder
Schizophrenia
Bipolar disorder
Deliberate self-harm

Children in institutions

Children in care, especially in children's homes, have increased rates of psychiatric disorder, notably conduct disorder, substance misuse, post-traumatic stress disorder (PTSD) and self-harm. This may be both a cause and a consequence of being in care.

- Teenagers in detention facilities have extremely high rates of psychiatric disorder, with conduct disorder, substance misuse and self-harm again prominent.

Children with physical illness

Children with any chronic illness are at increased risk of psychiatric disorder. This is especially true for organic brain syndromes and epilepsy. The associations may partly reflect a common aetiology, but also the effects of physical illness on the child's intellectual, psychological and social development.

- Close cooperation between those involved in the psychiatric and medical disorders is essential.

Children with psychiatrically ill parents

If a parent has a psychiatric disorder, the child is at risk of psychiatric problems via an increased likelihood of inadequate or abnormal parenting, as well as from inheritance of a genetic predisposition. Hence the mental health (and personality) of parents is part of the child psychiatric assessment (Table 16.1). Specific parental problems associated with particular outcomes in the child include:

- Maternal substance misuse affects foetal development.
- Paternal alcoholism and development of conduct disorder.
- Maternal depression may impair the formation of secure infant attachments.
- Maternal eating disorder and abnormal feeding of the child.
- Fabricated and induced illness (sometimes called *Munchausen syndrome by proxy* or *Meadows' syndrome*) – the parent fabricates symptoms or signs in the child.

Abused children

Children can be abused sexually, physically or emotionally. The abuse has psychiatric as well as medical and legal repercussions. Key points concerning the psychiatric aspects of child abuse are:

- Take specialist advice whenever abuse is suspected. This may be obtained from paediatricians, child psychiatrists and social services' child protection teams.
- Your responsibility is first and foremost to protect the child. This may override the usual duty of confidentiality.
- Children who are being abused may show physical, psychological or behavioural signs.
- Managing abused children is difficult and needs multidisciplinary input. Child psychiatrists have particular roles in identifying and treating the psychological consequences of the abuse. It is unknown whether intervention alters the long-term prognosis.
- Physical abuse (non-accidental injury) causes significant morbidity and mortality. Either the child or the abuser may need to be removed from the home. Physical abuse leads to higher rates of emotional and behavioural disorder.
- Children who are emotionally abused or neglected have delayed psychological and physical development and increased rates of emotional disturbance. In extreme cases, they may present with failure to thrive (*deprivation dwarfism*).

The effects of child abuse may continue into adulthood:

- Women who were sexually abused have double the risk of psychiatric disorder and five times higher rates of psychiatric admission. Borderline personality disorder and possibly bulimia nervosa appear to be particularly common.
- There are no good data on the outcome of sexually abused boys, apart from an increased risk of becoming abusers and perpetuating the cycle.
- Emotional abuse may lead to persistent low self-esteem, relationship difficulties and personality disorder.

 Clinical scenario

Jade is a 15-year-old girl who was taken into foster care 2 years ago following allegations of sexual abuse by her father. She has moved through eight foster placements in 2 years and her current placement is at risk of breakdown owing to her challenging behaviour. She has started drinking alcohol heavily and smokes cannabis at weekends, and has self-harmed on a number of occasions. The first two times you meet Jade with her foster mother, she swears at you and leaves the room when you 'ask too many questions'. Jade agrees to meet you at her school for her next appointment. When you see Jade alone, she reveals she is very distressed by bad dreams at night and 'videotapes' playing during the day of the abuse by her father. She feels detached from people she used to be close to and avoids going back to her family home for contact visits, even though her father is no longer living there. You diagnose post-traumatic stress disorder, and Jade starts individual sessions with the team's psychologist, who uses trauma-focused cognitive behavioural therapy to address Jade's symptoms. Jade is sleeping a lot better, seems to be focusing better on her school work, and is drinking less often. She still has bad dreams and self-harms regularly now by cutting, but has had no suicidal ideation. You are concerned that in the longer term she may have persisting difficulties with emotion regulation as a consequence of the long-term sexual abuse, and offer her a place on a group programme to address emotional regulation problems. Jade is not keen to be involved and says she would rather 'get on with life'. You agree to review her in 2 months and explain you would be happy to refer her again if she changes her mind.

Refugee children

Children who find themselves in a foreign country, with strange customs, a language they may not understand, and often with major social deprivation and other stressors, are a vulnerable and neglected group. Their psychiatric needs are not well met by most services. Depression, PTSD, and anxiety disorders are particularly common.

KEYPOINTS

- Conduct disorder and emotional disorder are the most common childhood psychiatric diagnoses.
- The principles of child psychiatry and psychiatric assessment are similar to the adult context. However, more attention must be paid to the child's developmental history, and to the home and school environment.
- The risk of child psychiatric disorder is greater in urban areas, in boys, in those in care and in children with learning disability or chronic illness.
- Most disorders arise from an interaction between genetic and environmental factors.
- Treatment is usually behavioural and, given the degree of influence the parents have on a child's behaviour, must be aimed at the family as well as at the child.
- Medication is used far less frequently than in adults, but can be effective for a number of conditions. Caution is required, especially with antidepressants.

FURTHER READING

National Institute for Health and Care Excellence (NICE) (2005) CG28 Depression in children and young people. Access at www.nice.org.uk/CG28

National Institute for Health and Care Excellence (NICE) (2008) CG72 Attention deficit hyperactivity disorder: Diagnosis and management of ADHD in children, young people and adults. Access at www.nice.org.uk/cg72

National Institute for Health and Care Excellence (NICE) (2009) CG89 When to suspect child maltreatment. Access at www.nice.org.uk/cg89

? SELF-ASSESSMENT

1 A 10-year-old is brought to clinic with school refusal. His mother reports that the boy has never had clear friendships at school, and tends to 'talk over' other children. He has been bullied frequently, but teachers also report that he sometimes is aggressive to other children without an identifiable reason. Which of the following psychiatric diagnoses is the best explanation for his difficulties?
   a Schizophrenia
   b Social phobia
   c Generalized anxiety disorder
   d Asperger's syndrome
   e Conduct disorder

2 A 17-year-old girl attends clinic with low mood and poor sleep and appetite. She always feels tired at school, and no longer enjoys her pastimes of netball and dancing. You diagnose a moderate depressive episode. She has not disclosed to her parents that she is attending a mental health service. Which is the most appropriate first-line treatment?
   a Family therapy
   b Cognitive analytic therapy
   c Citalopram
   d Cognitive behavioural therapy
   e Fluoxetine

Learning disability (mental retardation)

Learning objectives

✓ To understand and be able to describe the definition, classification, assessment and aetiology of learning disability

✓ To learn about common psychiatric presentations in individuals with a learning disability

Principles

Definition and key features

Mental retardation, mental handicap, developmental disability, intellectual disability and *learning disability* are all synonyms. *Mental retardation* is the term in ICD-10 and DSM-IV, while DSM-5 uses *intellectual disability*. *Learning disability* is usually preferred by patients and families, and is used here.

Learning disability is defined as:

- IQ below 70.
- Impairment across a wide range of functions.
- Onset before 18 years old.

The features of learning disability are shown in Table 17.1. It must be distinguished from:

- Lower than average intelligence but IQ >70.
- Specific developmental disorders (Chapter 16).
- Intellectual impairment secondary to an adult organic syndrome (Chapter 13).

The incidence of learning disability has declined because of medical advances (e.g. immunization) and termination of affected pregnancies. However, the prevalence is increasing because of improved survival.

Mild learning disability represents the tail end of the normal population distribution for intelligence and, as such, results from an interaction between multiple genetic and environmental factors. A specific cause is more often identifiable for severe cases.

Clinical features

Learning disability can be *mild, moderate, severe* or *profound* depending on IQ (Table 17.2). Its cause, if known, is coded separately.

Assessment of learning disability

The presence of learning disability may be suspected:

- Before birth – from antenatal tests or pregnancy complications.
- At birth – from the physical appearance.
- In infancy or childhood – as a result of developmental delay.

Assessment of a child with suspected learning disability encompasses:

- Making the diagnosis – establish its presence, severity and likely cause. This usually involves community paediatricians and sometimes paediatric neurologists and clinical geneticists.
- Evaluating the level of adaptive functioning.

Psychiatry Lecture Notes, Eleventh Edition. Gautam Gulati, Mary-Ellen Lynall and Kate Saunders. © 2014 John Wiley & Sons, Ltd. Published 2014 by John Wiley & Sons, Ltd.

Table 17.1 Features of learning disability

Mild, moderate, severe and profound forms

Prevalence is approximately 2%, with a male:female ratio of 3:2

Usually untreatable

Often accompanied by:
  Psychiatric disorder
  Challenging behaviour
  Medical problems (e.g. epilepsy)

Caused by:
  Chromosomal abnormalities
  Genetic mutations causing single gene disorders
  Environmental factors
  Most common specific causes are Down's syndrome and fragile X syndrome

- Evaluating comorbid psychiatric problems.
- Evaluating comorbid medical problems.

The areas of assessment are listed in Table 17.3. The procedures necessary depend on the child's age and the circumstances of the assessment. Compared with the standard psychiatric assessment there is a special emphasis on the obstetric and neurodevelopmental history and on the physical examination.

Psychiatric aspects of learning disability

Children and adults with learning disability have high rates (>40%) of challenging behaviour and psychiatric disorder. The risk of these problems is higher with coexistent epilepsy, and lower in Down's syndrome (save for depression, rates of which are higher in Down's syndrome partially due to hypothyroidism).

Psychiatric disorder in children with learning disability

All the main psychiatric disorders are more common in children with learning disabilities. The assessment of these follows the principles of the child psychiatric assessment, but modified according to intellectual level (Table 17.4).

Psychiatric disorder in learning-disabled adults

An adult with learning disability may require psychiatric assessment for a number of reasons:

- To assess the level of functioning and nature of current problems in order to help plan future management (e.g. placement).
- To investigate a suspected psychiatric disorder, such as schizophrenia and depression. These occur more commonly than in the general population. Their recognition may be difficult because of the learning disability. Various scales have been devised to help but sometimes the effect of a trial of medication may be needed.
- To assess and characterize a behavioural problem – called a *challenging behaviour* – such as shouting or inappropriate sexual activities, and to determine if it is secondary to a psychiatric diagnosis (e.g. depression), a physical illness (e.g. an infection) or seizure activity, which is especially common in this population.
- As part of a forensic or risk assessment.
- To assess a decline in abilities. This most commonly reflects a superimposed disorder (e.g. depression). Dementia is more common than expected in learning disability (not just in Down's syndrome) and especially in cases of severe epilepsy that is difficult to control.

Table 17.2 Comparison of mild, moderate, severe and profound learning disability

	Mild	Moderate	Severe/profound
IQ range	69–50	49–35	<35 (profound <20)
Percentage of cases	85%	10%	5%
Ability to self-care	Independent	Need some help	Limited
Communication	Reasonable	Limited	Basic or none
Reading and writing	Basic	Limited	Minimal or none
Ability to work	Semi-skilled	Unskilled, supervised	Supervised basic tasks
Social skills	Normal	Moderate	Few
Physical problems	Rare	Sometimes	Common
Aetiology discovered	Rarely	Often	Usually

Table 17.3 Assessment of a child with learning disability

History
Details of pregnancy:
   Foetal growth
   Infections, trauma, eclampsia
   Alcohol or substance misuse
   Exposure to other drugs, toxins
Delivery:
   Gestational age
   Complications
   Condition of baby
Child's development:
   Milestones
   Physical difficulties
Family history:
   Mental retardation
   Physical anomalies
   Consanguinity of parents

Examination
General:
   Overall health
Weight, height, head circumference
Physical anomalies
Skin
Neurological:
   Tone, posture, power, reflexes
   Cranial nerves
   Motor skills
   Comprehension and use of language

Neuropsychological testing
Intelligence quotient
Language development
Assessments for autism spectrum disorder

Laboratory investigations
Karyotyping and genetic testing
Biochemical studies
Brain imaging
EEG

Table 17.4 Psychiatric assessment in learning disability

Background
Overall level of functioning
Associated physical disability
Cause of learning disability
Methods of communication

Psychiatric history
Usual behaviours
Recent changes in environment
Recent changes in behaviour

Examination
Interactions
Behaviours
Mood
Usual presentation of emotional expression
Features of autism

Investigations
Behavioural rating scales
Autism rating scales

Physical investigation
Evidence of infection (especially urinary tract infection
   or lower respiratory tract infection)
Evidence of seizures
Evidence of constipation or gastrointestinal reflux

factors. The nature and amount of intervention needed is determined by:

- Overall level of functioning.
- Ability in specific domains (e.g. communication, socialization, daily living tasks).
- Physical disabilities (including epilepsy) and motor skills.
- Coexisting psychiatric disorder, especially autism, which is over-represented.
- Personality, behaviour and personal preferences.
- Ability of the family to care for the individual.

Psychiatric diagnoses in adults with learning disability follow ICD-10 criteria, in a modified, multiaxial approach (Table 17.5).

Management

Some individuals with learning disability do not require any specific service provision. This may be true for those at the mild end of the spectrum. Their psychiatric problems tend to be managed by general psychiatry services. However, the majority are cared for by specialist services due to the challenges faced by the individual, and this is usually due to a complex interplay between physical, social and psychological

Table 17.5 Diagnostic system for psychiatric disorders in adults with learning disabilities

Axis I: severity of learning disability

Axis II: cause of learning disability

Axis III: psychiatric disorders
   Level A: developmental disorders
   Level B: psychiatric illness
   Level C: personality disorders
   Level D: problem behaviours
   Level E: other disorders

The management of learning disability is based on the approaches employed elsewhere in psychiatry:

- The large majority of children with learning disability now live at home. Most adults with severe learning disability live in well-supported group homes. Long-stay institutional care has now virtually disappeared in the United Kingdom.
- Care is provided by multidisciplinary community learning disability teams using a framework similar to Community Mental Health Teams (Chapter 8).
- Most local services have some in-patient beds for the assessment and treatment of behavioural and psychiatric disorders. Forensic services for people with learning disability are provided regionally.
- Voluntary agencies play an important role.

Four principles guide the current strategy for care of people with learning disability:

- Legal and human rights – to a decent education, to marry, to have children, to vote, etc.
- The right to independence – independence, not dependence, is the default position.
- The right to choice – in where to live, what work to do, who cares for them.
- The right to inclusion – in mainstream services and local communities.

'*Essential lifestyle planning*' is one approach by which to find out what the person thinks about these decisions, and to provide the right package of care and support to help them achieve their goals.

 Clinical scenario

Aa 24-year-old man with severe learning disability is brought to his GP by his carer from a residential placement where he lives with three other residents. The carer reports a 6-month history of unpredictable aggression, which is always followed by urinary incontinence and the patient falling asleep. The doctor requests an EEG, which shows seizure activity. The incidents of aggression cease after the commencement of an antiepileptic.

Specific conditions associated with learning disability

The main individual causes of learning disability are mentioned here. Chromosomal and genetic factors predominate. By and large, the aetiology does not markedly affect management, but it may have major implications for prognosis, and the likelihood of similar problems arising in other family members, as well as secondary prevention.

- A useful concept is *behavioural phenotype* – that is, the association of a certain profile of behaviours with a genetic condition, such that recognition of the profile gives useful clues as to the cause of the learning disability. For example, self-injury suggests Lesch–Nyhan syndrome, and overeating suggests Prader–Willi syndrome.

Chromosomal abnormalities

A range of chromosomal microdeletions, translocations and aneuploidies can cause mental retardation. In total they explain 5–35% of cases.

- Many of the abnormalities can be detected by routine karyotyping. Others require specialist tests, such as subtelomeric analyses, which assess the ends of chromosomes (telomeres) that are relatively common sites of abnormality (5–10% of severe learning disability) and tests targeted at specific regions of the chromosomes known to be causative for a particular syndrome.
- Much smaller chromosomal abnormalities, called *copy number variants* (CNVs), as described for autism (Chapter 16), are also common in learning disability and may well account for many hitherto unexplained cases.

Down's syndrome

Down's syndrome (trisomy 21) produces learning disability with characteristic physical features (Table 17.6). The diagnosis is usually made at, or before, birth. It is the most common cause of learning disability. Its 'true' incidence is 1 in 650 live births (though this has fallen to 1 in 1000 in the United Kingdom due to antenatal testing and pregnancy termination). The risk is strongly dependent on maternal age, rising from <1/2000 at age 20 to 1/30 at age 45.

The aetiology in 95% of cases is triplication of chromosome 21, with the syndrome presumed to result from expression of the extra genes on the third copy of the chromosome. The remainder are due to a translocation involving chromosome 21 or to mosaicism (a mixture of normal and trisomic cells).

- The prognosis has improved with better medical management. Many now survive to middle age, when intellectual decline due to Alzheimer's disease is common. The association between the two

Table 17.6 Features of Down's syndrome

Moderate or severe learning disability
Placid temperament
Physical features:
  Down-slanting palpebral fissures and presence of epicanthic folds
  Small mouth with large protruding tongue
  Flat nasal bridge
  Flattened occiput
  Small hands with single transverse palmar (simian) crease
  Hypotonia

Associated medical problems:
  Cardiac septal defects
  Gastrointestinal obstruction
  Atlantoaxial instability
  Susceptibility to infection

Increased risk of:
  Leukaemia
  Hypothyroidism
  Autoimmune disorders
  Alzheimer's disease

Depression

Table 17.7 Features of fragile X syndrome

More common in males (~2:1)

All features are particularly variable

Learning disability:
  May be mild, moderate, severe or profound
  Deteriorates late in childhood
  Performance IQ affected more than verbal IQ
  Litany speech – repetitive, lacking in themes or content
  Poor attention and concentration
  Autistic features common

Physical features:
  Large, protruding ears
  Long face with high-arched palate
  Flat feet
  Lax joints
  Soft skin
  Large testes (after puberty)
  Mitral valve prolapse

disorders was crucial in the discovery of the latter's genetic basis.

 Clinical scenario

A 46-year-old man with Down's syndrome presents with his carer. The carer reports a year-long history of personality change with increased irritability, loss of skills citing inability to use a knife and fork, seizures (which have only begun recently) and that he is sleeping in the day but not at night. Psychological assessment and interviews with staff who have known the patient for many years confirm a diagnosis of Alzheimer's dementia.

Fragile X syndrome

Fragile X syndrome is so called because of a fragile site on the long arm of the X chromosome seen when cells are grown in a folate-deficient medium. It occurs in about 1/1500 births and is the second most common cause of learning disability (about 10% of cases). Its exact prevalence is uncertain because its phenotype (Table 17.7) is variable and accurate genetic testing has only recently become possible.

Most cases of fragile X syndrome are due to a trinucleotide (triplet) repeat mutation in the *FMR1* gene, impairing the gene's normal role in regulating expression of other genes. Being on the X chromosome, the syndrome is more common in boys than in girls. Along with several other X-linked disorders, it explains much of the higher rate of learning disability in males. However, the unusual nature of the *FMR1* mutation means that some males who have the mutation are normal, and more females are affected than would be expected. Female carriers also have an increased risk of psychiatric disorders.

- The disorder gets worse in succeeding generations (*anticipation*).
- Genetic detection of affected individuals and carriers is feasible.
- There is no specific treatment. *Methylphenidate* and *folic acid* may improve the attentional deficits.
- *FMR1* regulates genes involved in the formation of synapses and dendrites, and this function is impaired in fragile X syndrome because of the mutation.

Other chromosomal abnormalities

Severe learning disability is common with other autosomal abnormalities, but less frequent in sex chromosome aneuploidies.

- *Prader–Willi syndrome* is learning disability together with compulsive eating, obesity, challenging behaviour, hypogonadism and psychosis. It is due to deletion of part of chromosome 15.

Angelman syndrome (severe learning disability, puppet-like movements) is caused by the same abnormality when inherited from the mother rather than from the father ('imprinting').

- *Williams syndrome*, also known as infantile hypercalcaemia, affects 1 in 15 000 infants. Most cases are sporadic, and due to deletion of part of chromosome 7, including the elastin gene. Children show an 'elfin-like' appearance, and a moderate to severe learning disability. Verbal abilities are much better preserved – especially expressive language – than are visuospatial skills.
- *Velo-cardio-facial syndrome*, or *DiGeorge syndrome*, is due to deletion of part of chromosome 22q. It is usually sporadic, and is relatively common (1 in 2000 infants). The physical appearance is characteristic (prominent nose, small head or jaw, short stature, long hyperextensible fingers, plus cardiac and pulmonary abnormalities. Speech and language problems are common and 90% have learning disability. It is also a risk factor for schizophrenia.

Single gene disorders

There are over 1000 different genes known to cause learning disability, often via effects on metabolism or brain development. Most are very rare.

Phenylketonuria

Phenylketonuria (PKU) is the classic inborn error of metabolism (Table 17.8). The amino acid phenylalanine cannot be converted into paratyrosine because of a defective converting enzyme. It is autosomal recessive and affects 1 in 10 000 live births.

- PKU is one of the few treatable causes of severe learning disability. A rigorous low-phenylalanine diet must be started in the first months of life to prevent deterioration – hence the neonatal screening for phenylalanine levels. Carriers can be detected.

Other inherited errors of metabolism

Learning disability can result from disorders of other metabolic pathways (Table 17.9). The frequency of each is low and varies between ethnic groups. Most are associated with failure to thrive, and hepatic and/or renal dysfunction.

- In *Lesch–Nyhan syndrome*, self-mutilation by biting is the behavioural phenotype.

All the examples cited in Table 17.9 are recessive and most can be detected prenatally. A few can be ameliorated by diet.

Other genetic disorders

Neurofibromatosis and *tuberous sclerosis complex* are neurocutaneous syndromes. Both are autosomal dominant, but spontaneous mutations are also common.

- *Neurofibromatosis* (von Recklinghausen's disease) affects 1 in 4000 births. Diagnostic features are *café au lait* spots on the skin and multiple neurofibromas. Mild learning disability occurs in about 50% of cases of type 1 neurofibromatosis, which is due to mutations in the *NF1* (neurofibromin) gene on chromosome 17.
- *Tuberous sclerosis complex* occurs in 1 in 6000 births. There are several characteristic skin lesions and multiple tumours (hamartomas) in the brain

Table 17.8 Features of untreated phenylketonuria

Severe learning disability
Unpredictable aggression
Abnormal movements and mannerisms
Fair skinned
Short stature
Associated medical problems:
Eczema
Vomiting
Seizures

Table 17.9 Examples of metabolic disorders associated with learning disability

Metabolic category	Example
Amino acids	Homocysteinuria
Lipids	Tay–Sachs disease
Mucopolysaccharides	Hurler's syndrome
Carbohydrates	Galactosaemia
Purines	Lesch–Nyhan syndrome

and elsewhere. Epilepsy and progressive mental retardation occur in 60%. Autistic features are often seen. It is caused by two genes, *TSC1* (hamartin) on chromosome 9 and *TSC2* (tuberin) on chromosome 16, which affect cell growth and proliferation.

Environmental factors

Learning disability can be caused by a variety of environmental insults. Most act pre- or perinatally (Table 17.10) but postnatal factors are also recognized (Table 17.11).

Table 17.11 Postnatal causes of learning disability

Infections:
   Meningitis
   Encephalitis
Brain tumours
Head injury:
   Accidental
   Non-accidental
Hypoxia (e.g. anaesthetic accident)
Lead poisoning
Rare idiopathic syndromes:
   Disintegrative psychoses

Table 17.10 Pre- and perinatal environmental causes of learning disability

Category	Comment
Obstetric complications	
In utero infections:	
Rubella	Greatest risk (50%) if infection is in first trimester
HIV	Learning disability in 50% of infected children
Syphilis	
Cytomegalovirus	
Toxoplasmosis	
Foetal alcohol syndrome	In some offspring of mothers who drink heavily
Other drugs and toxins	For example, methylmercury
Placental insufficiency	
Placental abruption	
Eclampsia/toxaemia	
Birth complications	May be a consequence of earlier foetal abnormality
Ventricular haemorrhage	
Perinatal factors	
Hypothyroidism (cretinism)	An important cause in areas with low-iodine diets
Hyperbilirubinaemia	
Other factors	
Cerebral palsy	
Hydrocephalus	
Spina bifida	

 KEYPOINTS

- Learning disability (mental retardation) is defined as an IQ below 70, with functional impairments in several areas and a childhood onset. It affects about 2% of the population, boys more commonly than girls.
- Psychiatric and behavioural problems are common, especially in those who also have epilepsy.
- Severe learning disability is usually caused by genetic or chromosomal abnormalities (e.g. Down's syndrome, fragile X). Mild learning disability is often idiopathic and multifactorial.
- Learning disability is rarely treatable. Management is aimed at maximizing potential and quality of life, and at treating concurrent psychiatric and behavioural problems.
- Most people with learning disability live in the community.

 FURTHER READING

Bhaumik S, Branford D. (2005) *Frith Prescribing Guidelines for Adults With a Learning Disability.* Taylor & Francis, Oxford.

Department of Health (2008) Healthcare for all: report of the independent enquiry into access to healthcare for people with learning disabilities. Access at www.dh.gov.uk/en/publicationsandstatistics/publications/publicationspolicyandguidance/DH_099255

Royal College of Psychiatrists (2001) *OP48. CD-LD: Diagnostic Criteria for Psychiatric Disorders for Use with Adults with Learning Disabilities/Mental Retardation.* RC Psych, London.

? SELF-ASSESSMENT

1 A 16-year-old boy with learning disability presents with 'hearing voices' and 'strange' behaviour. His parents are concerned that he has unusual beliefs. They tell you that he was born with a cleft palate and has suffered repeatedly from infections since he was born. He has a heart murmur. Which of the following diagnostic entities would you suspect?

a Fragile X syndrome
b DiGeorge syndrome
c Down's syndrome
d Neurofibromatosis
e Williams syndrome

2 A 24-year-old man with severe learning disability has become increasingly agitated over the last few days. He is intermittently pyrexial. There is no history of seizures. There has been no change to his eating habits and his carer reports that he is defecating regularly. What would you do next?

a Wait and watch.
b Suggest a low-dose antipsychotic to help with the agitation.
c Admit the man to a general hospital.
d Ask for a urine dipstick.
e Admit him to a psychiatric in-patient unit.

Psychiatry in other settings

Learning objectives

✓ To have a working knowledge of the relevance of psychiatry in settings other than secondary care mental health.

One of the most important messages of this book is that psychiatry is an integral part of medicine – there is nothing unique about psychiatric patients or psychiatric disorders. Rather it is the traditional separation of psychiatric services from the rest of medicine that has made this appear to be the case. The conventional view of psychiatry, often gained from attachments to hospital based psychiatric teams, is potentially misleading: most people with psychiatric disorder present to, and are managed by, other doctors in other settings. All doctors must therefore have basic skills in psychiatric assessment and management. This chapter discusses the implications of the following facts:

- Psychiatric disorders are very common in the population, and thus in all areas of medical practice.
- Outside specialist psychiatric services, somatic symptoms are often the presenting feature of psychiatric disorder.
- Psychiatric disorders frequently coexist with medical illnesses.

Epidemiology of psychiatric disorder in different settings

In the population

Epidemiological surveys show that at least 20% of the adult population has a psychiatric disorder at any one time. Neuroses and substance misuse account for most of this morbidity, and psychosis is relatively rare (Table 18.1 summarizes key figures from the Adult Psychiatric Morbidity Survey in England). Overall psychiatric morbidity is strongly associated with social deprivation. Rates are twice as high in areas of deprivation.

Population prevalence is not the same as demand on services. Many of the individuals in Table 18.1 will never present to any service with their disorder. The difference between the population prevalence and the number who seek medical help is the first step on the pyramid, the peak of which is the tiny and unrepresentative percentage of cases that become psychiatric in-patients. Various 'filters' explain why so few make it to the top (Figure 18.1).

General practice

Most psychiatric disorder is seen and managed in general practice. The most common psychiatric disorders in general practice are the neuroses and somatoform disorders, depression and substance misuse. Patients with psychosis are rare – most GPs have only a few on their books, and these are usually also under specialist care.

Psychiatry as seen from general practice

Since psychiatrists and GPs see a different profile of psychiatric disorder it is not surprising that they may have differing views about priorities. For example,

Psychiatry Lecture Notes, Eleventh Edition. Gautam Gulati, Mary-Ellen Lynall and Kate Saunders. © 2014 John Wiley & Sons, Ltd. Published 2014 by John Wiley & Sons, Ltd.

Table 18.1 Approximate population prevalence of psychiatric disorders

Disorder	Prevalence in Men (%)	Prevalence (%) in Women
Mixed anxiety and depression	7.6	11.8
Alcohol dependence	8.7	3.3
Generalized anxiety disorder	3.6	5.8
Drug dependence	4.5	2.3
Depressive episode	2.2	3.0
Phobia	1.0	2.4
Obsessive-compulsive disorder	1.1	1.5
Panic disorder	1.0	1.4
Dementia (in age group 75–79)	5.04	6.67
Eating disorder	3.5	9.2
Psychotic disorder	0.3	0.5

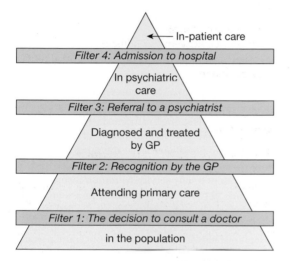

Figure 18.1 Psychiatric disorders in different settings and the filters to psychiatric care. Not everyone with a psychiatric disorder presents to a doctor. The decision to do so – the first filter to psychiatric care – depends on several factors; for example, awareness that the symptoms may signify psychiatric disorder, their severity, choosing to see a practitioner of alternative medicine, stigma, etc. Of those who do see a doctor (in the UK, usually a GP), the psychiatric disorder is recognized and treated in about half. This filter is determined by the doctor's diagnostic and treatment decisions. About 10% of patients are referred to psychiatric services; this filter depends on the nature of the disorder, the doctor's characteristics and the availability of resources. A tiny minority at some stage have a psychiatric admission. This last filter is based mainly upon the diagnosis, the risk of harm, and availability of psychiatric beds and alternative treatment options. This figure emphasizes that one's perspective on psychiatry depends largely on where on the pyramid you are standing.

a GP may wish to allocate resources to manage neurotic disorders that fill her surgeries, whereas her local psychiatrist will probably argue that rarer, but more severe, disorders – which dominate his caseload – take priority. This difference may cause tensions when psychiatrists and GPs are jointly involved in planning services in a cash-limited health service.

Integration and coordination between primary and secondary psychiatric care can be improved by:

- Regular meetings (e.g. psychiatrists regularly visiting general practices in their sectors).
- Trainee GPs spending time in psychiatry (and vice versa).
- Good communication, to ensure consistent management of cases by GPs and psychiatrists.
- Local guidelines for the management of common psychiatric disorders.

A&E departments

Deliberate self-harm is the major psychiatric problem in A&E departments. Although only a minority of these patients have persistent psychiatric disorder, many have stress-related disorders and some have depressive disorders. Intoxication and delirium related to alcohol and drugs are common, particularly in inner city hospitals and in people involved in accidents.

- Some patients with somatoform disorders and a few with factitious disorders are frequent users of A&E departments.

Medical and surgical out-patient clinics

One-third of medical and surgical out-patient clinic attendees have a psychiatric disorder. Half of these have depressive and anxiety disorders, and the remainder have somatoform disorders.

- Adequate recognition and treatment of their psychiatric disorder should be an integral part of management, since this has been shown to improve outcome.
- Depression is a common cause of apparent worsening of a medical condition.
- Panic disorder is an important cause of medically unexplained symptoms such as chest pain, dizziness and tingling.

Medical and surgical wards

About 20% of medical and surgical in-patients have a depressive or anxiety disorder coexisting with their medical disease; 10% have a significant alcohol misuse problem, and up to one-third of elderly in-patients have an episode of delirium.

- Some patients with severe somatoform disorders get admitted and undergo multiple investigations and even surgery before the diagnosis is made.
- Remember alcohol withdrawal as a possible cause of delirium in in-patients.

Psychiatric and medical comorbidity

Many patients with medical disease *also* have psychiatric disorder – the two occur together much more often than would be expected by chance. We have previously covered the situations where a medical condition such as hyperthyroidism or Cushing's disease can produce psychiatric symptoms as part of its pathophysiology. However, there are several other reasons why medical and psychiatric disorders frequently coexist:

- Psychiatric symptoms may be a response to the physical disease. For example, depression associated with cancer; sexual dysfunction after myocardial infarction; a body image disturbance after limb amputation.
- Psychiatric disorder may cause medical illness. For example, anorexia nervosa may cause osteoporosis.
- There may be a shared cause, such as a major life event precipitating both a stroke and depression.

The coexistence of a psychiatric disorder and a medical disorder is clinically important because it:

- Magnifies suffering and disability.
- Prolongs medical care and increases overall health costs.
- Worsens outcome. For example, the mortality of heart disease, cancer or stroke is higher in those with a comorbid depressive disorder.

Presentations of psychiatric disorder in a medical setting

Some cases of psychiatric disorders that present in medical settings do so with psychological symptoms or behavioural disturbance. However, many others present in ways that are less obviously 'psychiatric', with:

- somatic symptoms;
- a medical management problem;
- an apparent exacerbation of an established medical condition.

Presentation with somatic symptoms

Psychiatric disorder and somatic symptoms

A significant minority of patients seen in general practice and in hospital out-patient clinics have somatic symptoms that cannot be explained by medical disease; many of these have a psychiatric disorder. The important diagnoses are depressive, anxiety and somatoform disorders.

- Figure 18.2 shows a simple diagnostic approach to medically unexplained somatic symptoms.

Depression, anxiety and somatic symptoms

Depression is associated with somatic symptoms such as fatigue, weight loss and pain. Similarly, anxiety produces the bodily symptoms of autonomic arousal, which include palpitations, breathlessness and sensory symptoms.

For any patient who presents with bodily symptoms that are not adequately explicable by a medical diagnosis, consider the possibility that the patient may have a depressive or anxiety disorder. This psychiatric diagnosis may be the only diagnosis or it may be complicating a medical condition, in which case two diagnoses must be made. When assessing a patient with somatic

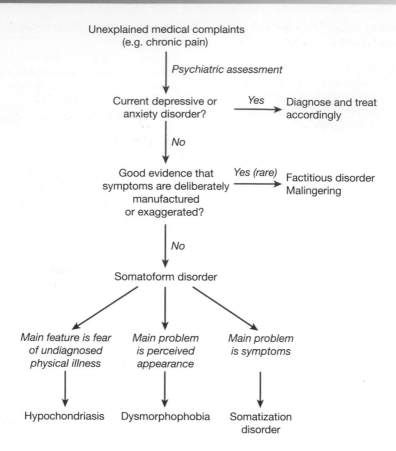

Figure 18.2 Psychiatric assessment and diagnostic pathways in people with unexplained medical complaints.

symptoms it is important not only to carry out the appropriate investigations to exclude physical disease but also to seek evidence of depression or anxiety.

- The converse situation – a misdiagnosis of depression or anxiety in a patient whose symptoms are caused by a medical disease – though much rarer, must not be overlooked.

 Clinical scenario

Ms M went to her doctor because of abdominal pain. She was upset, but both she and the doctor saw her distress as being a result of the pain. An urgent laparotomy was performed and a normal appendix removed. Only after she took an overdose the following month was a further history taken, which revealed that she had been having problems with her relationship with her mother and had developed symptoms of depressive disorder (low

mood, anhedonia and poor sleep) prior to the pain starting. She was given an antidepressant drug, helped to address the family conflict and made a full recovery.

Somatoform disorders and somatic symptoms

Patients with medically unexplained somatic symptoms who do *not* have a depressive or anxiety disorder may be regarded as having a somatoform disorder (Chapter 10).

Clinical scenario

Mr H has attended a gastroenterology clinic intermittently for years with abdominal discomfort and flatulence. No significant abnormalities have been found despite numerous investigations throughout the length of his gastrointestinal tract. Trials of antispasmodics, laxatives and antiulcer drugs have not produced sustained effects. A new junior doctor reviews his case and sees a connection between stresses at home or work and the exacerbation of abdominal as well as anxiety symptoms. Mr H is unwilling to countenance a psychological basis for his problems but agrees to see a liaison psychiatrist who works closely with the clinic. Mr H embarks on a course of problem-solving therapy and attends a stress management class. His irritable bowel syndrome improves markedly and he agrees (for the first time) that further medical interventions are not necessary.

Presentation with a medical management problem

Psychiatric disorders may also present as a problem in medical management. For example:

- An old lady repeatedly pulls out her drip in the orthopaedic ward.
- A young woman is repeatedly admitted with an infected operative wound.
- A woman with diabetes refuses to take adequate insulin.
- A young man has assaulted a doctor in surgical out-patients.

The diagnosis in all these cases proved to be psychiatric. It was, respectively: delirium, factitious disorder, depression and personality disorder. The cases illustrate that any psychiatric disorder can present with a medical management problem, and that a psychiatric assessment, even if brief, is essential.

Psychiatric disorder presenting as an apparent worsening of a medical disease

An exacerbation of symptoms or disability in a patient with a chronic medical condition may erroneously be attributed to a worsening of the disease process, when it is in fact due to the development of a comorbid psychiatric disorder. For example:

- A man with previously stable angina repeatedly presents with severe chest pain.
- A woman with previous hypothyroidism suffers a recurrence of severe lethargy.
- A woman with arthritis becomes housebound.

The diagnosis in these cases proved to be, respectively: panic disorder, depression and agoraphobia. The danger is that such patients are given unnecessary and potentially hazardous medical treatment instead of appropriate psychiatric management.

Management of psychiatric disorder in medicine

There are three main requirements for the effective management of psychiatric disorder in medical settings. These requirements serve to emphasize the knowledge, skills and attitudes that all doctors should have (Chapter 1):

- To be able to recognize it.
- To be able to treat it appropriately.
- To know how and when to refer to specialist psychiatric services.

Recognition

The diagnosis of psychiatric disorder in non-psychiatric settings is often missed. This error may be attributable to the doctor, the patient or the circumstances (Table 18.2).

Doctors will be better at the detection and assessment of psychiatric disorder if they:

- Realize that somatic symptoms are not always due to medical conditions.
- Always do a brief psychiatric assessment – even if just a few questions.
- Ask the patient about their worries and concerns.
- Enable the patient to express emotions.

Table 18.2 Reasons psychiatric diagnoses are missed in medical settings

Doctor
Failure to consider the possibility
Failure to ask about psychiatric symptoms – through lack of effort or skill

Patient
Reports only their somatic symptoms
Hides emotional distress and psychosocial stresses from the doctor

Circumstances
Lack of time
Lack of privacy
Clinics geared solely towards the detection of physical disease

Treatment

The treatment of psychiatric disorder in medical settings follows the same principles as treatment in psychiatric settings. It also requires that:

- The psychiatric diagnosis is explained to the patient in a way that they can accept. This is achieved by emphasizing that it is a real illness, that it is an understandable reaction and not a sign of weakness, and that it can be treated effectively.
- Effective evidence-based treatment is available. Some doctors will regularly use simple psychological therapies themselves. Others will have ensured that they have members of the clinical team, such as specialist nurses or counsellors, whom they can ask for assistance.
- The doctor has confidence in prescribing the main psychotropic drugs.

Referral to specialist psychiatric services

A small but important minority of patients will require a referral to specialist psychiatric services. The main indications for referral are:

- Request for second opinion.
- Failure of first-line management.
- Need for specialist treatment, such as ECT.
- Serious suicide risk.
- Presence of a condition such as psychosis requiring specialist services.
- Severe substance misuse.
- Need for compulsory treatment.

From primary care, referrals will usually be made to the local general psychiatric services, unless the problem falls into the remit of one of the subspecialties (Chapter 8). For patients in general hospitals there may be a hospital liaison psychiatry service that will assist both in management and in making appropriate referrals.

- Referrals, other than of exceptional emergencies, should only be made after the doctor has: (a) completed a basic assessment themselves; and (b) explained and agreed the referral with the patient.
- Following the referral, good communication between all the agencies involved is essential if problems are to be avoided.

 KEYPOINTS

- Patients with psychiatric disorders are encountered in all medical settings. Neurotic, somatoform, adjustment, depression and anxiety disorders are all common in general practice and general hospitals. In these settings they often present with somatic symptoms.
- Medical disease is frequently accompanied by psychiatric disorder. The combination worsens disability and prognosis if not effectively managed.
- Management of psychiatric disorder is based on the general principles described in this book, plus: (a) attention to the patient's medical condition and treatment; and (b) necessary adaptation to the medical setting.
- Because psychiatric disorders are so common in the general population, all doctors must be:
  - alert to the possibility of psychiatric disorder in all patients;
  - aware that psychiatric disorder often presents with somatic symptoms;
  - aware of the prevalence of psychiatric disorder in the physically ill;
  - able to screen for psychiatric disorder;
  - able to use simple psychological treatments;
  - able to use antidepressants;
  - aware when and how to refer to psychiatric services.

 FURTHER READING

Gask L, Lester H, Kendrick T, Peveler R (eds) (2009) *Primary Care Mental Health*. Royal College of Psychiatrists, London.

McManus S, Meltzer H, Brugha T, Bebbington P, Jenkins R (eds) (2009) Adult psychiatric morbidity in England, 2007. National Center for Social Research, London. Access at www.ic.nhs.uk/pubs/psychiatricmorbidity07

? SELF-ASSESSMENT

1 Ms A is a 42-year-old lady who works as a paramedic. She has presented to four different Emergency Departments over the last 3 months with abdominal pain. Ms A has been cooperative with staff following admission for investigations. Following normal results of all investigations, Ms A is discharged from hospital on each occasion and returns to work. Ms A's motivation for hospital admission is not connected to financial gain. Ms A's most likely psychiatric diagnosis is which of the following?

   a Hypochondriasis
   b Malingering
   c Factitious disorder
   d Somatization disorder
   e Conversion disorder

2 Mr B is a 48-year-old gentleman who is concerned that he has bowel cancer. He has presented to his GP on several occasions and complained of intermittent mild abdominal pain, 'stomach rumblings' and says that he can sometimes feel a mass in his abdomen. Following appropriate investigations, Mr B is reassured by his GP that no evidence of any serious physical disease has been found. Mr B continues to worry that he has bowel cancer. Mr F's most likely psychiatric diagnosis is which of the following?

   a Hypochondriasis
   b Malingering
   c Factitious disorder
   d Somatization disorder
   e Conversion disorder

3 Which of the following statements about the epidemiology of psychiatric disorders is incorrect?

   a Neuroses are more common in females.
   b Substance abuse is commoner in males
   c Psychiatric morbidity is associated with social deprivation.
   d Psychiatric morbidity is uncommon in prisons.
   e Psychiatric disorders commonly present in medical settings.

19

Mental health and the law

Learning objectives

✓ To understand the scope and purpose of the Mental Capacity Act
✓ To understand the scope and purpose of the Mental Health Act

Compulsory treatment

The nature of psychiatric disorders means that some people refuse treatment, even though to do so puts their health or the well-being of others at risk. In such circumstances psychiatrists may have to treat people against their will.

- There is continuing debate about balancing the benefits of treatment against infringement of civil liberties.
- The laws relating to mental health differ markedly between countries. They even differ between England and Wales, Scotland and Northern Ireland.

However, before considering mental health law specifically, we discuss the broader issue of how consent to treatment is determined, and the circumstances in which treatment may be given in the absence of informed consent: the key word is *capacity*.

- This applies to patients, and doctors, in all branches of medicine.

Common law and capacity

Treatment without informed consent is technically an assault. However, in an emergency, a doctor may treat a patient without consent if rapid action is called for to save life – for example, to maintain an airway in a comatose patient, or to sedate an uncontrollably delirious patient. Such actions were, until recently, carried out under the *common law* (law arising from court judgments as opposed to that enacted by parliament), applying the principle that a doctor can and should do what the public would consider reasonable in that situation (and where failing to act would be considered unreasonable). Most situations are now covered, in England and

Wales, by the *Mental Capacity Act (2005)* and in Scotland by the *Adults with Incapacity Act (2000)*.

- The Mental Capacity Act (MCA) applies to all of medicine, but has particular relevance to psychiatry because capacity can be affected by psychiatric disorders, and because psychiatrists may be seen as having particular expertise.
- The MCA is separate from the Mental Health Act (MHA), discussed below, and the two Acts use different criteria and standards. People detained under the MHA commonly but not always lack capacity, and you can enforce treatment in someone deemed to have capacity using the MHA.
- The MCA does not apply to those under the age of 16 and there are limits to its application for those aged 16 and 17. Treatment of under-16s who lack capacity is covered by the Children Act (1989).

Mental Capacity Act (2005) and the assessment of capacity

Some people, some of the time, lack the *capacity* to consent to (or refuse) treatment. The MCA aims to identify and protect these people. It has five key principles (Box 19.1). Whether working under the MCA jurisdiction or not, it is important to be able to assess capacity (see Figure 19.1).

- About 40% of in-patients on acute medical wards, and 60% on psychiatric wards, lack capacity.
- *Competency* is a concept closely related to capacity, and a widely used term (e.g. with regard to making a will), but it is not defined legally in the present context.

Psychiatry Lecture Notes, Eleventh Edition. Gautam Gulati, Mary-Ellen Lynall and Kate Saunders. © 2014 John Wiley & Sons, Ltd. Published 2014 by John Wiley & Sons, Ltd.

Box 9.1 Mental Capacity Act (2005)

Five key principles

1 Capacity is assumed until proven otherwise

2 The person must be helped to make decisions before capacity is judged to be absent (e.g. given time if capacity fluctuates; use of interpreters).

3 Patients are entitled to make unwise decisions. It is the process by which a decision is made, not the decision itself, that determines capacity.

4 Decisions made for people who lack capacity must be in their best interests.

5 Decisions must be the least restrictive option, in terms of their human rights.

Other elements

- Independent Mental Capacity Advocates – someone to advocate for those who lack capacity.

- Lasting power of attorney – a person can nominate someone authorized to make decisions for them if they ever lose capacity.

- Advance decisions (directives) – to specify interventions the person would not want if they lost capacity.

- Deprivation of liberty safeguards ('DOLS') introduced in 2009: designed to ensure that patients who lack capacity are not subject to undue restraints of their liberty. Particularly applies to patients in nursing homes with dementia.

- Expanded court of protection – to arbitrate on a wide range of capacity issues.

- Clinicians are expected to respect all the above elements.

- Failures to comply with the Act are potentially criminal offences.

Mental Health Act (1983, amended 2007)

Compulsory psychiatric admission and treatment in England and Wales is carried out under Sections of the 1983 MHA, amended in 2007 (Box 19.2 and Table 19.1).

- The 2007 Act is an amendment of the 1983 Act; many aspects remain unchanged.
- All doctors need to know about Section 5(2).
- GPs are involved in most Sections.
- Scotland has different regulations, and is covered by the Mental Health Care and Treatment Act (Scotland) 2003 (Table 19.2).

Reason to suspect mental incapacity
- Delirium
- Abnormal or inappropriate behaviour
- History of cognitive impairment
- Refusing treatment

Assess capacity.
Incapacity means demonstrating that the patient has:
- Impairment of reasoning ability
- Inability to retain, understand or apply relevant information
- Inability to communicate their decision

Figure 19.1 Assessing mental capacity. The starting assumption should always be that the person has capacity. If the assessment is being done under the Mental Capacity Act, demonstration of lack of capacity is followed by several steps before deciding on actions, following the principles of the Act (Box 19.1).

 Box 9.2 Key aspects of the Mental Health Act (1983/2007)

- The behaviour must be the result of a known or suspected 'mental disorder'. Disruptive behaviour, intoxication, drug abuse and dependence are not of themselves grounds for detention.

- The person must be at acute, significant risk of self-harm, self-neglect or harming others.

- The person must have refused voluntary treatment.

- Other options have been considered but are not appropriate.

- There must be an appropriate treatment available to the patient.

- Implementing most Sections involves an application from one of two people. (1) An Approved Mental Health Professional (AMHP), usually a senior social worker. (A nearest relative can apply instead of an AMHP, but this is very rare.). (2) Based on two medical recommendations, one a Responsible Clinician (RC), usually a senior psychiatrist, approved under Section 12 of the Act; the other doctor is usually the GP or another section 12 approved doctor.

- Detained patients can appeal to hospital managers or to a Mental Health Review Tribunal for the Section to be discharged. A Section is discharged by the RC once the patient's mental state no longer justifies it, and/or when he or she adheres consistently to treatment.

- There is an independent Mental Health Advocate scheme.
- There is a legal Code of Practice that all professionals must take note of.
- The Act only covers assessment and treatment for psychiatric disorder. It cannot be used if a patient refuses treatment for a medical problem unless it is a direct result of the mental disorder, e.g. refeeding in anorexia nervosa.

Section 2: admission for assessment

- *Uses*: Assessment of a suspected mental disorder. Drug treatment can be given without consent, but use Section 3 once compulsory treatment becomes the primary reason for in-patient care.
- *Applied for by*: AMHP (Box 19.2) in consultation with the nearest relative. Medical recommendation from an RC and another doctor (usually the GP). The AMHP must have seen the person within the past 14 days, the doctors within 5 days.
- *Duration*: 28 days.
- *Right of appeal*: in first 14 days, to the Mental Health Review Tribunal (MHRT).

Section 3: admission for treatment

- *Uses*. For an established mental disorder where admission is intended to alleviate the condition or prevent deterioration.
- *Applied for by*: as for Section 2. Cannot normally proceed if the nearest relative objects.

- *Duration*: 6 months, renewable. Section 3 patients can go on leave for up to 6 months in total on a *Section 17 but are required to be seen by their clinical team at fortnightly intervals*. Before discharge, a *Section 117 meeting* is held to discuss future management; there are statutory responsibilities for subsequent care.
- *Right of appeal*: one per 6 months to the MHRT. One per 6 months to the hospital managers. Reviews are instituted automatically if no appeal is made. At 3 months all treatment must be reviewed by a Second Opinion Appointed Doctor (SOAD) unless the patient consents to ongoing treatment.

Section 4: admission in an emergency

- *Uses*. For compulsory admission when it is urgent and a second medical recommendation cannot be obtained. Cannot be used just because it is easier to organize than a Section 2.
- *Applied for by*: AHMP or nearest relative. Medical recommendation by any doctor, usually GP.
- *Duration*: 72 hours, during which a full assessment for a Section 2 or 3 is made.
- *Right of appeal*: none.

Section 5(2): emergency detention of an in-patient

- *Uses*: A '5-2' prevents a patient leaving any hospital where to do so would place themselves or others at risk. For example, a voluntary patient on a psychiatric ward who is acutely suicidal and tries to run off the ward can be legally detained on the ward using Section 5(2). A Section 5(2) does not allow treatment to be enforced. [A Section 5(4) is used by psychiatric nurses to detain a

Table 19.1 Key Mental Health Act Sections and their uses		
Situation	**Section**	**Duration**
Psychiatric admission, for assessment	2	28 days
Psychiatric admission, for treatment	3	6 months
Psychiatric admission, when no second doctor is available	4	72 hours
Leave from hospital while a detained patient	17	Variable
'Holding powers' preventing an in-patient leaving a hospital	5(2) doctor 5(4) nurse	72 hours 6 hours
For police to enter a private residence and take person to a safe place (requires a warrant from a magistrate)	135	72 hours
For police to take a person from a public place to an approved place of safety	136	72 hours
Psychiatric assessment or treatment of prisoners and those on remand	35–38, 41	
Emergency treatment	62	

Table 19.2 Key Sections of the Scottish Mental Health (Care and Treatment) Act 2003

Situation	Section	Duration	Applicants
Emergency detention	36(1)	72 hours	Registered doctor,[a] plus MHO[b] if available
Nurses' holding power	299	2 hours	Registered specialist nurse
Short-term detention	44(1)	28 days	Approved doctor[c] and MHO
Compulsory treatment order	64(4)	6 months	Two doctors, one approved, plus MHO, plus approval of mental health review tribunal

[a]Registered doctor: any doctor registered with the General Medical Council.
[b]MHO: Mental Health Officer, a specially trained social worker.
[c]Approved doctor: a psychiatrist approved under the Act.

psychiatric in-patient for 6 hours if no psychiatrist is to hand.] Section 5(2) can only be used in in-patient environments and cannot be used to hold patients in emergency departments or outpatient departments.

- *Applied for by*: the doctor in charge of the treatment of the patient, or their nominee (in practice, a consultant or junior doctor in the team, but not a foundation doctor). In a general hospital, this means the physicians managing the patient, ideally in consultation with a liaison psychiatrist.
- *Duration*: 72 hours, during which a full MHA assessment is carried out. Once completed, the Section 5 is converted to a Section 2, or a Section 3 is instituted, or it lapses.
- *Right of appeal*: none.

Other Sections

- *Section 135* allows the police to enter private property and take a person to a nominated place of safety (e.g. a hospital or police station) for 72 hours. It is requested by an AMHP and granted by a magistrate. It can only be used once. If a patient is not at home and the police enter a further warrant is required.
- *Section 136* empowers the police to take someone in a public place whom they suspect has a mental disorder (e.g. because of bizarre behaviour) to a designated place of safety (police station, hospital). Lasts for 72 hours.
- *Sections 35–38* are used by a Court to send offenders to hospital for psychiatric assessment or treatment. *Sections 47* and *48* allow for transfer of a prisoner or other detainees to hospital.
- Electroconvulsive therapy (ECT) may not be given without consent to detained patients, unless it is necessary to prevent death or deterioration. A second opinion must be obtained and Section 58 completed before the course of ECT proceeds. In an emergency situation ECT can be given using provisions set out in Section 62 providing that the treatment is required to save the patient's life, prevent irreversible deterioration in the patient's condition or in very rare circumstances where patients are at such risk to themselves or others and no alternative treatment is available.

Supervised Community Treatment

The 2007 MHA amendment introduced *Community Treatment Orders (CTOs)*, allowing compulsory treatment in the community as well as in hospital – a controversial change. CTOs apply to a restricted set of patients and circumstances:

- The patient is currently detained under Section 3. Thus they have a severe and chronic psychiatric disorder, most commonly schizophrenia, which continues to meet the criteria for detention under the MHA.
- A CTO is designed for patients with cycles of relapse and readmission ('revolving door patients') associated with treatment non-compliance in the community, and for whom the structure and monitoring provided by a CTO may be valuable.
- A CTO is necessary for the patient's health or safety, or for the protection of others.
- The appropriate treatment does not require the patient to remain in hospital.
- A CTO lasts 6 months and is renewable.

Before initiating a CTO, a risk assessment is performed to assess the risk of relapse, and its consequences. The application is made by the RC, and an AHMP must agree. A CTO means that the patient must make themselves available for examination as requested by the RC (e.g. to attend clinic for review of their mental state, or to receive depot medication). The RC can also recall the person to hospital for treatment.

- A CTO does not include physical restraint to administer medication in the community without consent.
- It is unclear how many patients will be subject to CTOs, and their worth and ethics continue to be debated. Their use in practice is an alternative to the option of long-term hospital leave under Section 17 (see above).

Other aspects of the law and psychiatry

Forensic psychiatrists specialize in the law, but all psychiatrists find themselves involved with the law from time to time. Not all issues are strictly related to treatment, but they are summarized here for convenience.

- *The law and child psychiatry.* Children under 16 are subject to different laws and conventions, and there are additional safeguards for 16- and 17-year-olds. The main legislation is the Children's Act (1989). Consult a child psychiatric team or social services for advice.
- *Writing legal reports.* Psychiatrists may be asked to write a report on a patient who has been charged with an offence, usually to give an opinion as to whether psychiatric factors contributed to the offence or influence how it should be dealt with. They may also be asked to write a report concerning the psychiatric consequences of an accident as part of a compensation claim.
- *Fitness to enter into contracts.* Psychiatric opinion may be sought regarding the person's capacity (or competence) to make a will, get married, etc. These issues are now covered by the MCA.
- *Fitness to drive.* Psychiatric disorders and medications can impair driving by affecting judgement or concentration. Psychiatrists should warn patients of this and of their duty to inform the relevant authority. A person may not drive for 6 months after a psychotic episode. People with dementia (even mild cases) have an excess of accidents and should be discouraged from driving.
- *Confidentiality.* There are exceptional circumstances that override the principle of medical confidentiality in psychiatry. For example, if a patient tells you he is going to murder his wife (perhaps

because of morbid jealousy; Chapter 12), or if you suspect a colleague is unfit to practise, you have a duty to act. If unsure, always seek advice and keep notes.

 KEYPOINTS

- The Mental Capacity Act provides for the treatment and safeguarding of incapacitous individuals both in medical and psychiatric settings.
- The Mental Health Act allows individuals with mental disorders to be detained and treated against their will if there is a significant risk to their well-being or that of others.
- There are a number of safeguards in the Mental Health Act that ensure treatment is regularly reviewed, patients have the right to appeal their detention and are provided with appropriate aftercare.
- The police and nursing staff have some powers to detain under the Mental Health Act although the duration of these powers is limited.

 FURTHER READING

Department for Constitutional Affairs (2007) *Mental Capacity Act 2005 Code of Practice*. The Stationery Office, London.
Department of Health (2008) *Code of Practice Mental Health Act 1983*. The Stationery Office, London.

 SELF-ASSESSMENT

1 A gentleman is brought into A&E having ingested antifreeze. He is agitated, confused and resisting medical care and making attempts to leave. Staff are certain that he needs to be kept in hospital. What law would you use to keep him in hospital for treatment?
   a Section 5.2.
   b Mental Capacity Act.
   c Section 136 as he is in a public place.
   d Common law.
   e Request a mental health act assessment.

Self-assessment answers

Chapter 2

1 c The congruity statement is the only one that is true. The mental state examination is limited to those features present at the time of the interview, but includes both features noted by the patient (e.g. current thoughts of self-harm) and features noticed by the interviewer (e.g. thought disorder). The 'FAST' questions help to screen for hazardous drinking, but dependency is better identified by the 'CAGE' questions (p. 157). Derealization is a feeling of detachment from the external world, while depersonalization is a feeling of detachment from the normal sense of self. Both are described as 'dissociative' symptoms. Delusions are a *symptom*, that is, a phenomenon experienced by the patient which is a behavioural pattern considered to be a diagnostic entity, for example schizophrenia. The lack of consensus within and outside of psychiatry about which patterns of behaviour should count as 'disordered', and how to divide such patterns into discrete diagnoses, renders this definition circular. Thus, a 'psychiatric disorder' is simply whatever is defined as a disorder in your legal system or diagnostic manual of choice.

Chapter 3

1 a Thought disorder may occur in a number of psychiatric disorders. Alone, it is not strongly suggestive of the specific diagnosis of schizophrenia and is not considered a first-rank symptom. The other options are all first-rank symptoms (see Table 3.1).

2 a In psychiatry, thoughts, impulses or images must be intrusive in order to qualify as obsessions. They must also cause marked anxiety or distress. Obsessions are not diagnostic of obsessive-compulsive disorder, as they may also occur in other disorders, for example depression. Compulsive behaviours are often secondary to obsessions, but the reverse is not true. Obsessions may be a side effect of dopaminergic medication. The predisposing factors for this and other psychiatric side effects of dopaminergic medication remain unclear, but the risk is higher for patients with Parkinson's disease.

3 a Hallucinations may occur in severe depression. Visual hallucinations suggest an organic disorder. Voices talking *about* the person are characteristic of schizophrenia. Hypnopompic hallucinations are those that occur on waking. Like hypnagogic hallucinations (while falling asleep), they are normal. The etymology serves as an aide-memoire: waking up is like 'sending sleep away', which in Greek is *hypnos* (sleep) + *pompe* (sending away), related to ceremonial 'pomp', a 'sending-off'.

Chapter 4

1 d Individuals who repeatedly self-harm are at increased risk of further self-harm and subsequent suicide even if their method of harm is limited to cutting.

2 b It is the patient's responsibility to inform the DVLA as you would be breaching confidentiality in doing so. Only in very rare situations would this become necessary. Mania is associated with driving at high speeds so this advice should not be limited simply to situations where medication is being prescribed. If unsure, guidance for each disorder can be found online at www.dft.gov.uk/**dvla**/medical/~/media/pdf/medical/at_a_glance.ashx

Chapter 6

1 d Heritability is the proportion of a disorder in a population that is attributable to genes. It does not capture the effects of specific genes. It is usually calculated from twin studies. The heritability estimates for schizophrenia, depression and anxiety disorders are approximately 80%, 40% and 30% (see Table 6.3).

2 b Positron emission tomography (PET) does indeed use radioactive ligands to measure brain receptors or metabolites. fMRI does not directly measure neural activity, but rather measures changes

Psychiatry Lecture Notes, Eleventh Edition. Gautam Gulati, Mary-Ellen Lynall and Kate Saunders. © 2014 John Wiley & Sons, Ltd. Published 2014 by John Wiley & Sons, Ltd.

in blood oxygenation at different locations in the brain, from which some information about neuronal activity can be inferred. This is because oxygen delivery through the capillary beds in the brain is regulated to track local metabolic needs of neurons and glia. Biomarkers need not be molecules. For example, a pattern of neural activity detected by fMRI could also act as a biomarker. Adoption studies do not control for the prenatal environment, which could be driving the increased risk in the adopted-away child.

Chapter 7

1 **a** Olanzapine has an evidence base in the treatment of psychosis and can be used first line. Clozapine is only used in refractory psychosis given its side-effect profile. ECT is reserved for emergencies such as catatonia. There is no role for a mood stabilizer at this point. CBT is unlikely to be helpful in someone who is acutely unwell. It may play a role once the patient improves with antipsychotics.

2 **c** Psychotic depression where a patient has stopped eating and drinking is an emergency for which ECT is the preferred treatment. It has good efficacy. Drug treatments take weeks to work and are therefore unsuitable in this scenario.

3 **c** Either an SSRI or a course of CBT or both will
  or be appropriate in the treatment of a phobia.
  e It depends on the patient's preference. Benzodiazepines should be avoided, save for very short periods, as they carry a risk of addiction.

Chapter 8

Question 1:

  i a Mr D is likely suffering with a schizophrenic illness and therefore needs management by a CMHT in secondary care. He does not need specialist services at this point.

  ii c Moderate depression without associated risks can be managed in primary care in the first instance. Psychological resources are available in primary care.

  iii b Given that the patient's lifestyle is chaotic and presents with difficulties in engagement, an assertive outreach team would be ideal. These teams often support patients with coexisting substance misuse issues.

Question 2:

  i a Decisions around medication are taken by psychiatrists. Although non-medical prescribing is possible, this is not common.

  ii b The patient and help to think through her past experiences. Although this can, to some extent, be done by other members of the team, it is best done in a psychological setting.

  iii d Social workers integrated within CMHTs are invaluable resources when looking at issues around finances and accommodation. They have links to, and are sometimes seconded from, local councils.

  iv f Support workers are usually not professionally qualified but can provide skilled support rehabilitation.

Chapter 9

1 **e** This would be described as a recurrent depressive disorder as she has had a previous depressive episode. The fact that her previous episode related to the birth of her child has no bearing on the diagnosis in this instance.

2 **b** His history is suggestive of dysthymia whereas his current presentation is consistent with the presence of a psychotic depression. This presentation requires urgent treatment and ECT may be indicated.

3 **c** A diagnosis of bipolar disorder can apply in the absence of depressive episodes. Unopposed antidepressant treatment is not recommended. If hospital admission is required for mania this would suggest a diagnosis of bipolar 1 as the mania is clearly severe in nature. Post-puerperal psychosis is more common in women with bipolar disorder.

Chapter 10

1 **c** Obsessions are egodystonic (i.e. uncomfortable for the sufferer). They are repetitive and intrusive thoughts or images that are distressing to the patient. One only needs evidence of either obsessions or compulsions to make a diagnosis of OCD. Some patients have both symptoms. SSRIs and CBT are the current first-line treatments for OCD. Anankastic personality disorder is the personality disorder most commonly associated with obsessional thoughts.

2 **c** Disinhibition is not a feature of PTSD. The rest are typical features.

3 **c** Agoraphobia is more common in women. Primary and secondary gain are associated with dissociative disorders. Malingering is not a psychiatric disorder. Somatization disorder is more common in females but does also occur in males.

Chapter 11

1 **b** A preoccupation with weight often precedes the emergence of eating disorder behaviours, which to occur during puberty.

2 All of the parameters (a–e) should be monitored, particularly in individuals who are at a very low weight or have been eating very little in the preceding weeks, to reduce the risk of and to diagnose any emerging refeeding syndrome.

Chapter 12

1 **c** The young man probably has a schizophrenic illness which had a prodrome. Given the risks involved, i.e. his running away, fearing for his own safety or using a weapon to protect himself from perceived threat, it would be safest to admit him, if necessary using the Mental Health Act. Even a short period of observation/assessment without medication in hospital is helpful in establishing a diagnosis; in practice treatment is started relatively quickly in hospital.

2 **d** Physical causes such as a urinary tract infection (UTI) and other infections can cause new-onset confusion, agitation, disturbances in sleep cycle and psychotic symptoms in the elderly. This is delirium – an organic condition, but patients are often referred to psychiatry due to hallucinations and other psychotic symptoms that accompany the picture. Diagnosing and treating the underlying cause will reduce agitation as well as psychotic symptoms. In any case, it is worth remembering that the elderly are very prone to adverse effects from psychotropic medications.

3 **a** It is true that as a *population*, patients with schizophrenia are more likely to have a criminal or violent conviction than the general population. However, on an *individual* level, the majority are not violent. Individuals who commit violent offences often have comorbid dissocial personality disorder and/or substance misuse.

Chapter 13

1 **a** Alzheimer's accounts for 50–60% of all dementias.

2 **c** This is a classic description of dementia with Lewy bodies. There may also be a history of worsening when antipsychotics have been used.

3 **b** Memantine is an NMDA glutamate receptor antagonist licensed for use in moderate to severe Alzheimer's disease. It can also be used if cholinesterase inhibitors are contraindicated or not tolerated.

4 **e** This is the most important aspect of treatment without which the delirium is unlikely to resolve. The other aspects are symptomatic measures and may not be needed in every case.

5 **e** The rate of suicide is elevated. Depression is common alongside epilepsy.

Chapter 14

1 **a** Lofexidine is the most appropriate non-opioid (it is an alpha-adrenergic agonist) for symptomatic relief of opiate withdrawal. Methadone is the most common agent used for detoxification and maintenance in opioid dependence and can only be prescribed in specialist addiction clinics. Buprenorphine is a partial opiate agonist licensed, like methadone, for treatment of drug dependence. Naloxone is used in the treatment of opiate overdose. Naltrexone is used in the maintenance of abstinence in formerly dependent opiate addicts who have been drug free for over 7 days.

2 **d** Cocaine intoxication is the most likely diagnosis. Tachyarrhythmia and tachycardia are common toxic effects of cocaine. Picking at the skin may present a typical hallucinatory disorder of formication (bugs crawling under the skin) in a long-term cocaine user. Cannabis intoxication may present as tachycardia but there is also dryness of the mouth and reddening of the eyes. Heroin intoxication is characterized by constricted pupils, and CNS and respiratory depression. Cocaine withdrawal is not usually accompanied by significant physical symptoms. Ketamine intoxication is associated with nausea, ataxia, slurred speech, synaesthesia and hallucinations.

Chapter 15

1 **d** The pervasive nature of the symptoms is important, as there is a significant overlap of symptoms between personality disorder and other psychiatric disorders.

2 **c** The fact that the man has never moved out of home and never worked points to a pervasive rather than situational problem. There may, of course, be a superimposed depressive disorder related to an abnormal grief reaction and it would be useful to check for depressive symptoms as the same could coexist with the underlying personality disorder. 'Normal bereavement' is unlikely to last this long.

Chapter 16

1 **d** Asperger's syndrome fits best with the description given. Children with Asperger's are often targeted by bullies as they are noticeably 'different' in their interaction style and confidence and have few or no friends to support them. As in this case, they are sometimes involved in physical altercations with other children, and it can be hard for them to explain what has distressed them and led to the incident. Schizophrenia can be a cause of

school refusal in adolescence but is rare before the age of 16. Social phobia is a common cause, but affected children would rarely be aggressive to others, nor 'talk over' children, generally preferring to withdraw from situations. Generalized anxiety disorder is a cause of school refusal but there should be clear manifestations of anxiety present much of the time to make the diagnosis. Conduct disorder is linked to school truancy (which usually occurs without parents' knowledge) rather than school refusal (staying at home with parents' knowledge, though not necessarily their agreement).

2 d Cognitive behavioural therapy would be the recommended first-line treatment in this case. Family therapy could have been a valid choice if she had been willing to involve her family, as would interpersonal therapy if it was available locally. Fluoxetine would be an option if she declined psychological therapy or was too severely depressed to engage with a talking therapy first of all. Citalopram would not normally be used unless fluoxetine had been tried and found to be ineffective or poorly tolerated; sertraline would be the other second-line option if fluoxetine was unsuitable.

Chapter 17

1 b Schizophrenia is over-represented in DiGeorge syndrome, or velo-cardio-facial syndrome. This is thought to be because the *COMT* gene is present on 22q11, which is the site of deletion in this syndrome. The recurrent infections are due to an absent thymus.

2 d Physical causes such as a urinary tract infection (UTI), constipation and epilepsy must be considered when there is new-onset agitation in a patient with a learning disability. Diagnosing and treating the underlying cause will reduce agitation. Unplanned admissions must be avoided as patients will often destabilize in unfamiliar surroundings.

Chapter 18

1 c Factitious disorder. In this disorder, the only 'gain' is the 'sick-role', in contrast to malingering, in which compensation or other forms of financial gain are sought. Patients with factitious disorder are cooperative in behaviour and continue to function well and maintain jobs following discharge from hospital.

2 a Hypochondriasis. The patient is concerned with a particular diagnosis (bowel cancer in this case). In somatization disorder, rather than focusing on a diagnosis, the preoccupation is with symptoms, usually multiple, recurrent and frequently changing physical symptoms. In hypochondriasis, normal bodily sensations are often interpreted by patients as abnormal.

3 d There is considerable psychiatric morbidity in prisons, with rates of psychoses at approximately 4%, affective disorders around 10–12% and personality disorders as high as 60%.

Chapter 19

1 b Section 5.2 cannot be used as he is not admitted to hospital requesting a mental health act assessment will take too long unless staff are already on site s136 can only be used by the police and common law has largely been replaced by the Mental Capacity Act. Best practice would also involve requesting an urgent psychiatric assessment

Appendix 1

ICD-10 classification of psychiatric disorders

Category	Category	Example
F00–09	Organic disorders	F02.2 Huntington's disease
F10–19	Substance use disorders	F10.2 Alcohol dependence
F20–29	Schizophrenia and other psychoses	F20.0 Paranoid schizophrenia
F30–39	Mood disorders	F32.1 Moderate depressive episode
F40–49	Neurotic and stress-related disorders	F45.2 Hypochondriasis
F50–59	Eating, sleep and related syndromes	F50.2 Bulimia nervosa
F60–69	Disorders of personality and behaviour	F60.2 Dissocial personality disorder
F70–79	Mental retardation (Learning disability)	F72.0 Severe mental retardation
F80–89	Developmental disorders	F84.0 Autism
F90–99	Childhood disorders	F94.0 Elective mutism

Psychiatry Lecture Notes, Eleventh Edition. Gautam Gulati, Mary-Ellen Lynall and Kate Saunders. © 2014 John Wiley & Sons, Ltd. Published 2014 by John Wiley & Sons, Ltd.

Appendix 2

Keeping up to date and evidence-based

Textbooks and articles can be biased and outdated. The following are sources of up-to-date, good quality evidence in psychiatry.

Finding the evidence

Access to high quality evidence in psychiatry is improving all the time.

- NHS Evidence (www.evidence.nhs.uk) is a website maintained by NICE (now renamed the National Institute for Health and Care Excellence) that brings together many good resources including the Cochrane Database of Systematic Reviews, the British National Formulary, Clinical Evidence and MEDLINE. Access to these resources is free to practitioners in the UK.

- Emerging new evidence in psychiatry is summarized in *Evidence-based Mental Health* – a quarterly journal from the BMJ Publishing Group. The content of the journal is also available online (http://ebmh.bmjjournals.com/).

Clinical practice guidelines

Clinical guidelines (CGs) are recommendations on the appropriate treatment and care of people with specific disorders. CGs can be a useful help, but should augment rather than replace clinical expertise and experience.

In the UK, NICE prepares national evidence-based guidelines. We have referenced guidelines relevant to each chapter of the book under 'Further reading'. All NICE clinical guidelines are available at www.nice.org.uk.

Psychiatry Lecture Notes, Eleventh Edition. Gautam Gulati, Mary-Ellen Lynall and Kate Saunders. © 2014 John Wiley & Sons, Ltd. Published 2014 by John Wiley & Sons, Ltd.

Index

Psychiatry Lecture Notes, Eleventh Edition. Gautam Gulati, Mary-Ellen Lynall and Kate Saunders. © 2014 John Wiley & Sons, Ltd. Published 2014 by John Wiley & Sons, Ltd.

WITHDRAWN FROM LIBRARY